CHEMISTRY RESEARCH AND APPLICATIONS

# GAMMA-AMINOBUTYRIC ACID (GABA)

## BIOSYNTHESIS, MEDICINAL USES AND HEALTH EFFECTS

# Chemistry Research and Applications

Additional books in this series can be found on Nova's website
under the Series tab.

Additional e-books in this series can be found on Nova's website
under the e-book tab.

CHEMISTRY RESEARCH AND APPLICATIONS

# GAMMA-AMINOBUTYRIC ACID (GABA)

## BIOSYNTHESIS, MEDICINAL USES AND HEALTH EFFECTS

JOSIPA VLAINIĆ
AND
MAJA JAZVINŠĆAK JEMBREK
EDITORS

nova publishers
*New York*

For permission to use material from this book please contact us:
Telephone 631-231-7269; Fax 631-231-8175
Web Site: http://www.novapublishers.com



Additional color graphics may be available in the e-book version of this book.

**Library of Congress Cataloging-in-Publication Data**

ISBN: 978-1-63321-838-3

*Published by Nova Science Publishers, Inc. † New York*

# CONTENTS

# PREFACE

Gamma-amino butyric acid (GABA) is ubiquitous non protein amino acid which exerts various functions in different mamalian tissues and other organisms (e.g. bacteria, plants, fungi). Beyond its most investigated function as neurotransmitter in mammalian brain where it serves as an inhibitory neurotransmitter, GABA has a role as a hormone or trophic factor in non-neuronal peripheral and endocrine systems. Other effects of GABA include hypotensive, tranquilizing, diuretic and antidiabetic activity.

Most of its action neurotransmitter GABA exerts through $GABA_A$ receptors which are ubiquitous within the central nervous systems. These ionotropic receptors constituted as transmembrane ion channels that open or close in response to the binding of a ligand (among them most prominent is GABA) are playing an essential role in controlling neural inhibition and timing of neural networks.

Due to its numerous roles and functions the research on GABA has several lines. Therefore in this book several topics are covered starting from the beginning:

- To better understand described topics the process of GABA synthesis and transport have been reviewed. The metabolism of GABA and its importance in the budding yeast *Saccharomyces cerevisiae* has been reported. Moreover, the role of GABA in development and behavior is described.
- Prolonged exposure of $GABA_A$ receptors to its ligands could lead to different molecular changes affecting functioning of central nervous system: in a book the effects of persistent activation of these receptors by GABA are revealed.
- Since GABA regulates neuroendocrine functions and affects the activity of hypothalamic-pituitary-adrenal (HPA) axis the complex mechanisms of GABAergic drugs on the activity of HPA axis are described withing the book chapter presented here; with the emphasis on the possible implications for the human therapy.
- One of the objectives of the book was to review the therapeutic trials with GABAergic drugs (e.g. gabapentin, pregabalin, tiagabine and baclofen), in the treatment of various types of cerebellar ataxia and other motor disorders of the central nervous system. Moreover, involvement of GABA-mediated over inhibition in cognitive and neuromorphological phenotypes in Down syndrome is presented.
- GABAergic system appears to be important in the neuronal control of learning and memory. Dementias, and among them most recognized Alzheimer's disease lead to the loss of mental functions such as learning and memory. Here are several

hypotheses reviewed on the involvement of GABA system in the above mentioned diseases with the emphasis on behavioral and psychiological symptoms. Moreover, the implications for the treatment with GABAergic drugs are also discussed.

- Due to growing care for the animals there are numerous substances that potentiate the effect of GABA on $GABA_A$ receptors that have been commonly used in veterinary medicine. The species specific pharmacological properties with emphasis on adverse reactions and side effects are described within the book.

In: Gamma-Aminobutyric Acid (GABA)
Editors: Josipa Vlainić and Maja Jazvinšćak Jembrek
ISBN: 978-1-63321-838-3


*Chapter 1*

# REGULATION OF GABA SYNTHESIS AND TRANSPORT

***Jigar Pravinchandra Modi[1,2], Howard Prentice[1,2] and Jang-Yen Wu[1,2,3*]***

[1]College of Medicine, Florida Atlantic University; [2]Center for Complex Systems and Brain Sciences, Florida Atlantic University and [3]China Medical University, Taiwan

## ABSTRACT

GABA has been established as a major neurotransmitter in the vertebrate and invertebrate nervous systems from physiological, biochemical, pharmacological, and morphological studies. The rate-limiting step in GABA biosynthesis is the decarboxylation of glutamate by L-glutamic acid decarboxylase (GAD). Since the original purification of soluble GAD (sGAD) from mouse brain more than four decades ago much progress has been made in identification of GABA neurons and delineating GABAergic circuitry as well as in regulation of GAD activity and cloning and structural analysis of GAD. Genes encoding GAD have been cloned from several species. GAD65 and GAD67, referring to GAD with a molecular weight of 65 KDa and 67 KDa, respectively, are encoded by two separate genes and have distinct intraneuronal distributions and co-factor interactions. GAD67 is a soluble protein that is distributed evenly throughout the cell, whereas GAD65 is concentrated in the nerve terminals and can become membrane associated. In this review, we will discuss the role of post translational modifications including protein phosphorylation and proteolytic cleavage in regulation of both GAD65 and GAD67 activity. In addition, a novel mechanism, namely, a coupling mechanism between GABA synthesis by synaptic vesicle (SV)-associated GAD and GABA transport into SV by vesicular GABA transporter will also be discussed with special emphasis on its role in overall regulation of GABA neurotransmission.

**Keywords**: GABA, GAD 65 and 67, Protein phosphorylation, PKC epsilon and VGAT

---

* Corresponding author: Dr. Jang-Yen Wu, Professor of Biomedical Science, Florida Atlantic University, 777 Glades Road, BC # 71, Room- 325, Boca Raton, FL 33431. jwu@fau.edu.

## GABA Neurotransmission in Disease

Gamma-amino butyric acid (GABA) is the major inhibitory neurotransmitter in the mammalian central nervous system. It plays a key role in regulating neuronal excitability throughout the nervous system. Biosynthesis of GABA is carried out about by the decarboxylation of glutamate catalyzed by L-glutamic acid decarboxylase (GAD) (EC 4.1.1.15). Disruption of GABA neurotransmission is ascribed to many neurological diseases including epilepsy (Freichel, Potschka, Ebert, Brandt, & Löscher, 2006; Lloyd et al., 1986) Huntington's chorea (Gourfinkel-An et al., 2003; Spokes, Garrett, Rossor, & Iversen, 1980), Parkinson's disease (de Jong, Lakke, & Teelken, 1984) and general anxiety disorder (Kosel et al., 2004).

The level of GABA in the brain is controlled and regulated by the rate limiting step enzyme involved in GABA synthesis, namely, GAD. Interestingly, in the mammalian brain, GABA unlike any other neurotransmitters is the only neurotransmitter synthesized by two isoforms of enzymes, namely GAD65 and GAD67, with 65 and 67 denoting their respective molecular weights in KDa (Martin & Rimvall, 1993). 90% of GABA is synthesized by constitutively expressed GAD67 in the cytosol and channeled for non-neurotransmission related functions, synaptic vesicle (SV) membrane-associated GAD65 (mGAD) is transiently activated to synthesize GABA for release in high frequency bursts and fine-tuning of GABAergic neurotransmission at the synapse (Owens & Kriegstein, 2002; Pinal & Tobin, 1998).

In addition to its importance in regulating the GABA level in the central nervous system, GAD has also been implicated as an autoantigen in several autoimmune diseases, such as insulin dependent diabetes mellitus (IDDM) and Stiff–Person syndrome (Butler et al., 1993; Burbelo et al., 2008).

## GABA Synthesis and Packaging into Synaptic Vesicles

It is known that GAD67 is spread evenly throughout the neuronal cytoplasm and that the GABA generated by GAD67 may be utilized for purposes other than neurotransmission such as functioning as a trophic factor for synaptogenesis during early development, in protection after neuronal injury, as a source of energy via the GABA shunt and as a regulator of redox potential during oxidative stress (Lamigeon et al., 2001; Pinal and Tobin, 1998; Waagepetersen et al., 1999). On the other hand, GAD65 is concentrated in the nerve terminals where it synthesizes GABA for neurotransmission purposes (Martin and Rimvall, 1993). Previously, we have reported that GAD65 but not GAD67 forms a complex with heat shock cognate 70 (HSC70), cysteine string protein (CSP) and vesicular GABA transporter (VGAT) in the nerve terminal. This complex appears to be the necessary machinery required for efficient GABA synthesis and packaging into synaptic vesicles (SV) through VGAT (Jin et al., 2003).

In our earlier work, we demonstrated that a functional coupling exists between the vesicular GABA transporter (VGAT) and SV - associated GAD65 (Jin et al., 2003). Such an alignment in close proximity between these two molecules enables VGAT to preferentially load the newly synthesized GABA generated by the transiently activated membrane -

associated GAD65 (mGAD) into the SVs, with priority over the pre-existing GABA constitutively generated by GAD67 in the soma. This key phenomenon is disrupted in GAD65 knockout mice. Mice deficient in GAD65 appear normal but are highly susceptible to epilepsy and general anxiety disorder which can be spontaneously precipitated by fear or mild stress (Kash et al., 1997; Walls et al., 2010). These findings underscore the pivotal role played by membrane - associated GAD65 in regulating GABA for extra-synaptic tonic inhibition.

It is of interest that some studies suggest that GAD67 can also be targeted to intracellular organelles through its interaction with GAD65 or independent of GAD65 (Dirkx et al., 1995; J. Kanaani, 1999; Lernmark, 1996). However, the significance of membrane-associated GAD67 in GABA neurotransmission is not clear.

In our previous publications, we reported the presence of truncated GAD65 (tGAD65) during protein purification of human recombinant full length GAD65 (fGAD65) from a bacterial expression system in vitro (Wei et al., 2003). fGAD65 could be readily cleaved by mild trypsin treatment or incubation with Factor Xa to yield a 58 KDa tGAD65, confirming a previous report that a proteolytic hot-spot is contained within the first 100 amino acids of GAD65 (Christgau et al., 1992). Peptide fragment analysis revealed the identity of the cleavage site located precisely between Arg69 and Lys70 (Wei et al., 2003). Interestingly, in vitro biochemical characterization of fGAD65 versus tGAD65 indicated that the truncated form was 2–3 times more stable and stronger than the full length form (Wei et al., 2003). In addition, we demonstrated that rat brain fGAD65 could be cleaved upon neuronal stimulation in vivo to yield a cleaved product, which had similar electrophoretic mobility as the purified recombinant tGAD65 on SDS-PAGE (Wei et al., 2006). Furthermore, by biochemical approaches, we demonstrated that the enzyme calpain was responsible for the cleavage of fGAD65 to form tGAD65 (Wei et al., 2006). However, the conditions favoring calpain cleavage of fGAD65 and the implications this cleavage site may have on GABA neurotransmission have not been fully characterized.

# GAD Regulation

## Transcriptional Regulation

Over the past few decades, substantial progress has been made in understanding the regulatory mechanisms of GAD65 and GAD67 with analysis of transcriptional, translational and post-translational regulation of GADs. It has been shown that the expression of GAD65 and GAD67 genes and the synthesis of GAD65 and GAD67 proteins are differentially regulated during development (Somogyi et al., 1995). At the mRNA level, there is evidence of the existence of splice variants of GAD67, namely GAD44 and GAD25 arising during embryonic development, and only GAD44 is known to be enzymatically active (Behar et al., 1993).

However, no such splice variants are reported for GAD65. It has also been established that GAD67 is expressed early during development, and the later expression of GAD65 is consistent with their respective roles in synaptogenesis and as a source of neurotransmitter pool (Pinal & Tobin, 1998).

## Post-Translational Regulation

GAD67 and GAD65 are also known to undergo post-translational modifications including palmitoylation, proteolytic cleavage and phosphorylation (Wei and Wu, 2008) as detailed below.

## Palmitoylation

Palmitoylation, however, is unique to GAD65. GAD65 is primarily synthesized as a soluble cytosolic protein but undergoes palmitoylation catalyzed by a palmitoyl transferase (PAT) at cysteine residues 30 and 45, which is crucial for post-Golgi trafficking to presynaptic clusters in neurons (Kanaani et al., 2004). A depalmitoylation – repalmitoylation cycle serves to cycle GAD65 between Golgi and post-Golgi membranes and dynamically regulates the levels of the enzyme directed to the synapse (Jamil Kanaani, Patterson, Schaufele, Lippincott-Schwartz, & Baekkeskov, 2008).

The details of protein palmitoylation and the enzymes involved are still not clear. A large family of DHHC (Asp-His-His-Cys) proteins has emerged as protein PATs (Dietrich & Ungermann, 2004; Dirkx et al., 1995; J. Kanaani, 1999; Lernmark, 1996; Noritake et al., 2009). It is interesting that (Noritake et al., 2009) reported that a dendritically localized PAT, DHHC2, but not the Golgi resident PAT, DHHC3, mediates the activity-sensitive palmitoylation of PSD-95 suggesting that individual PAT DHHC members are differentially regulated and that dynamic recruitment of protein palmitoylation machinery enables compartmentalized regulation of protein trafficking in response to extracellular signals. There are four PATs including DHHC-3, DHHC-8, DHHC-13 and huntingtin interacting protein 14 (HIP14) have been reported to enhance the palmitoylation of GAD65 in co-transfected COS cells (Huang et al., 2009). Among these four PATs, HIP14 which was initially isolated as a huntingtin-interacting protein (Singaraja et al., 2002) and later proven to be a neuronal PAT due to the presence of a core DHHC (Asp-His-His-Lys) motif essential for PAT activity (Huang et al., 2004) appears to be the primary PAT responsible for palmitoylation of GAD65. This notion is supported from the observations that palmitoylation of endogenous GAD65 in neuronal culture is decreased by knocking down HIP14, but is not affected by DHHC-3 knockdown (Huang et al., 2009). Furthermore, overexpression of HIP14 enhances perinuclear accumulation of GAD65 in cultured neurons, whereas HIP14 small interfering RNA significantly reduces axonal clustering of GFP-tagged GAD65 (Huang et al., 2004). Recently Rush et al. (2012) also reported that palmitoylation of GAD65 is reduced in the Huntington's disease animal model and over-expression of HIP14 in vivo, could rescue GAD65 palmitoylation and SV-associated GAD65 trafficking suggesting that GAD65 palmitoylation is important for anchoring of GAD65 to GABAergic SV. Based on the evidence discussed above, we propose that the sequence of events leading from neuronal stimulation to an increase of GABA synthesis, packaging and release resulting in an increase of GABA transmission can be proposed as follows: 1). Upon neuronal stimulation, intracellular Ca2+ level is increased due to Ca2+influx; 2). Consequently, phospholipase A2 is activated, leading to the conversion of phospholipid to arachidonic acid (AA); 3). AA binds to PKCε and facilitates its translocation from cytosol to SV membrane; 4). This translocation brings activated PKCε close to GAD65, resulting in phosphorylation and activation of SV-associated

GAD65; 5). Increase of palmitoylation of GAD65 by HIP14 will also facilitate its anchoring to SV resulting in a synergistic effect on GABA synthesis by SV-associated GAD65 and its packaging into SV by VGAT through a coupling mechanism; 6). The refilled GABA in SV is ready to be released upon the arrival of a subsequent action potential.

## Regulation by Proteolytic Cleavage of Full Length GAD (fGAD) to Truncated GAD (tGAD)

With the purified recombinant human GAD preparation, we found that the recombinant human GAD65 could be cleaved into a more stable truncated form in vitro by Factor Xa or mild trypsin treatment. The enzyme activity assay indicated that this truncated form is more active than the full length GAD65 (fGAD65). N-terminal sequencing of the truncated form revealed that this cleavage occurs between Arginine 69 and Lysine 70 (Wei et al., 2003). This observation is consistent with the report that the region around 69-70 is a proteolytic hot spot in native GAD65 (Christgau et al., 1992). In addition to GAD65, we also found that GAD67 is cleaved at two specific sites, one at arginine 70 and another one at arginine 90 to produce two truncated forms of GAD67 (tGAD67) (Sha et al., 2005). However, contrary to tGAD65, tGAD67 is less active than the full length GAD67 (fGAD67) (Sha et al., 2005; Wei et al., 2003).

In addition to the recombinant human GAD65 and GAD67, we have also shown the presence of tGAD65 and tGAD67 in the brain and identified the endogenous protease responsible for the cleavage of fGAD65 and fGAD67 as μ-calpain (calpain-1) which is active at micromolar (μM) concentrations of calcium but not m-calpain (calpain-2) which requires millimolar (mM) levels of calcium for activation (Buddhala et al., 2012; Sha et al., 2008; Wei et al., 2006). It is of interest that although GAD65 is activated when it is cleaved to the tGAD65 by u-calpain under excessive stimulation or pathological conditions e.g., ischemic condition, the packaging of GABA into the SV and hence the GABA neurotransmission is reduced due to dissociation of GAD65 from the SV (Buddhala et al., 2012). Based on these observations, it is clear that the activity of GABA neurotransmission is not dependent on the GABA synthesizing activity of GAD alone but also dependent on whether GAD is associated with the SV and coupled with VGAT for efficient transport of GABA into the SV.

## Regulation by Protein Phosphorylation and Dephosphorylation

Reversible protein phosphorylation is a key regulatory post translational mechanism by which most signaling pathways such as cell growth, differentiation, migration and apoptosis in eukaryotes operate (de Graauw et al., 2006). We have shown that both GAD65 and GAD67 are regulated by phosphorylation and dephosphorylation (Wei et al., 2004). In vitro GAD65 was activated by phosphorylation mediated by protein kinase C-epsilon (PKC-epsilon) while GAD67 was inhibited by phosphorylation mediated by PKA (Wei et al., 2004). In addition, we identified T91 to be an important phosphorylation site for GAD67 by matrix-assisted laser desorption/ionization-time of flight (MALDI-TOF) mass spectrometry (Wei et al., 2004). Phosphorylation sites for GAD65 have not been identified yet. Efforts are underway in developing phosphorylation state specific antibodies to T91 of GAD67 to advance our functional studies on phosphorylation of GAD67. Out-with our own work, it was reported that phosphorylation of serine residues 3, 6, 10, and 13 in GAD65 is involved in its anchoring to the SV membrane and has no effect on GAD activity (Namchuk et al., 1997). Determining which kinases and phosphatases are involved in vivo in the regulation of GAD is crucial to understand how GABA biosynthesis is regulated.

### Role of Cysteine in GAD Activity

In pursuit of studying the role of structural residues that are crucial determinants for a favourable conformation of GAD enzymes, the importance of cysteine residues in the function of brain GAD activity has long been appreciated (Wu and Roberts, 1974). Cysteine residues 455 and 446 of GAD67 and GAD65, respectively have been reported to be very important structural residues in regulating GAD activity since mutation of this cysteine residue reduced GAD activity more than 90% (Wei and Wu, 2005). It was further confirmed by the recently reported crystallographic structure of GADs that these cysteine residues reside in the co-factor pyridoxal 50-phosphate (PLP) binding domain (Fenalti et al., 2007). Interaction with PLP is another means of short-term regulation of GADs. Post-translated GADs are highly regulated by shuttling between their active PLP-bound holoGAD form and an inactive PLP-unbound apoGAD form. Unlike 73% of GAD67 which is holoGAD, about 93% of GAD65 is largely apoGAD and responds to demand for GABA neurotransmission by converting transiently from apoGAD to holoGAD (Battaglioli et al., 2003). There have also been reports that GADs are influenced by hormones (Grattan et al., 1996), cytokines (Schmidli et al., 1996), neurotransmitters, e.g. dopamine (Laprade and Soghomonian, 1995a) and excitatory amino acids (Laprade and Soghomonian, 1995b). The levels of GAD65 and GAD67 protein are also differentially regulated by GABA (Rimvall and Martin, 1994).

## Role of VGAT (Vesicular GABA Transporter)

VGAT is an integral membrane protein with 10 transmembrane domains (Pinal and Tobin, 1998), whereas GAD65 and GAD67 are soluble proteins lacking any transmembrane regions (Watanabe et al., 2002). Although GAD65 is not considered to be an integral membrane protein because it lacks a stretch of hydrophobic amino acids long enough to span the membrane, it remains anchored to synaptic vesicle (SV) membranes. The nature of the anchoring mechanism remains elusive. Recently, we have shown that GAD65 anchored to synaptic vesicle (SV) membrane through protein-protein interaction, presumably involved heat shock protein 70 (HSP70) and cysteine string protein (CSP), a SV protein (Hsu et al., 2000). Vesicular GABA transporter (VGAT), as part of the protein complex associated with GAD65 (Jin et al., 2003). The identification of VGAT is part of GAD65 protein complex led us to propose a structural and functional coupling between GABA synthesis by SV-associated GAD65 and its packaging into SV by VGAT as depicted in Figure 1.

According to this model, when GABA neurons are stimulated, Ca2+ enters neuron triggering GABA release by exocytosis (step 1). Furthermore, PKC-epsilon could be translocated to the SV upon stimulation and activated by phospholipids (step 2).

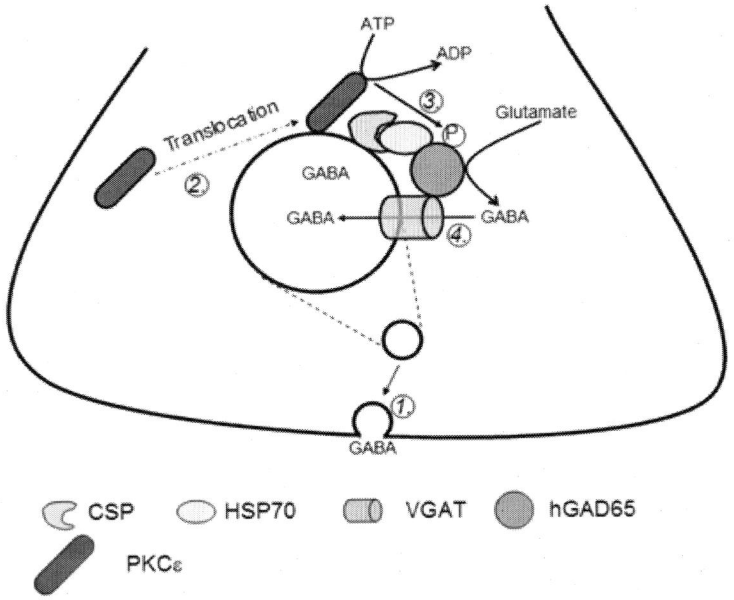


Figure 1. A model depicting a structural and functional coupling between GABA synthesis and vesicular GABA transport into SV. (See the text for details).

Activated PKC-epsilon could then phosphorylate SV-associated GAD65 resulting in activation of GAD65 (step 3). Newly synthesized GABA by SV-associated GAD65 is then transported into SV by VGAT through a coupling mechanism between GAD65 and VGAT as proposed (step 4). The refilled GABAergic SVs are ready to be released upon the arrival of the next stimulation. This model is supported by the following observations: First of all, the newly synthesized [$^3$H]GABA from [$^3$H]Glutamate by SV-associated GAD65 is taken up efficiently by VGAT. The VGAT activity is markedly inhibited when the GAD inhibitor, hydrazine or aminooxyacetate, is included in the reaction system, suggesting a functional coupling between SV-associated GAD and VGAT (Jin et al., 2003). Secondly, both vesicular uptake of GABA by VGAT (Jin et al., 2003) and activation of mGAD/GAD65 by ATP depend on the integrity of the proton gradient as well as V-type ATPase activity on SV (Hsu et al., 1999). Thirdly, although PKC-epsilon is a soluble protein, it can become membrane-associated and activated through translocation from cytosol to target membranes (Saitoh et al., 2001). Hence, it is proposed that when GABA neurons are stimulated, the stimulation will facilitate the translocation of PKC-epsilon to become membrane anchored where it can phosphorylate and activate SV-associated GAD65. In fact, our preliminary studies have demonstrated that the presence of PKC**ε** in the purified SV preparations and translocation to membrane fractions upon stimulation (Fig 2). Fourthly, although GAD is a soluble protein, it can anchor to SV through its interaction with HSP70 and several members of SV proteins including CSP and VGAT (Hsu et al., 2000; Jin et al., 2003). This protein machinery provides a structural basis for an efficient coupling between GABA synthesis by SV-associated GAD65 and GABA uptake into SV by VGAT.

In addition to GABAergic system, we have shown that similar mechanism may be responsible for neurotransmitter synthesis and packaging into SV in cholinergic and dopaminergic systems (Chen et al., 2003; Sha et al., 2004).

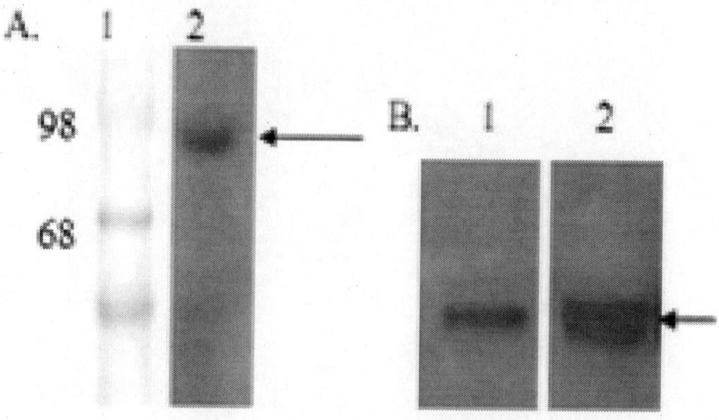


Figure 2. Translocation of PKCε to membrance fraction under stimulation. A. Immunoblotting showing the presence of PKCε in crude synaptic vesicles. Lane 1 protein marker; Lane 2: PKCε. B. Immunoblotting showing the translocation of PKCε to membrane fractions under stimulation. Lane 1, membrane fractions before stimulation; Lane 2, Membrane fractions after stimulation. Arrow indicates the position of PKCε.

## CONCLUSION

Free cytosolic fGAD67 in its dephosphorylated state, constitutively synthesizes GABA for nonneurotransmission purposes to meet the high energy requirements in the neuron (Pinal & Tobin, 1998; Wei et al., 2004).To summarize, here we bring forth a new viewpoint of the possible role of GAD65 associated with mitochondria in supplying the ATP required by synaptic vesicle membrane-associated GAD65 to synthesize GABA for uptake into SV to be released for GABA neurotransmission.

## REFERENCES

Battaglioli G, Liu H, Martin DL (2003) Kinetic differences between the isoforms of glutamate decarboxylase: implications for the regulation of GABA synthesis. *J. Neurochem.* 86(4):879–87.

Behar T, Schaffner A, Laing P, Hudson L, Komoly S, Barker J (1993) Many spinal cord cells transiently express low molecular weight forms of glutamic acid decarboxylase during embryonic development. *Brain Research. Developmental Brain Res.* 72(2):203–18.

Buddhala C, Suarez M, Modi J, Prentice H, Ma Z, Tao R, Wu, J-Y (2012) Calpain cleavage of brain glutamic acid decarboxylase 65 is pathological and impairs GABA neurotransmission. *PloS One.* 7(3), e33002.

Burbelo PD, Groot S, Dalakas MC, Iadarola MJ (2008) High definition profiling of autoantibodies to glutamic acid decarboxylases GAD65/GAD67 in stiff-person syndrome. *Biochem. Biophys. Res. Commun.* 366(1):1–7.

Butler MH, Solimena M, Dirkx R, Hayday A, De Camilli P (1993) Identification of a dominant epitope of glutamic acid decarboxylase (GAD-65) recognized by autoantibodies in stiff-man syndrome. *J. Exp. Med.* 178(6):2097–106.

Chen R, Wei J, Fowler SC, Wu J-Y (2003) Demonstration of functional coupling between dopamine synthesis and its packaging into synaptic vesicles. *J. Biom. Sci.* 10(6 Pt 2):774–81. doi:73965

Christgau S, Aanstoot HJ, Schierbeck H, Begley K, Tullin S, Hejnaes K, Baekkeskov S (1992) Membrane anchoring of the autoantigen GAD65 to microvesicles in pancreatic beta-cells by palmitoylation in the NH2-terminal domain. *J. Cell Biol.* 118(2):309–20.

De Graauw M, Hensbergen P, van de Water B (2006) Phospho-proteomic analysis of cellular signaling. *Electrophoresis*. 27(13):2676–86.

De Jong PJ, Lakke JP, Teelken AW (1984) CSF GABA levels in Parkinson's disease. *Adv. Neurol.* 40:427–30.

Dietrich LEP, Ungermann C (2004) On the mechanism of protein palmitoylation. *EMBO Rep.* 5(11):1053–7.

Dirkx R, Thomas A, Li L, Lernmark k, Sherwin RS, De Camilli P, Solimena M (1995) Targeting of the 67-kDa Isoform of Glutamic Acid Decarboxylase to Intracellular Organelles Is Mediated by Its Interaction with the NH(2)-terminal Region of the 65-kDa Isoform of Glutamic Acid Decarboxylase. *J. Biol. Chem.* 270(5):2241–2246.

Fenalti G, Law RHP, Buckle AM, Langendorf C, Tuck K, Rosado CJ, Whisstock, JC (2007) GABA production by glutamic acid decarboxylase is regulated by a dynamic catalytic loop. *Nat. Struct. Mol. Biol.* 14(4):280–6.

Freichel C, Potschka H, Ebert U, Brandt C, Löscher W (2006) Acute changes in the neuronal expression of GABA and glutamate decarboxylase isoforms in the rat piriform cortex following status epilepticus. *Neurosci.* 141(4):2177–94.

Gourfinkel-An I, Parain K, Hartmann A, Mangiarini L, Brice A, Bates G, Hirsch EC(2003) Changes in GAD67 mRNA expression evidenced by in situ hybridization in the brain of R6/2 transgenic mice. *J. Neurochem.* 86(6):1369–1378.

Grattan DR, Rocca MS, Strauss KI, Sagrillo CA, Selmanoff M, McCarthy MM (1996) GABAergic neuronal activity and mRNA levels for both forms of glutamic acid decarboxylase (GAD65 and GAD67) are reduced in the diagonal band of Broca during the afternoon of proestrus. *Brain Res.* 733(1):46–55.

Hsu CC, Davis KM., Jin H, Foos T, Floor E, Chen W, Wu J-Y (2000) Association of L-glutamic acid decarboxylase to the 70-kDa heat shock protein as a potential anchoring mechanism to synaptic vesicles. *J. Biol. Chem.* 275(27):20822–8.

Hsu CC, Thomas C, Chen W, Davis KM, Foos T, Chen JL, Wu J-Y (1999) Role of synaptic vesicle proton gradient and protein phosphorylation on ATP-mediated activation of membrane-associated brain glutamate decarboxylase. *J. Biol. Chem.* 274(34):24366–71.

Huang K, Sanders S, Singaraja R, Orban P, Cijsouw T, Arstikaitis P, El-Husseini A (2009) Neuronal palmitoyl acyl transferases exhibit distinct substrate specificity. *FASEB J.* 23(8):2605–15.

Huang K, Yanai A, Kang R, Arstikaitis P, Singaraja RR, Metzler M, El-Husseini A (2004) Huntingtin-interacting protein HIP14 is a palmitoyl transferase involved in palmitoylation and trafficking of multiple neuronal proteins. *Neuron.* 44(6):977–86.

Jin H, Wu H, Osterhaus G, Wei J, Davis K, Sha D, Wu J-Y (2003) Demonstration of functional coupling between gamma -aminobutyric acid (GABA) synthesis and vesicular GABA transport into synaptic vesicles. *Proc. Natl. Acad. Sci. U S A.* 100(7):4293–8.

Kanaani J (1999) The Hydrophilic Isoform of Glutamate Decarboxylase, GAD67, Is Targeted to Membranes and Nerve Terminals Independent of Dimerization with the Hydrophobic Membrane-anchored Isoform, GAD65. *J. Biol. Chem.* 274(52):37200–9.

Kanaani J, Diacovo MJ, El-Husseini AED, Bredt DS, Baekkeskov S (2004) Palmitoylation controls trafficking of GAD65 from Golgi membranes to axon-specific endosomes and a Rab5a-dependent pathway to presynaptic clusters. *J. Cell Sci.* 117(Pt 10):2001–13.

Kanaani J, Patterson G, Schaufele F, Lippincott-Schwartz J, Baekkeskov S (2008) A palmitoylation cycle dynamically regulates partitioning of the GABA-synthesizing enzyme GAD65 between ER-Golgi and post-Golgi membranes. *J. Cell Sci.* 121(Pt 4): 437–49.

Kash SF, Johnson RS, Tecott LH, Noebels JL, Mayfield RD, Hanahan D, Baekkeskov S (1997) Epilepsy in mice deficient in the 65-kDa isoform of glutamic acid decarboxylase. *Proc. Natl. Acad. Sci. U S A.* 94(25):14060–5.

Kosel M, Rudolph U, Wielepp P, Luginbühl M, Schmitt W, Fisch HU, Schlaepfer TE (2004) Diminished GABA(A) receptor-binding capacity and a DNA base substitution in a patient with treatment-resistant depression and anxiety. *Neuropsychopharmacol.* 29(2): 347–50.

Lamigeon C, Bellier JP, Sacchettoni S, Rujano M, Jacquemont B (2001) Enhanced neuronal protection from oxidative stress by coculture with glutamic acid decarboxylase-expressing astrocytes. *J. Neurochem.* 77(2):598–606.

Laprade N, Soghomonian JJ (1995a) MK-801 decreases striatal and cortical GAD65 mRNA levels. *Neurorep.* 6(14):1885–9.

Laprade N, Soghomonian, JJ (1995b) Differential regulation of mRNA levels encoding for the two isoforms of glutamate decarboxylase (GAD65 and GAD67) by dopamine receptors in the rat striatum. *Mol. Brain Res.* 34(1):65–74.

Lernmark A (1996) Glutamic acid decarboxylase-gene to antigen to disease. *J. Int. Med.* 240(5):259–77.

Lloyd KG, Bossi L, Morselli PL, Munari C, Rougier M, Loiseau H (1986) Alterations of GABA-mediated synaptic transmission in human epilepsy. *Adv. in Neurol.* 44:1033–44.

Martin DL, Rimvall K (1993) Regulation of gamma-aminobutyric acid synthesis in the brain. *J. Neurochem.* 60(2):395–407.

Namchuk M, Lindsay L, Turck CW, Kanaani J, Baekkeskov S (1997) Phosphorylation of serine residues 3, 6, 10, and 13 distinguishes membrane anchored from soluble glutamic acid decarboxylase 65 and is restricted to glutamic acid decarboxylase 65alpha. *J. Biol. Chem.* 272(3):1548–57.

Noritake J, Fukata Y, Iwanaga T, Hosomi N, Tsutsumi R, Matsuda N, Fukata M (2009) Mobile DHHC palmitoylating enzyme mediates activity-sensitive synaptic targeting of PSD-95. *J. Cell Biol.* 186(1):147–60.

Owens DF, Kriegstein AR (2002) Is there more to GABA than synaptic inhibition? *Nature Reviews. Neurosc.* 3(9):715–27.

Pinal CS, Tobin AJ (1998) Uniqueness and redundancy in GABA production. *Perspect. Dev. Neurobiol.* 5(2-3):109–18.

Rimvall K, Martin DL (1994) The level of GAD67 protein is highly sensitive to small increases in intraneuronal gamma-aminobutyric acid levels. *J. Neurochem.* 62(4):1375–81.

Rush DB, Leon RT, McCollum MH, Treu RW, Wei J (2012) Palmitoylation and trafficking of GAD65 are impaired in a cellular model of Huntington's disease. *Biochem. J.* 442(1):39–48.

Saitoh N, Hori T, Takahashi T (2001) Activation of the epsilon isoform of protein kinase C in the mammalian nerve terminal. *Proc. Natl. Acad. Sci. U S* A. 98(24):14017–21.

Schmidli R S, Faulkner-Jones BE, Harrison LC, James RF, DeAizpurua HJ (1996) Cytokine regulation of glutamate decarboxylase biosynthesis in isolated rat islets of Langerhans. *Biochem. J.* 317:713–9.

Sha D, Jin H, Kopke RD, Wu J-Y (2004) Choline acetyltransferase: regulation and coupling with protein kinase and vesicular acetylcholine transporter on synaptic vesicles. *Neurochem. Res.* 29(1):199–207.

Sha D, Jin Y, Wu H, Wei J, Lin C-H, Lee Y-H, Wu J-Y (2008) Role of mu-calpain in proteolytic cleavage of brain L-glutamic acid decarboxylase. *Brain Res.* 1207:9–18.

Sha D, Wei J, Wu H, Jin Y, Wu J-Y (2005) Molecular cloning, expression, purification, and characterization of shorter forms of human glutamic decarboxylase 67 in an E. coli expression system. *Brain Res. Mol. Brain Res.* 136(1-2):255–61.

Singaraja RR, Hadano S, Metzler M, Givan S, Wellington CL, Warby S, Yanai A, Gutekunst CA, Leavitt BR, Yi H, Fichter K, Gan L, McCutcheon K, Chopra V, Michel J, Hersch SM, Ikeda JE, Hayden MR (2002) HIP14, a novel ankyrin domain-containing protein, links huntingtin to intracellular trafficking and endocytosis. *Hum. Mol. Genet.* 11(23):2815–28.

Somogyi R, Wen X, Ma W, Barker JL (1995) Developmental kinetics of GAD family mRNAs parallel neurogenesis in the rat spinal cord. *J. Neurosci.* 15(4):2575–91.

Spokes EG, Garrett NJ, Rossor MN, Iversen LL (1980) Distribution of GABA in post-mortem brain tissue from control, psychotic and Huntington's chorea subjects. *J. Neurol. Sci.* 48(3):303–13.

Waagepetersen HS, Sonnewald U, Schousboe A (1999) The GABA paradox: multiple roles as metabolite, neurotransmitter, and neurodifferentiative agent. *J. Neurochem.* 73(4): 1335–42.

Walls AB, Nilsen LH, Eyjolfsson EM, Vestergaard HT, Hansen SL, Schousboe A, Waagepetersen HS (2010) GAD65 is essential for synthesis of GABA destined for tonic inhibition regulating epileptiform activity. *J. Neurochem.* 115(6):1398–408.

Watanabe M, Maemura K, Kanbara K, Tamayama T, Hayasaki H (2002) GABA and GABA receptors in the central nervous system and other organs. *Int. Rev. Cyt.* 213:1–47.

Wei J, Davis KM, Wu H, Wu J-Y (2004) Protein phosphorylation of human brain glutamic acid decarboxylase (GAD)65 and GAD67 and its physiological implications. *Biochem.* 43(20):6182–9.

Wei J, Jin Y, Wu H, Sha D, Wu J-Y (2003) Identification and functional analysis of truncated human glutamic acid decarboxylase 65. *J. Biom. Sci.* 10:617–24.

Wei J, Lin C-H, Wu H, Jin Y, Lee Y-H, Wu J-Y (2006) Activity-dependent cleavage of brain glutamic acid decarboxylase 65 by calpain. *J. Neurochem.* 98(5):1688–95.

Wei J, Wu J-Y (2005) Structural and functional analysis of cysteine residues in human glutamate decarboxylase 65 (GAD65) and GAD67. *J. Neurochem*. 93(3):624–33.

Wei J, Wu J-Y (2008) Post-translational regulation of L-glutamic acid decarboxylase in the brain. *Neurochem. Res*. 33(8):1459–65.

Wu J-Y, Roberts E (1974) Properties of brain L-glutamate decarboxylase: inhibition studies. *J. Neurochem*. 23(4):759–67.

In: Gamma-Aminobutyric Acid (GABA)
Editors: Josipa Vlainić and Maja Jazvinšćak Jembrek
ISBN: 978-1-63321-838-3


*Chapter 2*

# GABA METABOLISM IN *SACCHAROMYCES CEREVISIAE*

***Susana Correa-García*[*] *and Mariana Bermúdez-Moretti***
Departamento de Química Biológica, Facultad de Ciencias Exactas y Naturales, Universidad de Buenos Aires - IQUIBICEN, CONICET. Argentina

## ABSTRACT

The γ-aminobutyric acid (GABA) is a non protein amino acid present in bacteria, plants, fungi and even in vertebrates. The role of GABA in the budding yeast *Saccharomyces cerevisiae* is not fully understood. GABA can be used by yeast as the sole nitrogen source and its carbon backbone enters the tricarboxylic acid (TCA) cycle. Three permeases are involved in extracellular GABA uptake: the general amino acid permease Gap1, the proline-specific permease Put4 and the GABA-specific permease Uga4. Once, within the cell, GABA is deaminated by the enzyme GABA transaminase, yielding glutamate and succinate semialdehyde. Glutamate enters the central nitrogen metabolism, while succinate semialdehyde is converted to succinate by the succinate semialhehyde dehydrogenase. Then, succinate enters the TCA cycle. However, most of the incorporated GABA is not catabolized but accumulated in a subcellular compartment, like the vacuole.

On the other hand, GABA is synthesized in yeast cells by the decarboxylation of glutamate as an intermediate of the GABA shunt, by which α-ketoglutarate is converted to succinate. GABA shunt bypasses two steps of the TCA cycle and it is energetically less efficient than the direct oxidation of α-ketoglutarate at the TCA cycle. Strong evidence suggests that the GABA shunt plays a crucial role in protecting cells from stress.

**Keywords:** GABA, *Saccharomyces cerevisiae*, metabolism, transcriptional regulation

[*] Departamento de Química Biológica, Facultad de Ciencias Exactas y Naturales, CONICET, Universidad de Buenos Aires, Ciudad Universitaria, Buenos Aires, Argentina, Email: correa@qb.fcen.uba.ar.

## *SACCHAROMYCES CEREVISIAE* YEAST

Yeasts are fungi that grow as single cells, producing daughter cells either by budding (the budding yeasts) or binary fission (the fission yeasts). They grow typically in moist environments where a plentiful supply of simple, soluble nutrients, such as sugars and amino acids, are available. The most common budding yeast is the yeast *Saccharomyces cerevisiae*. *Saccharomyces* means "sugar fungus" because this yeast uses sugars as food, so they are found in the wild, growing on skin of grapes and other fruits; *cerevisiae* means "of beer". *S. cerevisiae* is used in industry for bread-making and for beer, wine and other alcoholic drinks production.

The yeast *S. cerevisiae* is certainly the best studied eukaryotic organism, which is very well genetically, biochemically, and physiologically characterized. It presents many advantages like fast doubling time, easy genetic manipulation and inexpensive cultivation. Its genome was the first to be sequenced (Goffeau et al., 1996) and many omic databases are available. It is one of the most intensively studied eukaryotic model organisms in molecular and cell biology and also serves as a biotechnology production organism (Krivoruchko et al., 2011; Otero et al., 2013). Many proteins important in human biology were first discovered by studying their homologues in yeast; these proteins include cell cycle proteins, signalling proteins, and protein-processing enzymes.

### GABA in Nature

The γ-aminobutyric acid (GABA) is a ubiquitous four-carbon non-protein amino acid that is widely distributed in nature. First discovered in potato tubers (Hulme and Arthington, 1950), it was found in both prokaryotic and eukaryotic organisms such as bacteria, yeast, plants and animals. To date, the role of GABA in most organisms has not been fully understood. The most well-known role of GABA is as a neurotransmitter in mammalian brain where it serves as an inhibitory neurotransmitter (Mody et al., 1994) and it also serves as a hormone or trophic factor in non-neuronal peripheral and endocrine systems (Gladkevich et al., 2006). Hypotensive, tranquilizing, diuretic and antidiabetic effects have been attributed to GABA (Dhakal et al., 2012; Hayakawa et al., 2004; Inoue et al., 2003; Jakobs et al., 1993; Li et al., 2010; Wong et al., 2003).

In plants, experimental evidence supports the involvement of GABA in pH regulation, nitrogen storage, plant development and defence. GABA acts as a compatible osmolyte and an intermediate in an alternative pathway for glutamate utilization (Bouche and Fromm, 2004; Shelp et al., 1999).

Yeast cells are able to use GABA as a nitrogen source (Ramos et al., 1985) and after being catabolized, its carbon skeleton enters the tricarboxylic acid (TCA) cycle as succinate. Several reports linked GABA with oxidative stress tolerance processes through the production of NADPH, an important antioxidant (Bach et al., 2009; Cao et al., 2013a; Cao et al., 2013b; Coleman et al., 2001).

## GABA Metabolism

GABA found in virtually all organisms is synthesized by the enzyme glutamate decarboxylase (GAD) (EC 4.1.1.15) from glutamate in a one-step irreversible reaction (Fig. 1). The enzyme from yeasts depends on pyridoxal 5′-phosphate (PLP) as a cofactor and is localized in the cytosol (Krishnaswamy and Giri, 1956). In *S. cerevisiae* cells, GAD (encoded by *GAD1* gene), that binds to calmodulin as the plant enzyme does, (Shelp et al., 1999) is required for tolerance to oxidative stress (Cao et al., 2013b; Coleman et al., 2001). It may be negatively regulating replicative lifespan in response to nutrient limitation and/or oxidative stress (Kamei et al., 2011). *GAD1* gene also displays significant induction by oxidants (Sulahian et al., 2006).

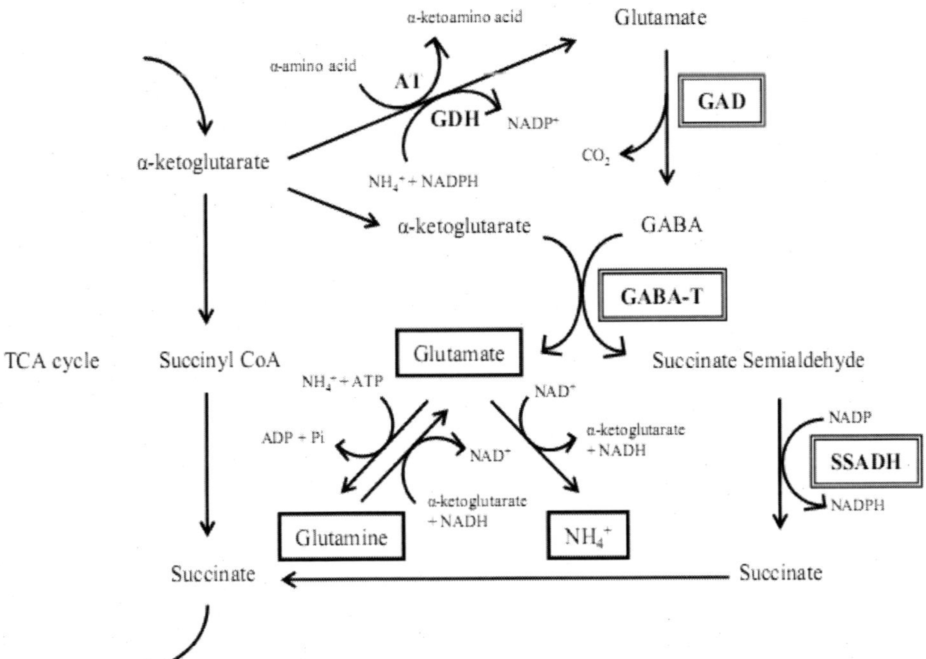


Figure 1. Schematic diagram of the GABA shunt in yeast that shows that this metabolic route links nitrogen and carbon metabolisms. Enzymes of this pathway are double framed. The main metabolites of the central nitrogen metabolism (CNM) are simple framed. GAD: glutamate decarboxylase; GABA-T: GABA transaminase; SSADH: succinate semialdehyde dehydrogenase; AT: α-aminotranferases; GDH: glutamate dehydrogenase.

The intracellular GABA synthesized by GAD or the GABA incorporated from extracellular medium (see below) is one of the thirty different compounds that yeast can use as nitrogen source (Godard et al., 2007). Cells convert these compounds into glutamate and ammonium which in turn form glutamine. These three metabolites form part of the central nitrogen metabolism (CNM) (Figure 1). Both amino acids, glutamate and glutamine, are the main nitrogen donors in the synthesis of all cellular nitrogen components.

Intracellular GABA is catabolized by two enzymes in *S. cerevisiae*: one is GABA transaminase (GABA-T) (EC 2.6.1.19) that deaminates GABA to succinate semialdehyde (SSA) and the other is SSA dehydrogenase (SSADH) (EC 1.2.1.16) that irreversibly catalyzes

SSA oxidation to succinate, which is supplied to TCA cycle (Figure 1). These enzymatic activities were early studied by Pietruszko and Fowden (Pietruszko and Fowden, 1961). Genetic analysis, directed to the search for mutant cells unable to grow in a medium containing GABA as the sole nitrogen source, revealed structural genes coding for both GABA-T and SSADH enzymes that were named *UGA1* and *UGA2*, respectively (Ramos et al., 1985). These names came from the ability to utilize GABA as the nitrogen source.

The fact that yeast cells deficient in *UGA2* gene were unable to grow on GABA as the sole nitrogen source and that these cells accumulate not only SSA but also secrete it to the extracellular medium led to the proposal that SSA could be a toxic metabolite to cells (Ramos et al., 1985). Moreover, SSA can also be reduced to γ-hydroxybutyric acid (GHB) by the enzyme γ-hydroxybutyric acid dehydrogenase (GHBDH) (EC 1.1.1.61). This enzyme has been detected in higher eukaryotes and in yeast (Andriamampandry et al., 1998; Bach et al., 2009; Breitkreuz et al., 2003). However, in this organism GHBDH activity has been only detected in the absence of SSADH and the amount of GHB formed is much lower than the amount of GABA consumed. Thus, GHB synthesis seems to play only a minor role in GABA degradation (Bach et al., 2009).

GABA-T and SSADH from *S. cerevisiae* are cytosolic enzymes (Cao et al., 2013a; Huh et al., 2003), unlike those of plants that are mitochondrial (Bouche and Fromm, 2004). *S. cerevisiae* GABA-T uses α-ketoglutarate (Ramos et al., 1985) as the amino acceptor, whereas both α-ketoglutarate or piruvate can be used in plants (Fait et al., 2008). It has been described that *S. cerevisiae* SSADH can use both $NAD^+$ or $NADP^+$, but it has higher affinity for $NADP^+$ (Ramos et al., 1985); however, Coleman et al. (Coleman et al., 2001) suggested that it is more likely that $NADP^+$ will serve as cofactor since the [NADPH + $NADP^+$]/[NADH + $NAD^+$] ratio is 35 in yeast (Anderlund et al., 1999).

The three enzymes required for GABA biosynthesis and catabolism: GAD, GABA-T and SSADH are involved in the GABA shunt that allows glutamate conversion to succinate via GABA (Figure 1). This pathway bypasses two enzymatic steps of the TCA cycle: α-ketoglutarate dehydrogenase complex (EC 1.2.4.2) and succinate CoA ligase (EC 6.2.1.4); these enzymes convert α-ketoglutarate into succinate. The amination of α-ketoglutarate to form glutamate is catalyzed by the enzyme glutamate dehydrogenase (GDH) encoded by yeast *GDH1* gene or by several α-ketoglutarate-dependent aminotransferases (AT) (Figure 1). This metabolic route, also called the GAD/GABA pathway, links nitrogen and carbon metabolisms and is conserved from bacteria, yeast, plants to vertebrates.

The role of the GABA shunt is not fully understood. In bacteria, it has been suggested that this pathway is involved in glutamate metabolism, anaplerosis and oxidative stress response (Feehily and Karatzas, 2012). In plants, the GABA shunt has been associated with various physiological responses, including the regulation of cytosolic pH, carbon fluxes into the TCA cycle, nitrogen metabolism, deterrence of insects, protection against oxidative stress, osmoregulation and signalling (Bouche and Fromm, 2004; Fait et al., 2008).

There is a limited number of reports studying the role of the GABA shunt in the yeast *S. cerevisiae*. *GAD1* is required for tolerance to oxidative stress and the loss of *UGA1* and *UGA2* genes reduces the tolerance to oxidative stress (Coleman et al., 2001). Recently, it has also been reported that yeast mutants deficient in *UGA1* or *UGA2* are sensitive to heat stress and it has been demonstrated that *uga1*Δ cells are more sensitive than *uga2*Δ cells (Cao et al., 2013b). A direct correlation between this thermosensitivity phenotype and the production of high levels of intracellular ROS was found (Cao et al., 2013b). However, it has not yet been elucidated whether in these mutant cells cytosolic NADPH is insufficient to abate ROS generation during heat stress.

GABA, which is widely distributed in nature and is one of thirty nitrogen sources used by yeast (Godard et al., 2007), is imported into *S. cerevisiae* cells by three proteins: the general amino acid permease (Gap1), the proline specific permease (Put4) and the GABA permease (Uga4) (Grenson, 1987). Uga4 also mediates the uptake of the δ-aminolevulinic acid, a precursor of porphyrins biosynthesis structurally related to GABA (Bermudez Moretti et al., 1996; Bermudez Moretti et al., 1995a; Bermudez Moretti et al., 1993; Bermudez Moretti et al., 1995b) and the uptake of putrescine (Uemura et al., 2004).

## Regulation of Genes Involved in GABA Utilization

The genes *UGA1*, *UGA2* and *UGA4* involved in GABA catabolism and its uptake form part of the *UGA* regulon. The expression of *UGA* genes is highly regulated and responds to changes in the availability of different kinds of nutrients. Transcription of these genes is induced by GABA and repressed by the presence of rich or preferred nitrogen sources, such as ammonium or glutamine, through a process known as Nitrogen Catabolite Repression (NCR). This mechanism implies the repression of several genes mainly involved in nitrogen metabolism.

The transcription factors Uga3 and Dal81/Uga35/DurL are essential in GABA induction of the three *UGA* genes. While Uga3 is specific for these genes (Andre, 1990), Dal81 is a regulator of genes in nitrogen utilization pathways, related to metabolisms of GABA, urea, arginine and allantoin pathways (Bricmont et al., 1991; Coornaert et al., 1991). Both factors positively act on *UGA4* promoter through a CG-rich sequence called $UAS_{GABA}$ (Andre et al., 1993). The central core of this DNA element is a perfect palindrome containing the sequence 5′-CCGCCGGCGG-3′ (Talibi et al., 1995). The central sequence *cis*-acting element present in the *UGA1* promoter contains an imperfect palindrome with the sequence 5′-CCGCGGGCGG-3′ (Talibi et al., 1995, Cunningham et al., 1994). The interaction between Uga3 and the $UAS_{GABA}$ from *UGA1* and *UGA4* was shown through electromobility shift assays (EMSA), in which the sequences of both elements were used as probes (Idicula et al., 2002). It has been determined that the consensus binding site for Uga3 is conformed by two independent elements with the sequence 5′-SGCGGNWWT-3′ and that the transcription is activated only if both binding sites are occupied (Idicula et al., 2002; Noel and Turcotte, 1998). In turn, in the regulatory region of *UGA2* gene, a single Uga3 consensus binding sequence 5′-SGCGGNWWT-3′ is found and there is not a $UAS_{GABA}$ element present. It has been demonstrated using *in vivo* binding assays (Chromatin Immunoprecipitation assays) that both transcription factors, Uga3 and Dal81, interact with *UGA* promoters in a GABA-dependent manner (Cardillo et al., 2010; Cardillo et al., 2012), in contrast with other results obtained from *in vitro* binding assays (Idicula et al., 2002). However, although the *UGA2* promoter contains a unique binding site for the Uga3 factor, *in vivo* interaction of this factor with the *UGA2* promoter was detected, indicating that, at least for this factor, the presence of one binding site is sufficient for transcriptional activation (Cardillo et al., 2012). It was also found that Uga3 needs Dal81 to interact with *UGA* promoters (Cardillo et al., 2012). In a similar way, *AGP1* gene (encoding an amino acid general permease) strictly depends on Dal81 for Stp1 binding to *AGP1* promoter and also for its proper induction in response to amino acids (Boban and Ljungdahl, 2007). Uga3 and Dal81 are also able to interact with different components of the SAGA complex and Uga3 is necessary for Dal81 interaction with *UGA1* promoter and for the transcriptional activation of this gene via SAGA and Gal11, components of the mediator complex for transcriptional activation (Sylvain et al., 2011).

The transcription factors Uga3 and Dal81 belong to the zinc binuclear cluster family and, like other members of this family, they contain a putative DNA-binding domain that consists of cysteine residues bound to two zinc atoms [$Zn(II)_2$-$Cys_6$]. This domain is essential for Uga3 activity (Talibi et al., 1995). In contrast, as urea amidolyase activity was measured, it was found that the DNA-binding domain of Dal81 is not essential for induction of *DUR1/2* gene (Bricmont et al., 1991). Similar observations were made for *Aspergillus nidulans* protein TamA, a protein closely related to Dal81 that is involved in nitrogen metabolism (Davis et al., 1996). For GABA induction of *UGA* genes, the [$Zn(II)_2$-$Cys_6$] domain of Dal81 is not required, even though Dal81 interact with *UGA* promoters (Cardillo et al., 2012). This interaction occurs through Uga3 that acts as a bridge between DNA and Dal81, since no interaction between Dal81 and the *UGA* promoters is detected in the absence of Uga3 or when the $UAS_{GABA}$ element is mutated (Cardillo et al., 2012). Dal81 also contains two polyglutamine stretches and one of them, the polyglutamine stretch between residues 73 and 94, is essential for both *UGA* genes induction (Cardillo et al., 2012) and also for the induction of *DUR1/2* (Bricmont et al., 1991); however, further studies should be carried out to elucidate the role of this polyglutamine domain.

To date, the mechanism leading to the activation of Uga3 and Dal81 in response to GABA remains unknown. As expression of these factors does not vary after the addition of GABA to the cells, activation may probably occur by some post-translational modification of the previously synthesized proteins (Andre, 1990).

Another transcription factor of the zinc binuclear cluster family involved in the transcriptional regulation of *UGA* genes is Leu3. This transcriptional regulator controls the expression of genes involved in the biosynthesis and in the transport of branched-chain amino acids (Friden and Schimmel, 1988; Nielsen et al., 2001; Zhou and Kohlhaw, 1990) and also in the regulation of *GDH1* gene, which is responsible for ammonium assimilation (Hu et al., 1995). Global transcriptional analysis revealed an increased *UGA4* transcription, among other genes, under ammonium limitation in a *leu3*Δ mutant (Boer et al., 2005). It has also been reported that Leu3 acts as a repressor on *UGA4* transcription (Cardillo et al., 2010). Although there is a putative Leu3 binding site within the $UAS_{GABA}$ element, *in vivo* binding of this factor to *UGA4* promoter was not detected, which suggests an indirect mechanism of regulation (Cardillo et al., 2010). *UGA1* but not *UGA2* is also negatively regulated by Leu3, in agreement with the fact that there is not a consensus binding site for Leu3 in *UGA2* promoter (Cardillo et al., 2011). This is in accordance with the physiological necessity of cells to rapidly and irreversibly catabolize the toxic product SSA formed by the enzyme GABA-T encoded by *UGA1* gene. However, the exact role of Leu3 in the regulation of *UGA* genes has not been elucidated yet.

The three genes of the *UGA* regulon are subject to NCR that mainly occurs through 5´-GAT(A/T)A-3´ sequences found in their promoter regions. *UGA4* promoter contains nine repeats of the sequence 5´-GAT(A/T)A-3´ or its complement reverse 5´-T(T/A)ATC-3´. Four of them form a cluster located 28 base pairs upstream the $UAS_{GABA}$, which constitute the $UAS_{GATA}$ element; while the other repeats are distributed downstream that element (Andre et al., 1995). *UGA1* promoter contains seven 5´-GAT(A/T)A-3´ repeats (Cunningham et al.,

1994) and in the regulatory region of *UGA2,* two close relatives of the GATAA sequence are present (Coleman et al., 2001). The four members of the ***GATA*** transcription factor family, Gln3 and Gat1/Nil1 activators and Dal80/Uga43 and Gzf3/Deh1 repressors, can act on a $UAS_{GATA}$ element. The two negative factors play different roles in the mechanisms of regulation of NCR-responsive genes: Dal80 impairs their activation in a non-preferred nitrogen source, whereas Gzf3 in a preferred one (Coffman et al., 1997; Cooper, 2002; Magasanik, 2005; Magasanik and Kaiser, 2002; Soussi-Boudekou et al., 1997). All four GATA factors are subject to an intricate cross-regulation network (Coffman et al., 1997; Soussi-Boudekou et al., 1997).

The $UAS_{GATA}$ element can potentially confer high levels of expression of *UGA4* in the absence of the inducer GABA. Nevertheless, this potential activity is inhibited in uninduced cells grown under conditions of nitrogen derepression, by a strong repression mechanism, which involves Dal80, a pleiotropic regulatory factor. Deletion of Dal80 produces high levels of expression of *UGA4* and *UGA1* genes in the absence of the inducer GABA (Andre et al., 1995; Cunningham and Cooper, 1991). Gln3 acts in the presence of inducer up-regulating the expression of *UGA4* by competing with Dal80 to bind to the $UAS_{GATA}$ sequence (Coffman et al., 1997; Soussi-Boudekou et al., 1997); however, Gln3 involvement in *UGA1* regulation is controversial (Daugherty et al., 1993; Talibi et al., 1995). The outcome of this competition influences basal levels of transcription. Availability of preferred nitrogen sources mediates the ability of Ure2, a pre-prionic cytoplasmic protein, to prevent Gln3 and Gat1 from nuclear localization, and consequently, their activity (Kulkarni et al., 2001). Gln3 activity not only depends on its subcellular localization, but also on its phosphorylation status and this phosphorylation depends on TORC1 kinase activity (target of rapamycin) (Beck and Hall, 1999). Therefore, the formation of the complex Ure2-Gln3 depends on the activity of TORC1, which in turn depends on the intracellular concentration of glutamine/glutamate (Crespo et al., 2002). As a result of this regulatory mechanism, in cells grown on any rich nitrogen source, Gln3 and Gat1 are localized in the cytoplasm and the expression of NCR sensitive genes is repressed. If the available nitrogen source is a poor one, such as proline, Gln3 and Gat1 become nuclear being the expression of such genes derepressed.

*In vitro* binding assays of GATA factors to *UGA* genes showed that Dal80 and Gln3 interact with *UGA4* promoter (Cunningham et al., 1994; Cunningham et al., 1996). Dal80 and Gat1 were detected bound *in vivo* to *UGA4* promoter in cells grown in a poor nitrogen source and competition between these two GATA factors was proposed (Georis et al., 2009). Recently, it has been demonstrated that Dal80 and Gln3 interact with *UGA4* and *UGA1* promoters, but not with *UGA2,* in a GABA-dependent manner (Cardillo et al., 2012). In cells grown on proline, Dal80 binds to these promoters and this binding is relieved when cells are pre-incubated with the inducer GABA. In contrast, no interaction of Gln3 was detected in cells grown on proline, but in the presence of GABA, Gln3 does interact with all *UGA* promoters (Cardillo et al., 2012). These observations are in agreement with the proposal that both GATA factors, Dal80 and Gln3, compete between each other for their DNA binding site (Andre et al., 1995; Cunningham et al., 1994).

Binding dynamics of Gln3 are opposite to those of Dal80 and interactions are dependent on GABA. This suggests that transcription factors acting on the $UAS_{GABA}$ element could influence the binding of GATA factors to *UGA* promoters. In fact, in cells deficient in Uga3 and Dal81 factors, Dal80 remains bound to *UGA4* and *UGA1* promoters, even in the presence of GABA (Cardillo et al., 2012). Interactions of Dal80 with *UGA2* promoter are different to those of the other two members of *UGA* regulon. Dal80 binding to *UGA2* promoter is barely detectable and this binding slightly increased in the absence of Uga3 and Dal81 (Cardillo et al., 2012). Taking into account that expression of *UGA2* is not negatively regulated by Leu3, which is in contrast with findings for *UGA4* and *UGA1* (Cardillo et al., 2011), it remains to be clarified whether Leu3 affects Dal80 interactions with promoters. Unfortunately, binding of Gln3 to *UGA* promoters has not been detected until now, since strains expressing tagged Gln3 and deficient in Uga3 and Dal81 grow poorly in proline and ChIPs experiments have not led to conclusive results (Cardillo et al., 2012). Studies on TamA of *A. nidulans*, a Dal81-related protein, demonstrated an interaction with AreA protein, a GATA-family transcription factor functionally related to Gln3 (Small et al., 2001), supporting the idea that Gln3 and Dal81 could be interacting. TamA also interacts with LeuB, an homologous to *S. cerevisiae* Leu3, and it has been proposed that TamA could have a function stabilizing AreA and LeuB interactions with DNA (Polotnianka et al., 2004). Therefore, it remains still a long way to elucidate the interplay between the major transcription factors (i.e. Gln3, Dal80, Uga3, Dal81 and Leu3) acting on the *UGA* promoters. Further research will get new insight into concerted interactions of those factors and DNA.

As it is stated above, expression of *UGA* genes depends on many environmental conditions. Among these, nitrogen and carbon sources, GABA, external amino acids and pH significantly affect the transcription of this regulon.

GABA induction of *UGA4* diminishes in the presence of extracellular amino acids and this effect is mediated by the SPS amino acid sensor system (Bermudez Moretti et al., 2005). The components of this sensor are three proteins: Ssy1, a nutrient receptor, and Ptr3 and Ssy5, two peripheral membrane-associated proteins. The homologous zinc finger transcription factors Stp1 and Stp2 are downstream effector components of the SPS sensor pathway (Ljungdahl, 2009). Inhibition of *UGA4* induction by leucine, an amino acid commonly used as an inducer of the SPS sensor, is relieved in cells deficient in Ssy1 protein or in both Stp1 and Stp2 transcription factors (Cardillo et al., 2010). Dal81 is not only required for the induction of *UGA* genes but also for the full induction of several amino acid permeases in response to signals triggered by the SPS sensor (Abdel-Sater et al., 2004; Boban and Ljungdahl, 2007). In cells pre-incubated with leucine, the GABA-dependent Dal81 binding to *UGA4* promoter is impaired, correlating with low levels of *UGA4* induction. Moreover, leucine also weakens Uga3 interaction with *UGA4* promoter (Cardillo et al., 2010). Taking into account that Uga3 is a specific transcription factor of *UGA* genes, this supports the finding that Uga3 and Dal81 need each other for their interaction with DNA (Cardillo et al., 2012). In the absence of Ssy1, both Dal81 and Uga3 binding to *UGA4* promoter is unaffected, which confirms that weak binding of these transcription factors to *UGA4* promoter in wild type cells pre-incubated with leucine is caused by the signal triggered by this amino acid through the SPS sensor system (Cardillo et al., 2010). The other members of the *UGA* regulon, *UGA1* and *UGA2*, are also subjected to amino acid regulation via the SPS sensor, as it occurs for *UGA4* (Cardillo et al., 2011).

*UGA4* expression is regulated by extracellular pH, being *UGA4* an acid-expressed gene (Moretti et al., 2001), as it is the *gabA* gene encoding GABA permease of *A. nidulans* (Espeso and Arst, 2000; Sarkar et al., 1996). In cells grown on the minimal medium described by Vavra and Johnson (Vavra and Johnson, 1956) buffered at a low pH (4.5), *UGA4* expression is very high and it does not depend on the presence of GABA, although it strictly depends on the transcription factors. Uga3 and Dal81, that act on the $UAS_{GABA}$ element (Bermudez Moretti et al., 1998; Garcia et al., 2000).

The quality of the carbon source also modulates *UGA4* gene expression through two parallel pathways: one of them acting on the Gln3 target sequence, the $UAS_{GATA}$ element, and the other acting on the $UAS_{GABA}$ element (Luzzani et al., 2007). In a non-fermentable carbon source, such as acetate, basal levels of *UGA4* expression are higher than in a fermentable carbon source, such as glucose. Besides, GABA induction is weaker in a non-fermentable carbon source than in a fermentable one (Levi et al., 2012; Luzzani et al., 2007). Studies on binding dynamics of transcription factors acting on the $UAS_{GATA}$ element demonstrated that, in acetate, no interaction between Gln3 and *UGA4* promoter is detected, even after incubating cells with GABA; and Dal80 remains bound, even in the presence of inducer (Levi et al., 2012). Moreover, Uga3 and Dal81 factors do not interact with *UGA4* promoter in cells grown in acetate even in the presence of GABA (Levi et al., 2012), in contrast with results obtained in cells grown in glucose (Cardillo et al., 2010). On the other hand, Gln3 nuclear localization and its phosphorylation status vary according to the carbon source (Bertram et al., 2002; Kuruvilla et al., 2001; Levi et al., 2012; Luzzani et al., 2007); however, it has not been demonstrated yet how nuclear localization and/or phosphorylation affect the binding of Gln3 to DNA. All together these findings support a cross-talk between factors acting on the $UAS_{GATA}$ and $UAS_{GABA}$ elements of *UGA4* promoter.

## Conclusion

GABA plays an important role in some industrial processes where the yeast *S. cerevisiae* participates. Wine acidity depends on the amount of the succinate obtained as the final product of the catabolism of GABA which represents a 20% of the nitrogen compounds available in grapes (Bach et al., 2009). GABA is also the main constituent of free amino acids in seed mash for sake brewing (Takahashi et al., 2004).

*S. cerevisiae* GAD and the *UGA* regulon play several important roles in cell physiology.

The main and best-known role of the *UGA* regulon is to supply metabolites useful for the CNM, since GABA can be used by yeast cells as the sole nitrogen source.

The GABA shunt pathway in yeast cells is involved in the assimilation of supplied glutamate and it is useful to feed the carbon skeleton from GABA into the respiratory chain within the mitochondria as succinate (Pietruszko and Fowden, 1961; Ramos et al., 1985). At the same time, this pathway is an important source of reduced cofactors required for the regeneration of two key components for resistance to oxidative stress, reduced glutathione and thioredoxin (Jamieson, 1998). Therefore, this shunt plays a crucial role in protecting yeast cells from stress by restricting ROS production (Cao et al., 2013b).

An important proportion of the synthesized or incorporated GABA undergoes no further metabolism and it is stored in a cellular component, most likely the vacuole (McKelvey et al., 1990), where it may also play a physiological function in stress tolerance mechanisms. The import of GABA to the vacuole seems to be mediated by the product of *UGA4* gene, the $H^+$/GABA symporter that has also been detected in the vacuolar membrane (Uemura et al., 2004), and may also help to regulate cytosolic pH. The fact that *UGA4* is a pH responsive gene (Moretti et al., 2001) is consistent with this hypothesis.

Further research on GABA metabolism and its regulation in *S. cerevisiae* cells will not only contribute to fully understand this process in yeast, but it will also be helpful to widen the knowledge of this pathway in other eukaryotic organisms and to improve biotechnological applications of yeasts.

## REFERENCES

Abdel-Sater F, Iraqui I, Urrestarazu A, Andre B (2004) The external amino acid signaling pathway promotes activation of Stp1 and Uga35/Dal81 transcription factors for induction of the AGP1 gene in Saccharomyces cerevisiae. *Genetics.* 166:1727-1739.

Anderlund M, Nissen TL, Nielsen J, Villadsen J, Rydstrom J, Hahn-Hagerdal B, Kielland-Brandt MC (1999) Expression of the Escherichia coli pntA and pntB genes, encoding nicotinamide nucleotide transhydrogenase, in Saccharomyces cerevisiae and its effect on product formation during anaerobic glucose fermentation. *Appl. Environ. Microbiol.* 65:2333-2340.

Andre B (1990) The UGA3 gene regulating the GABA catabolic pathway in Saccharomyces cerevisiae codes for a putative zinc-finger protein acting on RNA amount. *Mol. Gen. Genet.* 220:269-276.

Andre B, Hein C, Grenson M, Jauniaux JC (1993) Cloning and expression of the UGA4 gene coding for the inducible GABA-specific transport protein of Saccharomyces cerevisiae. *Mol. Gen. Genet.* 237:17-25.

Andre B, Talibi D, Soussi Boudekou S, Hein C, Vissers S, Coornaert D (1995) Two mutually exclusive regulatory systems inhibit UASGATA, a cluster of 5'-GAT(A/T)A-3' upstream from the UGA4 gene of Saccharomyces cerevisiae. *Nucleic Acids Res.* 23:558-564.

Andriamampandry C, Siffert JC, Schmitt M, Garnier JM, Staub A, Muller C, Gobaille S, Mark J, Maitre M (1998) Cloning of a rat brain succinic semialdehyde reductase involved in the synthesis of the neuromodulator gamma-hydroxybutyrate. *Biochem. J.* 334(Pt 1):43-50.

Bach B, Meudec E, Lepoutre JP, Rossignol T, Blondin B, Dequin S, Camarasa C (2009) New insights into {gamma}-aminobutyric acid catabolism: Evidence for {gamma}-hydroxybutyric acid and polyhydroxybutyrate synthesis in Saccharomyces cerevisiae. *Appl. Environ. Microbiol.* 75:4231-4239.

Beck T, Hall MN (1999) The TOR signalling pathway controls nuclear localization of nutrient-regulated transcription factors. *Nature.* 402:689-692.

Bermudez Moretti M, Correa Garcia S, Batlle A (1998) UGA4 gene expression in Saccharomyces cerevisiae depends on cell growth conditions. *Cell Mol. Biol.*(Noisy-le-grand). 44:585-590.

Bermudez Moretti M, Correa Garcia S, Ramos E, Batlle A (1996) delta-Aminolevulinic acid uptake is mediated by the gamma-aminobutyric acid-specific permease UGA4. *Cell Mol. Biol.* (Noisy-le-grand). 42:519-523.

Bermudez Moretti M, Correa Garcia S, Ramos EH, Batlle A (1995a) GABA uptake in a Saccharomyces cerevisiae strain. *Cell Mol. Biol.* (Noisy-le-grand). 41:843-849.

Bermudez Moretti M, Correa Garcia S, Stella C, Ramos E, Batlle AM (1993) Delta-aminolevulinic acid transport in Saccharomyces cerevisiae. *Int. J. Biochem.* 25:1917-1924.

Bermudez Moretti M, Correa Garcia SR, Chianelli MS, Ramos EH, Mattoon JR, Batlle A (1995b) Evidence that 4-aminobutyric acid and 5-aminolevulinic acid share a common transport system into Saccharomyces cerevisiae. *Int. J. Biochem. Cell Biol.* 27:169-173.

Bermudez Moretti M, Perullini AM, Batlle a, Correa Garcia S (2005) Expression of the UGA4 gene encoding the delta-aminolevulinic and gamma-aminobutyric acids permease in Saccharomyces cerevisiae is controlled by amino acid-sensing systems. *Arch. Microbiol.* 184:137-140.

Bertram PG, Choi JH, Carvalho J, Chan TF, Ai W, Zheng XF (2002) Convergence of TOR-nitrogen and Snf1-glucose signaling pathways onto Gln3. *Mol. Cell Biol.* 22:1246-1252.

Boban M, Ljungdahl PO (2007) Dal81 enhances Stp1- and Stp2-dependent transcription necessitating negative modulation by inner nuclear membrane protein Asi1 in Saccharomyces cerevisiae. *Genetics.* 176:2087-2097.

Boer VM, Daran JM, Almering MJ, de Winde JH, Pronk JT (2005) Contribution of the Saccharomyces cerevisiae transcriptional regulator Leu3p to physiology and gene expression in nitrogen- and carbon-limited chemostat cultures. *FEMS Yeast Res.* 5:885-897.

Bouche N, Fromm H (2004) GABA in plants: just a metabolite? *Trends Plant Sci.* 9:110-115.

Breitkreuz KE, Allan WL, Van Cauwenberghe OR, Jakobs C, Talibi D, Andre B, Shelp BJ (2003) A novel gamma-hydroxybutyrate dehydrogenase: identification and expression of an Arabidopsis cDNA and potential role under oxygen deficiency. *J. Biol. Chem.* 278:41552-41556.

Bricmont PA, Daugherty JR, Cooper TG (1991) The DAL81 gene product is required for induced expression of two differently regulated nitrogen catabolic genes in Saccharomyces cerevisiae. *Mol. Cell Biol.* 11:1161-1166.

Cao J, Barbosa JM, Singh N, Locy RD (2013a) GABA transaminases from Saccharomyces cerevisiae and Arabidopsis thaliana complement function in cytosol and mitochondria. *Yeast.* 30:279-289.

Cao J, Barbosa JM, Singh NK, Locy RD (2013b) GABA shunt mediates thermotolerance in Saccharomyces cerevisiae by reducing reactive oxygen production. *Yeast.* 30:129-144.

Cardillo SB, Bermudez Moretti M, Correa Garcia S (2010) Uga3 and Uga35/Dal81 transcription factors regulate UGA4 transcription in response to gamma-aminobutyric acid and leucine. *Eukaryot Cell.* 9:1262-1271.

Cardillo SB, Correa Garcia S, Bermudez Moretti M (2011) Common features and differences in the expression of the three genes forming the UGA regulon in Saccharomyces cerevisiae. *Biochem. Biophys. Res. Commun.* 410:885-889.

Cardillo SB, Levi CE, Bermudez Moretti M, Correa Garcia S (2012) Interplay between the transcription factors acting on the GATA- and GABA-responsive elements of Saccharomyces cerevisiae UGA promoters. *Microbiology.* 158(Pt 4):925-935.

Coffman JA, Rai R, Loprete DM, Cunningham T, Svetlov V, Cooper TG (1997) Cross regulation of four GATA factors that control nitrogen catabolic gene expression in Saccharomyces cerevisiae. *J. Bacteriol.* 179:3416-3429.

Coleman ST, Fang TK, Rovinsky SA, Turano FJ, Moye-Rowley WS (2001) Expression of a glutamate decarboxylase homologue is required for normal oxidative stress tolerance in Saccharomyces cerevisiae. *J. Biol. Chem.* 276:244-250.

Cooper TG (2002) Transmitting the signal of excess nitrogen in Saccharomyces cerevisiae from the Tor proteins to the GATA factors: connecting the dots. *FEMS Microbiol. Rev.* 26:223-238.

Coornaert D, Vissers S, Andre B (1991) The pleiotropic UGA35(DURL) regulatory gene of Saccharomyces cerevisiae: cloning, sequence and identity with the DAL81 gene. *Gene.* 97:163-171.

Crespo JL, Powers T, Fowler B, Hall MN (2002) The TOR-controlled transcription activators GLN3, RTG1, and RTG3 are regulated in response to intracellular levels of glutamine. *Proc. Natl. Acad. Sci. USA*. 99:6784-6789.

Cunningham TS, Cooper TG (1991) Expression of the DAL80 gene, whose product is homologous to the GATA factors and is a negative regulator of multiple nitrogen catabolic genes in Saccharomyces cerevisiae, is sensitive to nitrogen catabolite repression. *Mol. Cell Biol.* 11:6205-6215.

Cunningham TS, Dorrington RA, Cooper TG (1994) The UGA4 UASNTR site required for GLN3-dependent transcriptional activation also mediates DAL80-responsive regulation and DAL80 protein binding in Saccharomyces cerevisiae. *J. Bacteriol.* 176:4718-4725.

Cunningham TS, Svetlov VV, Rai R, Smart W, Cooper TG (1996) G1n3p is capable of binding to UAS(NTR) elements and activating transcription in Saccharomyces cerevisiae. *J. Bacteriol.* 178:3470-3479.

Daugherty JR, Rai R, el Berry HM, Cooper TG (1993) Regulatory circuit for responses of nitrogen catabolic gene expression to the GLN3 and DAL80 proteins and nitrogen catabolite repression in Saccharomyces cerevisiae. *J. Bacteriol.* 175:64-73.

Davis MA, Small AJ, Kourambas S, Hynes MJ (1996) The tamA gene of Aspergillus nidulans contains a putative zinc cluster motif which is not required for gene function. *J. Bacteriol.* 178:3406-3409.

Dhakal R, Bajpai VK, Baek KH (2012) Production of gaba (gamma - Aminobutyric acid) by microorganisms: a review. *Braz. J. Microbiol.* 43:1230-1241.

Espeso EA, Arst Jr. HN (2000) On the mechanism by which alkaline pH prevents expression of an acid-expressed gene. *Mol. Cell Biol.* 20:3355-3363.

Fait A, Fromm H, Walter D, Galili G, Fernie AR (2008) Highway or byway: the metabolic role of the GABA shunt in plants. *Trends Plant Sci.* 13:14-19.

Feehily C, Karatzas KA (2012) Role of glutamate metabolism in bacterial responses towards acid and other stresses. *J. Appl. Microbiol.* 114:11-24.

Friden P, Schimmel P (1988) LEU3 of Saccharomyces cerevisiae activates multiple genes for branched-chain amino acid biosynthesis by binding to a common decanucleotide core sequence. *Mol. Cell Biol.* 8:2690-2697.

Garcia SC, Moretti MB, Batlle A (2000) Constitutive expression of the UGA4 gene in Saccharomyces cerevisiae depends on two positive-acting proteins, Uga3p and Uga35p. *FEMS Microbiol. Lett.* 184:219-224.

Georis I, Feller A, Vierendeels F, Dubois E (2009) The yeast GATA factor Gat1 occupies a central position in nitrogen catabolite repression-sensitive gene activation. *Mol. Cell Biol.* 29:3803-3815.

Gladkevich A, Korf J, Hakobyan VP,. Melkonyan KV (2006) The peripheral GABAergic system as a target in endocrine disorders. *Auton Neurosci.* 124:1-8.

Godard P, Urrestarazu A, Vissers S, Kontos K, Bontempi G, van Helden J, Andre B (2007) Effect of 21 different nitrogen sources on global gene expression in the yeast Saccharomyces cerevisiae. *Mol. Cell Biol.* 27:3065-3086.

Goffeau A, Barrell BG, Bussey H, Davis RW, Dujon B, Feldmann H, Galibert F, Hoheisel JD, Jacq C, Johnston M, Louis EJ, Mewes HW, Murakami Y, Philippsen P, Tettelin H, Oliver SG (1996) Life with 6000 genes. *Science.* 274:546, 563-547.

Grenson M (1987) 4-Aminobutyric acid (GABA) uptake in Baker's yeast Saccharomyces cerevisiae is mediated by the general amino acid permease, the proline permease and a GABA specific permease integrated into the GABA-catabolic pathway. *Life Sci. Adv. Biochem.* 6:35-39.

Hayakawa K, Kimura M, Kasaha K, Matsumoto K, Sansawa H, Yamori Y (2004) Effect of a gamma-aminobutyric acid-enriched dairy product on the blood pressure of spontaneously hypertensive and normotensive Wistar-Kyoto rats. *Br. J. Nutr.* 92:411-417.

Hu Y, Cooper TG, Kohlhaw GB (1995) The Saccharomyces cerevisiae Leu3 protein activates expression of GDH1, a key gene in nitrogen assimilation. *Mol. Cell Biol.* 15:52-57.

Huh WK, Falvo JV, Gerke LC, Carroll AS, Howson RW, Weissman JS, O'Shea EK (2003) Global analysis of protein localization in budding yeast. *Nature.* 425:686-691.

Hulme AC, Arthington W (1950) rho-AMINO-butyric acid and alanine in plant tissues. *Nature.* 165:716.

Idicula AM, Blatch GL, Cooper TG, Dorrington RA (2002) Binding and activation by the zinc cluster transcription factors of Saccharomyces cerevisiae. Redefining the UASGABA and its interaction with Uga3p. *J. Biol. Chem.* 277:45977-45983.

Inoue K, Shirai T, Ochiai H, Kasao M, Hayakawa K, Kimura M, Sansawa H (2003) Blood-pressure-lowering effect of a novel fermented milk containing gamma-aminobutyric acid (GABA) in mild hypertensives. *Eur. J. Clin. Nutr.* 57:490-495.

Jakobs C, Jaeken J, Gibson KM (1993) Inherited disorders of GABA metabolism. *J. Inherit Metab. Dis.* 16:704-715.

Jamieson DJ (1998) Oxidative stress responses of the yeast Saccharomyces cerevisiae. *Yeast.* 14:1511-1527.

Kamei Y, Tamura T, Yoshida R, Ohta S, Fukusaki E, Mukai Y (2011) GABA metabolism pathway genes, UGA1 and GAD1, regulate replicative lifespan in Saccharomyces cerevisiae. *Biochem. Biophys. Res. Commun.* 407:185-190.

Krishnaswamy PR, Giri KV (1956) Glutamic acid decarboxylase in Rhodotorula glutinis. *Biochem. J.* 62:301-303.

Krivoruchko A, Siewers V, Nielsen J (2011) Opportunities for yeast metabolic engineering: Lessons from synthetic biology. *Biotechnol. J.* 6:262-276.

Kulkarni AA, Abul-Hamd AT, Rai R, El Berry H, Cooper TG (2001) Gln3p nuclear localization and interaction with Ure2p in Saccharomyces cerevisiae. *J. Biol. Chem.* 276:32136-32144.

Kuruvilla FG, Shamji AF, Schreiber SL (2001) Carbon- and nitrogen-quality signaling to translation are mediated by distinct GATA-type transcription factors. *Proc. Natl. Acad. Sci. USA.* 98:7283-7288.

Levi CE, Cardillo SB, Bertotti S, Rios C, Correa Garcia S, Moretti MB (2012) GABA induction of the Saccharomyces cerevisiae UGA4 gene depends on the quality of the carbon source: role of the key transcription factors acting in this process. *Biochem. Biophys. Res. Commun.* 421:572-577.

Li H, Qiu T, Huang G, Cao Y (2010) Production of gamma-aminobutyric acid by Lactobacillus brevis NCL912 using fed-batch fermentation. *Microb. Cell Fact.* 9:85.

Ljungdahl, P.O. 2009. Amino-acid-induced signalling via the SPS-sensing pathway in yeast. *Biochem. Soc. Trans.* 37:242-247.

Luzzani C, Cardillo SB, Bermudez Moretti M, Correa Garcia S (2007) New insights into the regulation of the Saccharomyces cerevisiae UGA4 gene: two parallel pathways participate in carbon-regulated transcription. *Microbiology.* 153:3677-3684.

Magasanik B (2005) The transduction of the nitrogen regulation signal in Saccharomyces cerevisiae. *Proc. Natl. Acad. Sci. USA.* 102:16537-16538.

Magasanik B, Kaiser CA (2002) Nitrogen regulation in Saccharomyces cerevisiae. *Gene.* 290:1-18.

McKelvey J, Rai R, Cooper TG (1990) GABA transport in Saccharomyces cerevisiae. *Yeast.* 6:263-270.

Mody I, De Koninck Y, Otis TS, Soltesz I (1994) Bridging the cleft at GABA synapses in the brain. *Trends Neurosci.* 17:517-525.

Moretti MB, Batlle A, Garcia SC (2001) UGA4 gene encoding the gamma-aminobutyric acid permease in Saccharomyces cerevisiae is an acid-expressed gene. *Int. J. Biochem. Cell Biol.* 33:1202-1207.

Nielsen PS, van den Hazel B, Didion T, de Boer M, Jorgensen M, Planta RJ, Kielland-Brandt MJ, Andersen HA (2001) Transcriptional regulation of the Saccharomyces cerevisiae amino acid permease gene BAP2. *Mol. Gen. Genet.* 264:613-622.

Noel J, Turcotte B (1998) Zinc cluster proteins Leu3p and Uga3p recognize highly related but distinct DNA targets. *J. Biol. Chem.* 273:17463-17468.

Otero JM, Cimini D, Patil KR, Poulsen SG, Olsson L, Nielsen J (2013) Industrial systems biology of Saccharomyces cerevisiae enables novel succinic acid cell factory. *PLoS One.* 8:e54144.

Pietruszko R, Fowden L (1961) 4-Aminobutyric acid metabolism in plants. Metabolism in yeast. *Annals of Botany.* 25:491-511.

Polotnianka R, Monahan BJ, Hynes MJ, Davis MA (2004) TamA interacts with LeuB, the homologue of Saccharomyces cerevisiae Leu3p, to regulate gdhA expression in Aspergillus nidulans. *Mol. Genet Genomics.* 272:452-459.

Ramos F, el Guezzar M, Grenson M, Wiame JM (1985) Mutations affecting the enzymes involved in the utilization of 4-aminobutyric acid as nitrogen source by the yeast Saccharomyces cerevisiae. *Eur. J. Biochem.* 149:401-404.

Sarkar S, Caddick MX, Bignell E, Tilburn J, Arst Jr. HN (1996) Regulation of gene expression by ambient pH in Aspergillus: genes expressed at acid pH. *Biochem. Soc. Trans.* 24:360-363.

Shelp BJ, Bown AW, McLean MD (1999) Metabolism and functions of gamma-aminobutyric acid. *Trends Plant Sci.* 4:446-452.

Small AJ, Todd RB, Zanker MC, Delimitrou S, Hynes MJ, Davis MA (2001) Functional analysis of TamA, a coactivator of nitrogen-regulated gene expression in Aspergillus nidulans. *Mol. Genet Genomics.* 265:636-646.

Soussi-Boudekou S, Vissers S, Urrestarazu A, Jauniaux JA, Andre B (1997) Gzf3p, a fourth GATA factor involved in nitrogen-regulated transcription in Saccharomyces cerevisiae. *Mol. Microbiol.* 23:1157-1168.

Sulahian R, Sikder D, Johnston SA, Kodadek T (2006) The proteasomal ATPase complex is required for stress-induced transcription in yeast. *Nucleic. Acids Res.* 34:1351-1357.

Sylvain MA, Liang XB, Hellauer K, Turcotte B (2011) Yeast Zinc Cluster Proteins Dal81 and Uga3 Cooperate by Targeting Common Coactivators for Transcriptional Activation of {gamma}-aminobutyrate Responsive Genes. *Genetics.* 188(3):523-534.

Takahashi T, Furukawa A, Hara S, Mizoguchi H (2004) Isolation and characterization of sake yeast mutants deficient in gamma-aminobutyric acid utilization in sake brewing. *J. Biosci. Bioeng.* 97:412-418.

Talibi D, Grenson M, Andre B (1995) Cis- and trans-acting elements determining induction of the genes of the gamma-aminobutyrate (GABA) utilization pathway in Saccharomyces cerevisiae. *Nucleic Acids Res.* 23:550-557.

Uemura T, Tomonari Y, Kashiwagi K, Igarashi K (2004) Uptake of GABA and putrescine by UGA4 on the vacuolar membrane in Saccharomyces cerevisiae. *Biochem. Biophys. Res.* Commun. 315:1082-1087.

Vavra JJ, Johnson MJ (1956) Aerobic and anaerobic biosynthesis of amino acids by bakers' yeast. *J. Biol. Chem.* 220:33-43.

Wong CG, Bottiglieri T, Snead 3$^{rd}$ OC (2003) GABA, gamma-hydroxybutyric acid, and neurological disease. *Ann. Neurol.* 54 Suppl 6:S3-12.

Zhou KM, Kohlhaw GB (1990) Transcriptional activator LEU3 of yeast. Mapping of the transcriptional activation function and significance of activation domain tryptophans. *J. Biol. Chem.* 265:17409-17412.

In: Gamma-Aminobutyric Acid (GABA)
Editors: Josipa Vlainić and Maja Jazvinšćak Jembrek
ISBN: 978-1-63321-838-3


*Chapter 3*

# The Effects of Persistent Activation of GABA$_A$ Receptors by Neurotransmitter GABA

***Josipa Vlainić[1†], Dubravka Švob Štrac[†] and Maja Jazvinšćak Jembrek***

Rudjer Boskovic Institute, Department of Molecular Medicine, Laboratory of Molecular Neuropharmacology, Zagreb, Croatia

## Abstract

Gamma-aminobutyric acid (GABA) has an important role in the transmission of neural information throughout all brain regions, and is involved directly and/or indirectly in the control of many vital functions. In particular, various brain functions depend on the balance between excitatory and inhibitory neurotransmission. Given that GABA is the main inhibitory neurotransmitter, changes in its level might lead to numerous neurological and psychiatric disorders.

GABA achieves its physiological actions mostly through GABA$_A$ receptors. Persistent activation of GABA$_A$ receptors by GABA, as well as by agonists and drugs facilitating the action of GABA, triggers regulatory changes in receptor expression and/or function that are relevant to physiological, pathological and pharmacological conditions. Therefore, the aim of our study was to better understand the effects and mechanisms that underlie adaptive changes at GABA$_A$ receptors following their prolonged exposure to neurotransmitter GABA itself.

Prolonged exposure of human embryonic kidney (HEK 293) cells stably expressing recombinant $\alpha_1\beta_2\gamma_{2S}$ GABA$_A$ receptors to GABA (1 mM) enhanced the maximum number of [$^3$H]flunitrazepam, [$^3$H]muscimol and [$^3$H]TBOB binding sites without affecting their affinity. The GABA-induced enhancement in the maximum number of benzodiazepine binding sites was reduced by bicuculline (100 μM), GABA$_A$ receptor antagonist, and by cycloheximide (10 μL/mL), a protein synthesis inhibitor. In parallel,

[1] Corresponding author: Rudjer Boskovic Institute, Division of Molecular Medicine, Bijenicka cesta 54, 10 000 Zagreb, Croatia. Email: josipa.vlainic@irb.hr.

[†] These authors equally contributed to the manuscript.

prolonged GABA treatment has not produced allosteric uncoupling of GABA and benzodiazepine binding sites as evidenced by unaltered GABA-induced potentiation of [$^3$H]flunitrazepam binding.

In conclusion, prolonged exposure of recombinant $GABA_A$ receptors to GABA results in enhancement of total receptor number, probably due to increased synthesis rather than decreased degradation of receptor proteins. Moreover, persistent activation of receptors by GABA has not resulted in functional uncoupling of GABA and benzodiazepine binding sites. Additional studies are needed to determine the functional implications of such changes, as well as relevance of obtained results to the development of tolerance and dependence.

**Keywords**: Recombinant $GABA_A$ receptor, GABA, radioligand binding studies, cell culture

## INTRODUCTION

Gamma-aminobutyric acid (GABA) has an important role in the transmission of neural information throughout all brain regions and is involved in the control of many vital functions. Namely, brain function depends on the balance between inhibitory and excitatory signals and thereby GABA is involved directly or indirectly in majority aspects of normal brain function. Given that GABA is major inhibitory neurotransmitter, changes in its level lead to numerous neuropsychiatric disorders such as insomnia, anxiety, panic disorders, epilepsy, schizophrenia, autism, hepatic encephalopathy, Huntington and Parkinson disease, etc (for review see Mohler, 2006).

GABA achieves its physiological action by acting on three major classes of GABA receptors: $GABA_A$, $GABA_B$, and $GABA_C$ (ρ receptors). Gamma-aminobutyric acid type A receptors ($GABA_A$-R) mediate most of the fast inhibitory neurotransmission in the central nervous system. These receptors are transmembrane glycoproteins forming central anion channel and classified to the superfamily of ligand gated ion channels. They appear in different forms depending on subunit association. Namely, so far 19 subunits of the mammalian $GABA_A$-R have been sequenced and classified into 8 groups: $\alpha_{1\text{-}6}$, $\beta_{1\text{-}3}$, $\gamma_{1\text{-}3}$, δ, ε, π, θ, and $\rho_{1\text{-}3}$ (Olsen and Sieghart, 2008). Moreover, the heterogeneity of $GABA_A$-Rs is further increased by the fact that some subunits (e.g. $\gamma_2$), appear also in the spliced forms ($\gamma_{2S}$, $\gamma_{2L}$ and $\gamma_{2XL}$). Additionally, it appears that the pentameric $GABA_A$-R assembly can also be formed from the combination of two, four, or even five different subunits. Although a variety of $GABA_A$-R complexes exist in the brain, the subunit composition of the most common type of the receptor found in the brain is 2α:2β:1γ (Sieghart, 2000).

The regulation of the neurotransmitter GABA is achieved by several specialized molecular mechanisms mediating its transport, sequestration, synthesis, and degradation. In addition to different regulatory mechanisms, GABA exerts its signalling role by acting on receptors located only on the surface of the cells/neurons. The transmitter concentration in the surrounding extra-cellular fluid determines the extent of receptor stimulation; therefore it is of exceptional importance that the extra-cellular concentrations are kept low (Farrant and Kaila, 2007). This is also required for a high signal in synaptic as well as in extra-synaptic transmission. Whereas GABA released into synapse may reach transient concentrations of ~1.5–3 mM, extra-synaptic transmitter concentration has been estimated to low micromolar range (~0.2–2.5 μM) (Glykys and Mody, 2007).

Since $GABA_A$-Rs and neurotransmitter GABA have tremendous importance in the normal brain functioning, as well as in various pathological conditions (Mohler, 2006), there are numerous drugs and substances in clinical use that modulate GABAergic function. Drugs that act as allosteric modulators of $GABA_A$-Rs (also known as GABAergic drugs) typically have relaxing, anti-anxiety, and anti-convulsive effects. The GABAergic drugs are widely used in the treatment of anxiety disorders, insomnia, epilepsy, restlessness, and aggressive behaviors and other various states and diseases. Moreover, $GABA_A$-Rs are the target for many intravenous and inhalational anesthetics, and substances of abuse, such as alcohol. Given that GABAergic drugs are used for prolonged period of time, the regulatory mechanisms which do appear at $GABA_A$-Rs are extremely important and are the subject of numerous studies. Namely, there are several unwanted effects related to the prolonged therapeutic use of drugs affecting the GABA system. Among those the most significant are the loss of drug efficacy, development of tolerance and/or dependence, as well as abuse and addiction.

Prolonged occupancy of $GABA_A$-Rs by GABA agonists and drugs facilitating the action of GABA leads to regulatory homeostatic changes in the number, localization and/or receptor function. Thus, chronic exposure of cultured cerebral cortical neurons to GABA decreases the number of benzodiazepine binding sites without affecting their affinity (Lyons et al., 2001; Mehta and Ticku, 1992; Tehrani and Barnes, 1988). Several groups of authors reported decrease in $GABA_A$-R subunit protein levels (Brown and Bristow, 1996; Mhatre and Ticku, 1994) and also GABA-stimulated $Cl^-$ uptake (Tehrani and Barnes, 1988) following prolonged GABA treatment. Moreover, following such treatment the reduction of mRNAs encoding different subunits of $GABA_A$-R was also found in cultured chick and mammalian neurons (Mhatre and Ticku, 1994; Montpied et al., 1991). Decrease in receptor number following prolonged GABA treatment was also observed in rat cortical slices by Shaw and Scarth (1991).

Although similar changes were found in animal models, the obtained results are often contradictory. It is reported that long-term treatment of rats with a GABA transaminase inhibitor or GABA agonist muscimol, down-regulate GABA-induced chloride influx but also to up-regulate cerebral GABA levels and number of benzodiazepine and GABA binding sites (for review see Barnes, 1996). Augmentation of GABA binding sites was also observed in cultured cerebellar granule cells (Meier et al., 1983). Moreover, Kim and colleagues (1993) reported that prolonged GABA treatment specifically stimulate an enhancement in the levels of mRNAs for $\alpha_1$ and $\beta_2$ $GABA_A$-R subunits and triggers an increase in the number of GABA binding sites. In an immunocytochemical study, Hansen and colleagues (1991) found that the density of the $GABA_A$-Rs was significantly increased in the cultures treated with 4,5,6,7-tetrahydroisoxazolo[5,4-c]pyridin-3-ol (THIP), a selective $GABA_A$ receptor agonist, when compared to the control cultures. Mentioned results suggest the induction of $GABA_A$-Rs gene expression as the mechanism involved in up-regulation of their density and/or function.

In addition, Mehta and Ticku (1992) and Roca and his colleagues (1990a) reported that prolonged treatment of cortical cultures with GABA also induces an allosteric uncoupling of GABA and benzodiazepine binding sites, characterized by a decrease in the GABA enhancement of benzodiazepine binding. These changes are independent of channel activation (Lyons et al., 2000; Russek et al., 2000). This notion is also supported by the research of Friedman and colleagues (1996), who hypothesized that the decrease of receptor number and uncoupling are produced by separate mechanisms since the exposure of neurons to benzodiazepines, barbiturates and neurosteroids causes uncoupling without altering the receptor number. Holt and colleagues (1999a) showed that even a single dose of diazepam produces a decrease in GABA potentiation of benzodiazepine binding. These results imply that uncoupling can occur in vivo under pharmacologically relevant conditions. It has been suggested that allosteric uncoupling of GABA and benzodiazepine binding sites which appear in animals and humans following prolonged treatment with GABA and several other drugs (benzodiazepines, barbiturates and steroids) may be related to the development of tolerance and physical dependence (Friedman et al., 1996; Gallager et al., 1984; Pericic et al., 2003; Pericic et al., 2007; Roca et al., 1990b; Svob Strac et al., 2008; Vlainic et al., 2010; Vlainic et al., 2012b). Although many in vitro and in vivo studies are performed, the exact mechanism(s) of uncoupling has not yet been elucidated (for review see Bateson, 2002 and Wafford, 2005).

The functional and pharmacological properties of $GABA_A$-Rs are determined by their subunit composition (Korpi et al., *2002*). Whereas certain subtypes are widely distributed in the brain, the expression of others is restricted to specific brain regions (Sieghart, 2000). Moreover, multiple subtypes of $GABA_A$-Rs occur within brain regions, or even on a single neuron (Barnard et al., 1998), what makes the research of pharmacological properties of a particular receptor subtype rather complex. Therefore, transient and stably transfected cells offer some advantages over the native receptors. Namely, cultured cells are a relatively homogenous cell population that can be well characterized with respect to receptor subunit composition, structure and function. Culture conditions can be tightly controlled, which facilitates the study of the mechanism of neurotransmitter receptor regulation (Klein and Harris, 1996). Moreover, the use of transient and stably transfected cells, which are devoid of neuronal gene products, allow the assessment of agonist - receptor interactions without possible changes in the neuronal environment. However, reports related to prolonged exposure of these cells to GABA and/or its agonists are relatively rare (Gutierrez at al., 2014; Klein et al., 1995; Klein and Harris, 1996; Pericic et al., 2003). More numerous are the reports (Ali and Olsen, 2001; Klein et al., 1996; Pericic et al., 2007; Primus et al., 1996; Svob Strac et al., 2008; Vlainic et al., 2010; Vlainic et al., 2012a; Wong et al., 1994) of prolonged effects of drugs such as benzodiazepines. Given acutely, benzodiazepines facilitate GABA-mediated transmission at the $GABA_A$ receptor, while chronic treatment with these drugs leads to development of side effects such as tolerance and physical dependence, which mechanisms have not been elucidated yet.

In our study, stably transfected human embryonic kidney (HEK) 293 cells (Besnard et al., 1997) were used as a model to study the effects of prolonged GABA exposure of the recombinant $\alpha_1\beta_2\gamma_{2S}$ $GABA_A$–Rs, the most common type of $GABA_A$ receptor found in the brain (Sieghart, 2000), with the aim to better understand the mechanisms that underlie adaptive changes in $GABA_A$ receptors following their prolonged exposure to neurotransmitter GABA and at a larger scale to drugs acting at $GABA_A$ receptors.

# MATERIALS AND METHODS

## Chemicals

The chemicals used in the study were purchased from a variety of suppliers. Culture medium, antibiotics and foetal bovine serum were supplied from Invitrogen/Gibco (Grand Island, NY, USA). GABA, bicuculline and cycloheximide were from Sigma (St. Louis, MO). Unlabeled TBOB was a gift from Prof. H.I. Yamamura. [$^3$H]flunitrazepam (specific activity 85 Ci/mmol) and [$^3$H]TBOB (**t**-[$^3$H]butylbicycloorthobenzoate, specific activity 24 Ci/mmol) were purchased from Amersham. [$^3$H]muscimol (specific activity 36.5 Ci/mmol) was from PerkinElmer (Boston, MA, USA).

## Cell Culture

The human embryonic kidney (HEK) 293 cell line stably expressing the $\alpha_1\beta_2\gamma_{2S}$ subtype of GABA$_A$ receptor was kindly donated by dr. David Graham (Sanofi-Synthélabo Research, France). The cells were maintained in 75 cm$^2$ flasks according to standard cell culture techniques at 37°C in humidified air with 5 % $CO_2$. They were cultured in Dulbecco's modified Eagle's medium (DMEM) supplemented with 10 % heat-inactivated foetal bovine serum, 2 mM L-glutamine, 100 units/ml penicillin and 100 μg/ml streptomycin.

## Drug Treatment

Three days prior to drug exposure the cells were transferred to new flasks and grown in the above medium. Three days after seeding, the medium was removed and replaced with fresh medium containing drugs or vehicles. GABA (final concentration 1 mM) and cycloheximide (final concentration 10 μg/ml) were dissolved in distilled water and bicuculline (final concentration 100 μM) in warm 0.1 N HCl. Control cells were treated with the corresponding vehicles. The cells were treated with GABA for 24, 48 and 96 h, with bicuculline for 96 h, and with cycloheximide 12 h before membrane isolation. When treatment lasted for 96 h, the drugs were replaced after 36 h in culture.

## Membrane Preparation

Membranes from stably transfected HEK 293 cells were prepared by the method previously described (Pericic et al., 2004). The cells were washed with phosphate-buffer saline (PBS), scraped from falcon flasks into ice-cold PBS and centrifuged at 12000 × g for 12 min. The cell pellet was homogenized in 50 mM Tris-citrate buffer, pH 7.4 using teflon pestle and a glass homogeniser (10 strokes up and down at 1250 rpm) and than centrifuged at 200000 × g for 20 min. The pellet was re-suspended and centrifuged at 200,000 × g for 20 min two more times. Finally, the pellet was re-suspended and stored in aliquots at -20°C. The suspension of the cell membranes was centrifuged on the day of binding assay once more at 200000 × g for 20 min.

For [$^3$H]muscimol binding assay, membranes were prepared by a method previously described (Pericic et al., *2005)*. Briefly, cell membrane suspension was thawed and incubated for 15 min at 4°C in 50 mM Tris-citrate buffer, pH 7.4 containing 0.05 % Triton X-100, and then centrifuged at 200,000×g for 20 min. The pellet was re-suspended in 50 mM Tris-citrate buffer and centrifuged at 17000×g for 10 min three times before use in the [$^3$H]muscimol binding assay.

## [$^3$H]flunitrazepam Binding Assay

Benzodiazepine binding was performed on membrane preparations as previously described using [$^3$H]flunitrazepam as radioligand (labelling benzodiazepine binding sites) (Pericic et al., 2004). Aliquots of cell membrane preparations (~100 μg protein) were incubated in 50 mM Tris-citrate buffer supplemented with 150 mM NaCl at 4°C for 90 min, either with various concentrations of [$^3$H]flunitrazepam (0.2–16 nM) or with a fixed concentration (1 nM) of [$^3$H]flunitrazepam in addition of varying concentrations of non-radioactive flunitrazepam (ten concentrations in the range 0.4–50 nM).

In stimulation studies, varying concentrations of GABA (1 nM–1 mM) were incubated with [$^3$H]flunitrazepam (1 nM).

Non-specific binding was taken as [$^3$H]flunitrazepam bound to the cell membranes in the presence of 100 μM diazepam.

Total assay volume of all binding studies was 0.5 ml. After rapid vacuum filtration, filters (Whatman GF/C) were dried overnight and then soaked in a liquid scintillation cocktail. Bound radioactivity was quantified on β-scintillation counter (Perkin Elmer, Wallace 1409DSA).

## [$^3$H]muscimol Binding Assay

[$^3$H]muscimol binding (labelling GABA binding sites) to cell membrane preparation (~ 150 μg protein) was performed at 4°C for 60 min in 50 mM Tris-citrate buffer with addition of 250 mM NaCl. For saturation studies, ten increasing concentrations of non-radioactive muscimol were added (3–150 nM) to a fixed concentration of [$^3$H]muscimol (4 nM). The total assay volume was 0.5 ml. Non-specific binding was determined in the presence of 1 M GABA.

## [3H]TBOB Binding Assay

[$^3$H]TBOB binding (labelling convulsant binding sites) was performed using aliquots of the cell membrane preparation (~90 μg protein) that were incubated in 50 mM Tris–citrate buffer supplemented with 200 mM NaCl at 25 °C for 90 min. Binding data were obtained by adding varying concentrations of non-radioactive TBOB to a fixed concentration (8 nM) of

$[^3H]$TBOB (ten final concentrations in the range 8–200 nM). The total assay volume was 0.5 ml. Non-specific $[^3H]$TBOB binding was defined in the presence of 100 μM picrotoxine.

## Protein Concentration Determination

Membrane protein concentrations were determined in 10 μl of membrane suspension according to Lowry el al. (1951), using bovine serum albumin as standard.

## Data Analysis

The analysis of binding data was performed using GraphPad Prism version 4.00 for Windows (GraphPad Software, San Diego, CA, USA). $K_d$ and $B_{max}$ values were obtained by nonlinear regression using the equation for a hyperbola (one binding site):

$$Y=B_{max}\times X/(K_d+X),$$

where $K_d$ is the dissociation constant presenting concentration of ligand required to reach half-maximal binding and $B_{max}$ is the maximum number of binding sites.

The GABA shift was defined as the $\mathbf{K_d}$ of $[^3H]$flunitrazepam binding measured in the absence of GABA divided by $\mathbf{K_d}$ measured in the presence of 100 μM GABA.

Results are presented as means ± SEM of at least three independent experiments. Statistical analysis of results was by Student's **t**-test or by one-way analysis of variance (ANOVA) followed by the Newman–Keuls multiple comparison test. The results were analyzed by two-way ANOVA, when the effects of two different treatments were studied in the same experiment. P-values of less than 0.05 were considered significant.

# RESULTS

## The Effect of Prolonged GABA Treatment on $[^3H]$flunitrazepam Binding

As shown in Table 1, prolonged exposure of HEK 293 cells stably transfected with $\alpha_1\beta_2\gamma_{2S}$ subunits of $GABA_A$-Rs to 1 milimolar GABA enhanced $[^3H]$flunitrazepam binding to cell membranes in a time-dependent manner. One-way ANOVA ($\mathbf{F}(3,20) = 21.30$; $\mathbf{P} = 0.0001$) indicated the significant enhancement of maximum number of benzodiazepine binding sites ($\mathbf{B_{max}}$) following GABA treatment. Namely, the exposure for 24, 48 and 96 h enhanced the maximum number of $[^3H]$flunitrazepam binding sites by 25%, 67% and 125%, respectively. The observed augmentation in the number of benzodiazepine binding sites reached significance for 48 and 96 h treatment ($\mathbf{P} = 0.01$, Newman–Keuls test). In addition, the affinity of benzodiazepine binding sites ($K_d$) was not affected.

**Table 1. The maximum number and affinity of benzodiazepine binding sites in control and GABA-treated cells**

| | | $B_{max}$ (pmol/mg protein) | $K_d$ (nM) |
|---|---|---|---|
| **Control** | | **5.93 ± 0.41** | **2.69 ± 0.38** |
| **1 mM GABA** | **24 h** | **7.41 ± 0.88** | **2.94 ± 0.46** |
| | **48 h** | **9.88 ± 0.29*** | **3.13 ± 0.28** |
| | **96 h** | **13.37 ± 0.98*** | **2.71 ± 0.29** |

***P** = 0.01, ANOVA followed by Newman–Keuls test.

## The Effect of Prolonged GABA Treatment on [$^3$H]muscimol Binding

We determined the kinetic properties of GABA binding sites using [$^3$H]muscimol as a ligand, to test the influence of prolonged GABA exposure of HEK 293 cells stably transfected with $\alpha_1\beta_2\gamma_{2S}$ subunits of $GABA_A$-Rs. As shown in Table 2, prolonged GABA treatment (1 mM, 96 h) also augments the number of [$^3$H]muscimol binding sites at the receptor, similar to that observed for benzodiazepine binding sites. Namely, following exposure to GABA the maximum number of [$^3$H]flunitrazepam binding sites was enhanced by 125%, while the number of binding sites for GABA, labelled with [$^3$H]muscimol, was enhanced by 123%. This enhancement also reached statistical significance (P = 0.05, Student's **t**-test). At the same time, the dissociation constant (**$K_d$**) of [$^3$H]muscimol binding sites was unaffected by prolonged exposure to GABA.

**Table 2. The maximum number and affinity of [$^3$H]muscimol binding sites in control and GABA-treated cells**

| | $B_{max}$ (pmol/mg protein) | $K_d$ (nM) |
|---|---|---|
| Control | 1.12 ± 0.58 | 29.67 ± 4.59 |
| 1 mM GABA 96 h | 2.50 ± 0.7* | 25.77 ± 4.38 |

P = 0.05, Student's *t*-test,

## The Effect of Prolonged GABA Treatment on [$^3$H]TBOB Binding

To test whether long-term GABA exposure of HEK 293 cells stably transfected with $\alpha_1\beta_2\gamma_{2S}$ subunits of $GABA_A$-Rs also affects the number of other receptor binding sites, we determined the kinetic properties of binding sites for convulsants. Following exposure to GABA (1 mM, 96 h) the number of binding sites labelled with the convulsant [$^3$H]TBOB was enhanced by 93% (**P** = 0.0009, Student's **t**-test). The alteration in the maximum number of convulsant binding sites (96%) was accompanied by a parallel enhancement of [$^3$H]flunitrazepam (125%) and [$^3$H]muscimol (123%) binding sites, respectively. The dissociation constant (**$K_d$**) of the same binding sites was unaffected by prolonged exposure to neurotransmitter GABA (Table 3).

**Table 3. The maximum number and affinity of [$^3$H]TBOB binding sites in control and GABA-treated cells**

| | $B_{max}$ (pmol/mg protein) | $K_d$ (nM) |
|---|---|---|
| Control | 6.81 ± 0.58 | 46.67 ± 4.59 |
| 1 mM GABA 96 h | 13.12 ± 1.10* | 53.47 ± 4.38 |

***P** = 0.0009, Student's **t**-test.

## The Effect of GABA Antagonist Bicuculline on the Up-regulation of [$^3$H]flunitrazepam Binding Induced by Prolonged GABA Treatment

To test whether GABA binding sites and their occupation with 1 milimolar GABA for 96 h are responsible for the enhancement of [$^3$H]flunitrazepam binding, we treated the cells simultaneously with GABA and bicuculline, the competitive antagonist of GABA binding sites. As shown in Figure 1 and indicated by one-way ANOVA ($\mathbf{F}(3,6) = 215.3$; $\mathbf{P} = 0.0001$), the maximum number of [$^3$H]flunitrazepam binding sites between the four treated groups (control, GABA, bicuculline, GABA + bicuculline) was different. GABA (1 mM) again produced a significant enhancement of [$^3$H]flunitrazepam binding sites. Bicuculline alone had no effect on the expression levels of binding sites for benzodiazepines at $GABA_A$-Rs. Nevertheless, simultaneous treatment of cells with GABA and bicuculline showed that bicuculline (100 μM) decreased the effect produced by prolonged GABA treatment ($\mathbf{P} = 0.001$). Two-way ANOVA also indicated a very significant effect of GABA ($\mathbf{F}(1,6) = 97.6$, $\mathbf{P} = 0.0001$) and bicuculline ($\mathbf{F}(1,6) = 28.5$, $\mathbf{P} = 0.005$), as well as a significant GABA × bicuculline interaction ($\mathbf{F}(1,6) = 29.3$, $\mathbf{P} = 0.005$). The affinity of benzodiazepine binding sites was affected by neither of these treatments (data not shown).

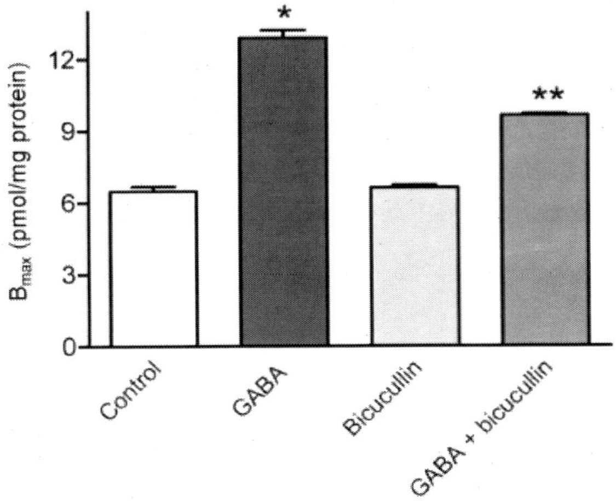


Figure 1. The ability of bicuculline to counteract the up-regulation of [$^3$H]flunitrazepam binding induced by chronic GABA (1 mM, 96 h) in HEK 293 cells stably transfected with $\alpha_1\beta_2\gamma_{2S}$ subunits of $GABA_A$ receptors.

HEK 293 cells were treated for 96 h with 1 mM GABA or 100 μM bicuculline, the combination of both drugs, or with their vehicles. Cell membranes were prepared as described in Materials and methods, and incubated with increasing concentrations of [$^3$H]flunitrazepam. Results are expressed as means ± SEM from three individual experiments performed in duplicate. *P = 0.01 vs. control; **P = 0.01 vs. all other groups (ANOVA followed by the Newman–Keuls test).

## The Effect of Protein Synthesis Inhibitor Cycloheximide on the Up-Regulation of [3H]Flunitrazepam Binding Induced by Prolonged GABA Treatment

The ability of GABA (1 mM, 96 h) to increase the density of [$^3$H]flunitrazepam binding sites in HEK 293 cells stably transfected with $\alpha_1\beta_2\gamma_{2S}$ subunits of $GABA_A$ receptors was also tested in the presence of an inhibitor of protein synthesis cycloheximide (10 μg/ml; present in culture for the last 12 h). One-way ANOVA (**F**(3,8) = 58.0) indicated significant differences (**P** = 0.0001) between four treated groups (control, GABA, cycloheximide, GABA + cycloheximide). The GABA effect was again significant (**P** = 0.01, Newman–Keuls test). The treatment of cells with cycloheximide abolished the enhancement of benzodiazepine binding sites produced by prolonged GABA (**P** = 0.001), whereas the effect of cycloheximide alone was not significantly different from control (Figure 2). These results indicate that the augmentation in the receptor number induced by prolonged GABA treatment is rather due to de novo synthesis of receptor proteins than to posttranslational regulatory mechanisms. Two-way ANOVA also indicated a significant effect of GABA (**F**(1,8) = 38.260, **P** = 0.0003), and cycloheximide (**F**(1,8) = 9.672, **P** = 0.01), as well as a significant GABA × cycloheximide interaction (**F**(1,8) = 11.256, **P** = 0.01). As indicated by one-way ANOVA (**F**(3,8) = 0.96), neither of these treatments affected the dissociation constant (**K**$_d$) of [$^3$H]flunitrazepam binding (data not shown).

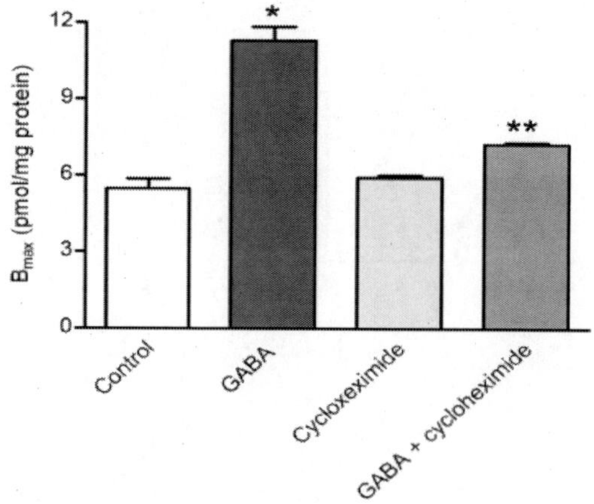


Figure 2. The ability of cycloheximide to counteract the up-regulation of [$^3$H]flunitrazepam binding induced by chronic GABA (1 mM, 96 h) in HEK 293 cells stably transfected with $\alpha_1\beta_2\gamma_{2S}$ subunits of $GABA_A$ receptors.

HEK 293 cells expressing $\alpha_1\beta_2\gamma_{2S}$ $GABA_A$ receptors were treated with 1 milimolar GABA, cycloheximide (10 µg/ml; present in cell culture for the last 12 h), the combination of both drugs, or with their vehicles. Cell membranes were prepared as described in Materials and methods, and incubated with increasing concentrations of [$^3$H]flunitrazepam. Results are expressed as means ± SEM from three individual experiments performed in duplicate. *P = 0.01 vs. control; **P = 0.01 vs. GABA-treated group (ANOVA followed by the Newman–Keuls test).

## The Effects of Prolonged GABA Treatment on the GABA-induced Enhancement of [$^3$H]flunitrazepam Binding

The addition of GABA (100 µM) enhanced the affinity of [$^3$H]flunitrazepam binding to membranes from control HEK 293 cells stably transfected with $\alpha_1\beta_2\gamma_{2S}$ subunits of $GABA_A$ receptors. Namely, the $\mathbf{K_d}$ value in the presence was significantly lower than in the absence of 100 µM GABA (GABA shift = 1.83 ± 0.27, **P** = 0.02). Moreover, GABA (100 µM) added to membranes from HEK 293 cells expressing $\alpha_1\beta_2\gamma_{2S}$ $GABA_A$ receptors pretreated for 48 h with 1 mM GABA also enhanced the affinity of [$^3$H]flunitrazepam binding (GABA shift = 1.81 ± 0.15, **P** = 0.01). Therefore, we can conclude that the GABA shift determined in membranes of HEK 293 cells expressing $\alpha_1\beta_2\gamma_{2S}$ $GABA_A$ receptors, chronically treated with GABA was not different from that obtained on control cells (Table 4). GABA shift was obtained by dividing $K_d$ of [$^3$H]flunitrazepam binding measured in the absence of GABA by $K_d$ measured in the presence of 100 µM GABA. Hence, the reduction in $\mathbf{K_d}$ value with no apparent effect on $\mathbf{B_{max}}$ following addition of 100 micromolar GABA can be seen in the control, as well as in GABA-treated HEK 293 cells stably transfected with $\alpha_1\beta_2\gamma_{2S}$ subunits of $GABA_A$ receptors. (Table 4).

**Table 4. The effects of prolonged GABA treatment on the GABA-shift**

| | $K_d$ (nM) | GABA-shift |
|---|---|---|
| Control | 2.41 ± 0.35 | 1.83 ± 0.27 |
| Control + 100 µM GABA | 1.31 ± 0.11* | |
| 1 mM GABA 96 h | 2.62 ± 0.31 | 1.81 ± 0.15 |
| 1 mM GABA + 100 µM GABA | 1.45 ± 0.12* | |

***P** = 0.01 (Student *t*-test).

# DISCUSSION

Although GABA was identified in brain tissue in the 1950s, it lasted several decades to identify that GABA inhibits the ability of neurons to fire potentials (Curtis and Watkins, 1965). Now it is known that almost one third of the synapses in the brain use GABA as neurotransmitter. Therefore, GABA is involved directly and/or indirectly in most aspects of normal brain functioning. Given the numerous specific functions of GABA and with respect to network homeostasis there are several hypotheses on how GABAergic signalling is regulated (for review see Ben Ari, 2012). Namely, the regulation of GABA concentration is achieved through several molecular processes regulating its transport, synthesis, sequestration and degradation (Roth and Draguhn, 2012). In addition, GABA exerts its role by acting on receptors located on the cell surface. Therefore its concentration in the extracellular matrix and time availability determines the extent of $GABA_A$-R stimulation (Farrant and Kaila, 2007). At the same time, Ben-Ari and his colleagues (2007) described long-term potentiation and long-term depression of GABAergic synapses in the neonatal and adult brain. Clements (1996) reports that GABA released as a result of a single action potential reaches relatively high synaptic concentrations of 1-5 mM, while Czurko and colleagues (1999) described basal firing rates that in the neocortex last for many minutes. Moreover, increase in extracellular GABA concentration as a result of cerebral ischemia through reversal of the GABA transporters was also reported (*Hutchinson et al., 2002*). Enhanced GABA concentrations were also observed during development (for review see *Takayama and Inoue, 2004)*. These results suggest that the release of GABA may be increased as well as present for prolonged period in the synaptic cleft during both physiological and pathological conditions. Moreover, it is hypothesized that the persistent activation of a substantial fraction (~30 %) of post-synaptic $GABA_A$-Rs over several minutes by milimolar GABA concentrations (Jones and Westbrook, 1995) requires the existence of regulatory mechanism(s) that negatively regulate GABA action. In the recently published paper it is also suggested that the uncoupling of allosteric sites at $GABA_A$-R is particulary relevant at the persistently activated $GABA_A$-Rs (Gutierrez et al., 2014).

Our presented results demonstrate that prolonged exposure of stably transfected HEK 293 cells, expressing recombinant $\alpha_1\beta_2\gamma_{2S}$ $GABA_A$-Rs, to neurotransmitter GABA increases the number of [$^3$H]flunitrazepam binding sites. The augmentation of benzodiazepine binding sites was accompanied by an analogous enhancement of binding sites for [$^3$H]TBOB and [$^3$H]muscimol, suggesting that prolonged exposure to GABA up-regulates the total number of $GABA_A$-Rs. At the same time, chronic treatment with GABA has not affected the affinity of [$^3$H]flunitrazepam, [$^3$H]TBOB or [$^3$H]muscimol binding sites. Consistent with our previous study (Pericic et al., 1998), stably transfected HEK 293 cells (Besnard et al., 1997) possess a relatively high density of $GABA_A$-Rs.

The observed up-regulation of $GABA_A$-Rs is in agreement with the study of Klein and colleagues (1995), who reported an enhanced (45%) binding of [$^3$H]flunitrazepam to recombinant bovine $\alpha_1\beta_1\gamma_{2L}$ $GABA_A$ receptors stably expressed in mouse $Ltk^-$ (PA3) cells following prolonged exposure to GABA (50 μM, 96 h). Moreover, following prolonged exposure of recombinant $GABA_A$-Rs to GABA agonist, muscimol (100 μM, 96 h) similar augmentation of total $GABA_A$-R number was observed (Pericic et al., 2003). Using the same model, the enhancement of benzodiazepine, GABA and convulsant binding sites was observed following prolonged treatment with benzodiazepine diazepam (Pericic et al., 2007; Svob Strac et al., 2008), imidazopyridine zolpidem (Vlainic et al., 2010; Vlainic et al., 2012b) and antagonist flumazenil (Jazvinscak Jembrek et al., 2008; Pericic et al., 2004; Pericic et al., 2005). However, the data presented for the recombinant $GABA_A$-Rs are in contrast with most of the data obtained for neurons demonstrating down-regulation of receptors after their prolonged exposure to GABA or GABA receptor agonists (Hablitz et al., 1989; Lyons et al., 2001; Mehta and Ticku, 1992; Montpied et al., 1991; Roca et al., 1990a; Tehrani and Barnes, 1988). It is also consistent with the reported down-regulation of mRNAs encoding different subunits of the $GABA_A$-R following GABA treatment of chick or mammalian brain neurons in culture (Mhatre and Ticku, 1994; Montpied et al., 1991). Down-regulation of $GABA_A$-R subunits has also been observed by Brown and Bristow (1996) and Calkin and Barnes (1994).

The density of the $GABA_A$-Rs was significantly increased following prolonged treatment of cell cultures with $GABA_A$-R agonist – THIP (Hansen et al., 1991). The discrepancy between the results obtaining decrease versus increase of receptor binding sites could be, at least partially, explained by the proposed biphasic effect of GABA on $GABA_A$-Rs (Platt et al., 1996). Namely, the two-day GABA exposure decreased $\alpha_1$, $\beta_{2,3}$ and $\alpha_6$ subunit protein expression while an eight-day treatment increased $\alpha_1$ and $\beta_{2,3}$ subunit protein expression, whereas $\alpha_6$ subunit protein expression remained below control levels. However, after ten-day GABA exposure, $\alpha_6$ subunit protein expression was also increased. The change in the expression of $GABA_A$-Rs and/or change in the proportion of receptors containing different subunits can influence $GABA_A$-R function (Sieghart, 2000). The reduced $GABA_A$-R function would presumably be favorable to neurons in a high GABA environment (Pistoia et al., 2013). One might assume that in our model the up-regulated $GABA_A$-R number could account for reduced GABA activity, and may presumably be one of the regulatory mechanisms developed to maintain homeostasis (for review see Ben-Ari, 2012).

The obtained increase in the number of benzodiazepine, GABA and convulsant binding sites (implicating the enhancement of total number of $GABA_A$-Rs) is nevertheless consistent with the results of experiments in which rats chronically treated with ethanolamine **O**-sulphate (a GABA transaminase inhibitor) showed up-regulation of GABA binding sites (Sykes et al., 1984). In immature cerebellar granule cells GABA, presumably due to its trophic effects (Meier et al., 1983; Schousboe and Redburn, 1995), induced up-regulation of GABA binding sites and mRNAs encoding for $\alpha_1$ and $\beta_2$ $GABA_A$-R subunits (Kim et al., 1993). Similar enhancement of the number of cerebellar $GABA_A$-Rs has been observed *in vivo* during postnatal development (Meinecke and Rakic, 1990). Trophic effects of GABA are probably mediated by both synaptic and non-synaptic mechanisms (Owens and Kriegstein, 2002). However, the trophic action of GABA seems unlikely to underline the observed increase in the number of $GABA_A$-Rs, as the subtype of these receptors expressed in HEK 293 cells corresponds to postnatal receptors located on the membrane of post-migratory/mature neuronal cells.

The observed GABA-induced up-regulation of $[^3H]$flunitrazepam binding sites was inhibited by bicuculline, a competitive $GABA_A$-R antagonist, indicating that this effect is mediated through the GABA recognition site. Simultaneous treatment with bicuculline alone failed to modify $[^3H]$flunitrazepam binding. Similar was observed in cultured cerebellar granule neurons where the effect produced by prolonged GABA treatment was prevented by the simultaneous administration of bicuculline (Kim et al., 1993). Moreover, the agonist-induced changes in the $\alpha_1$, $\alpha_2$ and $\alpha_3$ subunit mRNA and polypeptide expression were abolished by the concomitant exposure of cultured cortical neurons to R 5135, which is also an antagonist of $GABA_A$-R (Mhatre and Ticku, 1994; Platt et al., 1996).

To determine whether an increased synthesis versus decreased degradation of receptor proteins, an enhanced rate of receptor incorporation into membranes, and/or other factors (Maksay and Ticku, 1984) were responsible for the GABA-induced increase of $GABA_A$-Rs, we co-treated the cells with cycloheximide, a protein synthesis inhibitor. As shown in this chapter (Figure 2), cycloheximide abolished the GABA-induced up-regulation of benzodiazepine binding sites without affecting the maximum number of these sites in control cells. A significant interaction between GABA and cycloheximide (two-way ANOVA) indicated a different effect of cycloheximide on the receptor protein in the control and the GABA-treated group. The obtained results might suggest that prolonged GABA treatment up-regulates $GABA_A$-Rs by stimulating their synthesis. Nevertheless, to address this hypothesis and to determine whether the observed stimulation occurs at the translation and/or transcription level additional studies are needed. In addition, a general trophic effect of GABA treatment on the growth of HEK 293 cells could presumably be excluded because total cellular proteins did not vary between the control and GABA-treated group (data not shown). Additionally, in our experiments using membranes from non-transfected HEK 293 cells [$^3$H]TBOB or [$^3$H]flunitrazepam failed to bind after prolonged GABA treatment, excluding the likelihood that up-regulated, possibly endogenously present, $GABA_A$-R subunits interfere with stably expressed recombinant receptors (data not shown). It has been suggested that $GABA_A$-R subunit expression is independent of changes in mRNA levels and that the regulation of the $GABA_A$-R expression by chronic agonist treatment involves post-transcriptional and/or post-translational processes (Platt et al., 1996).

It has been demonstrated that chronic treatment of $GABA_A$-Rs with GABA agonists results in uncoupling or decreased coupling of allosteric interactions between GABA and benzodiazepine binding sites. This change in the so-called GABA shift is evidenced by a decrease in the enhancement of benzodiazepine binding by GABA and has been observed in chick (Lyons et al., 2001; Roca et al., 1990a) and mouse cerebral cortical cultured neurons (Mehta and Ticku, 1992). Prolonged treatment with GABA also reduced the GABA enhancement of [$^3$H]flunitrazepam binding to mouse Ltk$^-$ cells stably transfected with recombinant $\alpha_1\beta_1\gamma_{2L}$ $GABA_A$-Rs (Klein et al., 1995). On the other hand Wong and colleagues observed no change in WSS-1 cells stably transfected with $\alpha_1\gamma_2$ subunits. As shown in this chapter (Table 4), the analysis of [$^3$H]flunitrazepam binding to membranes of control and GABA (1 mM, 96 h)- treated cells, performed in the absence and presence of 100 μM GABA, failed to reveal differences in the GABA shift, suggesting the existence of functional coupling between GABA and benzodiazepine binding sites following persistent activation of $GABA_A$-Rs by neurotransmitter GABA.

Ali and Olsen (2001) proposed that prolonged benzodiazepine treatment induces internalization of surface $GABA_A$ receptors into intracellular vesicles, where the potentiation by GABA is impaired but the normal benzodiazepine binding can occur. However, internalisation of surface receptors was not observed by Primus and his colleagues (1996). Moreover, following lyses of internal vesicles of cortical neurons, uncoupling is not prevented (Gravielle et al., 2005). This suggests that uncoupling in mammalian neurons may occur via a different process than in insect cell lines. Whether a different expression milieu or the intensive up-regulation of receptors observed in our study explains why we could not see the change in GABA shift following chronic GABA exposure remains to be determined. On the other hand, as previously discussed, following chronic diazepam or flumazenil treatment, almost all GABA and benzodiazepine binding sites are expressed on the cell surface, suggesting that chronic exposure to diazepam (Pericic et al., 2007; Svob Strac et al., 2008) or flumazenil (Jazvinscak Jembrek et al., 2008) does not result in internalization of benzodiazepine binding sites in our experimental model. It is suggested that the uncoupling mechanism involves an initial receptor internalisation step followed by activation of signalling pathway(s) that might lead to selective changes in receptor subunit assembly (Gutierrez et al., 2014). However, functional uncoupling of GABA and benzodiazepine binding sites following prolonged treatment with benzodiazepines (Klein et al., 1994; Klein et al., 1995; Pericic et al., 2007; Primus et al., 1996; Svob Strac et al., 2008; Wong et al., 1994) or zolpidem (Vlainic et al., 2010; Vlainic et al., 2012a), but not with antagonist flumazenil (Jazvinscak Jembrek et al., 2008) was observed also with recombinant $GABA_A$-Rs. These receptors possess a defined subunit composition where subunit switch could not occur. Therefore, we hypothesize that uncoupling of GABA and benzodiazepine binding sites at recombinant $GABA_A$-Rs in engineered cell line can occur without the changes in the composition of receptor with additional novel subunits, and could involve either post-translational modification of $GABA_A$-R proteins or changes in subunit stoichiometry.

Although Shaw and coleagues (*2002*) demonstrated that HEK 293 cells contain many proteins typically found in neurons and concluded that these cells resemble more to neurons than to kidney epithelial cells, it has to be emphasized that the expression mechanisms in HEK 293 cells might be different. On the other hand there is possibility that $GABA_A$-Rs expressed on the membranes of HEK 293 cells respond to chronic GABA exactly as the receptors in immature cerebellar granule cells (Schousboe and Redburn; 1995) although the receptor formation accounts for $GABA_A$-Rs that could be found on the membranes of mature post-migratory neurons. Nevertheless the expression profile in these cells might still be different due to a lack of a normal neuronal environment, the absence of synapses, the absence of accessory proteins or proteins affecting trafficking of receptors, etc. (Birnir and Korpi, 2007).

In conclusion, prolonged exposure of HEK 293 cells stably expressing recombinant $\alpha_1\beta_2\gamma_{2S}$ $GABA_A$-R to neurotransmitter GABA results in an up-regulation of receptor number. The up-regulated number of $GABA_A$-Rs appears to be due to increased synthesis rather than decreased degradation of receptor proteins. On the other hand, prolonged GABA exposure failed to produce allosteric uncoupling of benzodiazepine and GABA binding sites. Further studies are needed to determine the relevance of these results to the phenomena of tolerance and dependence produced by prolonged treatment with GABA and other positive allosteric modulators of $GABA_A$-R, such as benzodiazepines; as well as determination of involvement of such process in the maintenance of brain homeostasis. Moreover, electrophysiological studies would be needed to determine the functional consequences of GABA-induced enhancement in the number of $GABA_A$-R.

## Acknowledgments

This study was conducted under the supervision of PI Danka Pericic, PhD and supported by the Croatian Ministry of Science, Education and Sports (Project: Stress, $GABA_A$ receptors and mechanisms of action of neuropsychoactive drugs). The assistance of Dr. Ivana Rajcan Spoljaric and Mrs. Zlatica Tonsetic is gratefully acknowledged.

## References

Ali NJ, Olsen RW (2001) Chronic benzodiazepine treatment of cells expressing recombinant GABA(A) receptors uncouples allosteric binding: studies on possible mechanisms. *J Neurochem.* 79:1100–1108.

Bateson AN (2002) Basic pharmacological mechanisms involved in benzodiazepine tolerance and withdrawal. *Curr Pharm. Des.* 8:5–21.

Ben-Ari Y (2012) The yin and yen of GABA in brain development and operation in health and disease. *Front Cell Neurosci.* 45.

Ben-Ari Y, Gaiarsa JL, Tyzio R, Khazipov R (2007) GABA: a pioneer transmitter that excites immature neurons and generates primitive oscillations. *Physiol Rev.* 87(4):1215-1284.

Besnard F, Even Y, Itier V, Granger P, Partiseti M, Avenet P, Depoortere H, Graham, D (1997) Development of stable cell lines expressing different subtypes of $GABA_A$ receptors. *J Recept Signal Transduct Res.* 17:99–113.

Birnir B, Korpi ER (2007) The impact of sub-cellular location and intracellular neuronal proteins on properties of GABA(A) receptors. Curr Pharm Des. 13(31):3169-3177.

Brown MJ, Bristow DR (1996) Molecular mechanisms of benzodiazepine-induced down-regulation of $GABA_A$ receptor $\alpha_1$ subunit protein in rat cerebellar granule cells. *Br J Pharmacol.* 118:1103–1110.

Calkin PA, Barnes EM (1994) γ-Aminobutyric acid ($GABA_A$) agonists down-regulate $GABA_A$/benzodiazepine receptor polypeptides from the surface of chick cortical neurons. *J Biol Chem.* 269:1548–1553.

Clements JD (1996) Transmitter timecourse in the synaptic cleft: its role in central synaptic function. *Trends Neurosci.* 19(5):163-171.

Curtis DR, Watkins JC (1965) The pharmacology of amino acids related to gamma-aminobutyric acid. *Pharmacol Rev.* 17(4):347-391.

Czurkó A, Hirase H, Csicsvari J, Buzsáki G (1999) Sustained activation of hippocampal pyramidal cells by 'space clamping' in a running wheel. *Eur J Neurosci.* 11(1):344-352.

Farrant M, Kaila K (2007) The cellular, molecular and ionic basis of GABA(A) receptor signalling. *Prog Brain Res.* 160:59-87.

Friedman LK, Gibbs TT, Farb DH (1996) gamma-aminobutyric $acid_A$ receptor regulation: heterologous uncoupling of modulatory site interactions induced by chronic steroid, barbiturate, benzodiazepine, or GABA treatment in culture. *Brain Res.* 707:100–109.

Gallager DW, Lakoski JM, Gonsalves SF, Rauch SL (1984) Chronic benzodiazepine treatment decreases postsynaptic GABA sensitivity. *Nature* 308:74–77.

Glykys J, Mody I (2007) Activation of $GABA_A$ receptors: views from outside the synaptic cleft. *Neuron* 56(5):763-770.

Gravielle MC, Faris R, Russek SJ, Farb DH (2005) GABA induces activity dependent delayed-onset uncoupling of GABA/benzodiazepine site interactions in neocortical neurons. *J Biol Chem.* 280(22):20954-20960.

Gutiérrez ML, Ferreri MC, Gravielle MC (2014) GABA-induced uncoupling of GABA/benzodiazepine site interactions is mediated by increased $GABA_A$receptor internalization and associated with a change in subunit composition. *Neuroscience* 257C:119-129.

Hansen GH, Belhage B, Schousboe A (1991) Effect of a GABA agonist on the expression and distribution of $GABA_A$ eceptors in the plasma membrane of cultured cerebellar granule cells: an immunocytochemical study. *Neurosci Lett.* 124(2):162-165.

Hablitz JJ, Tehrani MH, Barnes Jr. EM (1989) Chronic exposure of developing cortical neurons to GABA down-regulates GABA/benzodiazepine receptors and GABA-gated chloride currents. *Brain Res.* 501:332–338.

Holt RA, Bateson AN, Martin IL (1999) Decreased GABA enhancement of benzodiazepine binding after a single dose of diazepam. *J Neurochem.* 72(5):2219-2222.

Hu XJ, Ticku MK (1994) Chronic benzodiazepine agonist treatment reduces functional uncoupling of the γ-aminobutyric acid-benzodiazepine receptor ionophore complex in cortical neurons. *Mol Pharmacol.* 45:618–625.

Jazvinscak Jembrek M, Svob Strac D, Vlainic J, Pericic D (2008) The role of transcriptional and translational mechanisms in flumazenil-induced up-regulation of recombinant GABA(A) receptors. *Neurosci Res.* 61:234–241.

Jones MV, Westbrook GL (1995) Desensitized states prolong $GABA_A$ channel responses to brief agonist pulses. *Neuron* 15(1):181-191.

Kim HY, Sapp DW, Olsen RW, Tobin AJ (1993) GABA alters $GABA_A$ receptor mRNAs and increases ligand binding. *J Neurochem.* 62:2334–2337.

Klein RL, Harris RA (1996) Regulation of $GABA_A$ receptor structure and function by chronic drug treatments in vivo and with stably transfected cells. *Jpn J Pharmacol.* 70:1–15.

Klein RL, Whiting PJ, Harris RA (1994) Benzodiazepine treatment causes uncoupling of recombinant $GABA_A$ receptors expressed in stably transfected cells. *J Neurochem.* 63:2349–2352.

Klein RL, Mascia MP, Harkness PC, Hadingham KL, Whiting PJ, Harris RA (1995) Regulation of allosteric coupling and function of stably expressed γ-aminobutyric acid $(GABA)_A$ receptors by chronic treatment with $GABA_A$ and benzodiazepine agonists. *J Pharmacol Exp Ther.* 274:1484–1492.

Korpi ER, Grunder G, Lüddens H (2002) Drug interactions at GABA(A) receptors. *Prog Neurobiol.* 67:113-159.

Lowry OH, Rosebrough NJ, Farr AL, Randall RJ (1951) Protein measurement with the folin phenol reagent. *J Biol Chem.* 193:265-275.

Lyons HR, Land MB, Gibbs TT, Farb DH (2001) Distinct signal transduction pathways for GABA-induced $GABA_A$ receptor down-regulation and uncoupling in neuronal culture: a role for voltage-gated calcium channels. *J Neurochem.* 78:1114–1125.

Maksay G, Ticku MK (1984) Pretreatment with GABA and modulatory ligands enhances GABA receptor binding. *Eur J Pharmacol.* 104:185–188.

Mehta AK, Ticku MK (1992) Chronic GABA exposure down-regulates GABA–benzodiazepine receptor–ionophore complex in cultured cerebral cortical neurons. *Mol Brain Res.* 16:29–36.

Meier E, Dreier J, Schousboe A (1983) Trophic actions of GABA on the development of physiologically active GABA receptors. *Adv Biochem Psychopharmacol.* 37:47–58.

Meinecke D, Rakic P (1990) Developmental expression of GABA and subunits of the $GABA_A$ receptor complex in an inhibitory synaptic circuit in the rat cerebellum. *Dev Brain Res.* 55:73–86.

Mhatre MC, Ticku MK (1994) Chronic GABA treatment downregulates the $GABA_A$ receptor alpha 2 and alpha 3 subunit mRNAs as well as polypeptide expression in primary cultured cerebral cortical neurons. *Brain Res Mol Brain Res.* 24:159–165.

Möhler H (2006) $GABA_A$ receptors in central nervous system disease: anxiety, epilepsy, and insomnia. *J Recept Signal Transduct Res.* 26(5-6):731-740.

Montpied P, Ginns EI, Martin BM, Roca D, Farb DH, Paul SM (1991) Gamma-aminobutyric acid (GABA) induces a receptor-mediated reduction in $GABA_A$ receptor alpha subunit messenger RNAs in embryonic chick neurons in culture. *J Biol Chem.* 266:6011–6014.

Olsen RW, Sieghart W (2008) International Union of Pharmacology. LXX. Subtypes of gamma-aminobutyric acid(A) receptors: classification on the basis of subunit composition, pharmacology, and function. *Pharmacol Rev.* 60:243–260.

Owens DF, Kriegstein AR (2002) Is there more to GABA than synaptic inhibition? *Nat Rev Neurosci.* 3:715–727.

Pericic D, Jazvinscak Jembrek M, Svob Strac D, Lazic J, Spoljaric IR (2005) Enhancement of benzodiazepine binding sites following chronic treatment with flumazenil. *Eur J Pharmacol.* 507:7-13.

Pericic D, Lazic J, Jazvinscak Jembrek M, Svob Strac D, Rajcan I (2004) Chronic exposure of cells expressing recombinant $GABA_A$ receptors to benzodiazepine antagonist flumazenil enhances the maximum number of benzodiazepine binding sites. *Life Sci.* 76:303-317.

Pericic D, Mirkovic K, Jazvinscak M, Besnard F (1998) [3H]t-butylbicycloorthobenzoate binding to recombinant alpha1beta2gamma2s GABA(A) receptor. *Eur J Pharmacol.* 360(1):99-104.

Pericic D, Strac DS, Jembrek MJ, Rajcan I (2003) Prolonged exposure to gamma-aminobutyric acid up-regulates stably expressed recombinant alpha 1 beta 2 gamma 2s $GABA_A$ receptors. *Eur J Pharmacol.* 482(1-3):117-125.

Pericic D Svob Strac D, Jazvinscak Jembrek M, Vlainic J (2007) Allosteric uncoupling and up-regulation of benzodiazepine and GABA recognition sites following chronic diazepam treatment of HEK 293 cells stably transfected with alpha1beta2gamma2S subunits of GABA (A) receptors. *Naunyn Schmiedebergs Arch Pharmacol.* 375:177-187.

Pistoia F, Sarà M, Sacco S, Franceschini M, Carolei A (2014) Silencing The Brain May Be Better Than Stimulating it. *The GABA Effect. Curr Pharm Des.* 2013 *In press*

Platt KP, Zwartjes RE, Bristow DR (1996) The effect of GABA stimulation on $GABA_A$ receptor subunit protein and mRNA expression in rat cultured cerebellar granule cells. *Br J Pharmacol.* 119:1393–1400.

Primus RJ, Yu J, Xu J, Hartnett C, Meyyappan M, Kostas C, Ramabhadran TV, Gallager DW (1996) Allosteric uncoupling after chronic benzodiazepine exposure of recombinant γ-aminobutyric $acid_A$ receptors expressed in Sf9 cells: ligand efficacy and subtype selectivity. *J Pharmacol Exp Ther.* **276:**882–890.

Roca DJ, Rozenberg I, Farrant M, Farb DH (1990a) Chronic agonist exposure induces down-regulation and allosteric uncoupling of the γ-aminobutyric acid/benzodiazepine receptor complex. *Mol Pharmacol.* 37:37–43.

Roca DJ, Schiller GD, Friedman L, Rozenberg I, Gibbs TT, Farb DH (1990b) γ-Aminobutyric $acid_A$ receptor regulation in culture: altered allosteric interactions following prolonged exposure to benzodiazepines, barbiturates, and methylxanthines. *Mol Pharmacol.* 37:710–719.

Roth FC, Draguhn A (2012) GABA metabolism and transport: effects on synaptic efficacy. *Neural Plast.* 2012:805830.

Russek SJ, Bandyopadhyay S, Farb DH (2000) An initiator element mediates autologous downregulation of the human type A gamma -aminobutyric acid receptor beta 1 subunit gene. *Proc Natl Acad Sci USA.* 97(15):8600-8605.

Schousboe A, Redburn DA (1995) Modulatory actions of gamma aminobutyric acid (GABA) on GABA type A receptor subunit expression and function. *J Neurosci Res.* 41:1–7.

Shaw G, Morse S, Ararat M, Graham FL (2002) Preferential transformation of human neuronal cells by human adenoviruses and the origin of HEK 293 cells. *FASEB J.* **16:**869–871.

Shaw C, Scarth BA (1991) Characterization and differential regulation of $GABA_A$ and benzodiazepine receptors in rat neocortex. Brain Res Mol Brain Res. 11(3-4):273-282.

Sieghart W (2000) Unraveling the function of GABA(A) receptor subtypes. *Trends Pharmacol Sci.* 21(11):411-413.

Svob Strac D, Vlainic J, Jazvinscak Jembrek M, Pericic D (2008) Differential effects of diazepam treatment and withdrawal on recombinant $GABA_A$ receptor expression and functional coupling. *Brain Res.* 1246:29-40.

Sykes C, Prestwich S, Horton R (1984) Chronic administration of the GABA-transaminase inhibitor ethanolamine *O*-sulphate leads to up-regulation of GABA binding sites. *Biochem Pharmacol.* 33:387–393.

Takayama C, Inoue Y (2004) Extrasynaptic localization of GABA in the developing mouse cerebellum. *Neurosci Res.* 50(4):447-458.

Tehrani MH, Barnes EMJ (1988) GABA down-regulates the GABA/benzodiazepine receptor complex in developing cerebral neurons. *Neurosci Lett.* 87:288–292.

Vlainic J, Jazvinscak Jembrek M, Svob Strac D, Pericic D (2010) The effects of zolpidem treatment and withdrawal on the in vitro expression of recombinant alpha1beta2gamma2s GABA(A) receptors expressed in HEK 293 cells. *Naunyn Schmiedebergs Arch Pharmacol.* 382:201-212.

Vlainic J, Jembrek MJ, Vlainic T, Strac DS, Pericic D (2012a) Differential effects of short- and long-term zolpidem treatment on recombinant $\alpha_1\beta_2\gamma_{2S}$ subtype of GABA(A) receptors in vitro. *Acta Pharmacol Sin.* 33(12):1469-1476.

Vlainic J, Svob Strac D, Jazvinscak Jembrek M, Vlainic T, Pericic D (2012b) The effects of zolpidem treatment on GABA(A) receptors in cultured cerebellar granule cells: changes in functional coupling. *Life Sci.* 90(23-24):889-894.

Wafford KA (2005) $GABA_A$ receptor subtypes: any clues to the mechanism of benzodiazepine dependence? *Curr Opin Pharmacol.* 5:47-52.

Wong G, Lyon T, Skolnick P (1994) Chronic exposure to benzodiazepine receptor ligands uncouples the γ-aminobutyric acid type A receptor in WSS-1 cells. *Mol Pharmacol.* 46:1056–1062.

In: Gamma-Aminobutyric Acid (GABA)
Editors: Josipa Vlainić and Maja Jazvinšćak Jembrek
ISBN: 978-1-63321-838-3


*Chapter 4*

# THE ROLE OF GABA IN DEVELOPMENT AND BEHAVIOUR: EMPHASIS ON THE EFFECTS OF GABA RECEPTOR AGONISTS AND ANTAGONISTS

***Maja Jazvinšćak Jembrek***[1,2,*]***, Josipa Vlainić***[1]
***and Vedrana Radovanović***[1]
[1]Laboratory for Molecular Neuropharmacology, Division of Molecular Medicine, Rudjer Boskovic Institute, Zagreb, Croatia
[2]Department of Psychology, Croatian Catholic University, Zagreb, Croatia

## ABSTRACT

Normal brain functioning is characterized by the balance between excitatory and inhibitory neurotransmission. Gamma-aminobutyric acid (GABA) acts as the major inhibitory neurotransmitter in the mammalian brain and is found throughout the central nervous system. Ionotropic $GABA_{A/C}$ and metabotropic $GABA_B$ receptors, both of which mediate the effects of GABA, are also extensively distributed in the brain. As a result GABA affects numerous physiological processes. This review will briefly summarize some of the major functions of GABA, including the role of GABA in development and brain masculinization, and the effects of GABA on circadian rhythms, sleep, feeding, aggressive behavior, and learning and memory, primarily deduced from studies using GABA receptor agonists and antagonists.

**Keywords**: GABA, development, circadian rhythms, sleep, feeding, aggressive behavior, learning and memory

* Corresponding author: Department of Psychology, Croatian Catholic University, Zagreb, Croatia. Email: jazvin@irb.hr.

## INTRODUCTION

Behavior can be defined as the internally coordinated responses of whole living organisms to internal and/or external stimuli (Levitis et al., 2009). The biological approach of studying behavior, also called behavioral neuroscience or biological psychology, applies the principles of biology to the study of physiological, genetic, and developmental mechanisms of behavior at the level of neurons, neurotransmitters, brain circuits and basic biological processes that underlie normal and abnormal behavior. Neurotransmitters have central roles in synaptic communication and convey most of the information required for the operation of the brain and its networks.

Neuronal networks in the adult cerebral cortex are built out of two main classes of neurons which have opposite effects on postsynaptic membranes. Excitatory projection neurons constitute the vast majority of neurons, primarily use glutamate as a neurotransmitter, cause membrane depolarization and promote generation of action potentials. On the other hand, inhibitory local-circuit interneurons constitute about 20% of all cortical neurons, predominantly use GABA as the neurotransmitter, cause membrane hyperpolarization and depress action potential generation resulting in inhibition. Coordination between glutamatergic excitatory neurons and GABAergic inhibitory interneurons is fundamental to the regulation of neuronal firing rates in the cerebral cortex and generation of behaviorally relevant patterns. Various types of interneurons control the fine discharge of glutamatergic neurons, and the patterns that networks will generate. Cortical interneurons control neuronal excitability, integration and plasticity, and regulate generation of temporal synchrony and oscillatory behavior among networks of glutamatergic neurons. It is believed that such oscillations serve numerous complex functions, including perception, movement and memory (Ben-Ari, 2006; Buzsaki et al., 2007; Chattopadhyaya and Di Cristo, 2012).

## PHARMACOLOGY OF GABA RECEPTORS

Three major types of GABA receptors have been identified across the central nervous system. $GABA_A$ and $GABA_C$ receptors are ligand-gated ion channels, while $GABA_B$ receptors are seven transmembrane receptors that are coupled to G-proteins. GABA exerts most of its physiological effects after activation of $GABA_A$ receptors, $Cl^-$ channels composed of five subunits that are encoded from a pool of 19 different variants. These hetero-oligomeric ion channels are selectively blocked by the competitive antagonist bicuculline, and modulated by the channel blocker picrotoxin and a variety of clinically important drugs, such as anxiolytics, anticonvulsants, general anesthetics, barbiturates, ethanol and neuroactive steroids (Korpi et al., 2002; Sigel and Steinmann, 2012). In addition, muscimol, the principal psychoactive constituent of the mushroom *Amanita muscaria*, acts as a potent, selective agonist of $GABA_A$ receptors. GABA modulates behavior by increasing $GABA_A$ receptor activity which leads to anxiolysis, ataxia, myorelaxation, sedation, hypnosis, anesthesia and anterograde amnesia, whereas a decrease in $GABA_A$ receptor activity leads to increased vigilance, memory enhancement, anxiety and seizures (Korpi et al., 2002). The GABA system is therefore widely used in the treatment of anxiety disorders, insomnia, epilepsy, restlessness, and aggressive behaviors (Uusi-Oukari and Korpi, 2010).

GABA, the GABA analog baclofen and 3-aminopropylphosponous acid (3-APPA; CGP27492) are characteristic $GABA_B$ receptor agonists. They exhibit a number of pharmacological effects, including central muscle relaxation, epileptogenesis, suppression of drug craving, antinociception, cognitive impairment and inhibition of hormone release. Saclofen, phaclofen and 2-hydroxysaclofen act as $GABA_B$ receptor antagonists (Bowery et al., 2002).

$GABA_C$ receptors, expressed predominantly in the retina, are activated by *cis*- and *trans*-enantiomers of GABA analog 4-aminocrotonic acid (CACA and TACA, respectively), and blocked by TPMPA [(1,2,5,6-tetrahydropyridin-4-yl)methylphosphinic acid]. The sensitivity of $GABA_C$ receptors to GABA is much higher than that of $GABA_A$ receptors (Zhang et al., 2001). GABAc receptors are insensitive to bicuculline and baclofen, and are not modulated by barbiturates, benzodiazepines or neuroactive steroids. However, based on the recommendation of the International Union of Basic and Clinical Pharmacology, $GABA_C$ receptors are now generally assumed to be one of the isoforms of $GABA_A$ receptors (Sigel and Steinmann, 2012).

## TROPHIC ACTIONS OF GABA

During development, before synapse formation, GABA displays trophic actions in neuronal maturation. It is now well known that tonic GABAergic activity is critically involved in the generation of both physiological and pathophysiological activity patterns before and after establishment of functional GABAergic synapses (Kilb et al., 2013). GABAergic synapses precede glutamate synapses (Tyzio et al., 1999). The sequential formation of GABAergic synapses and circuits before glutamatergic ones indicates that, at least at an early stage, all the excitatory drive is GABAergic (Ben-Ari, 2006). The developmental excitatory action of GABA appears to be universal, and is observed in the cortex, hippocampus, thalamus, hypothalamus, cerebellum and spinal cord. Namely, $GABA_A$ receptors are permeable for $Cl^-$ ions in both directions. Timing of the depolarizing-hyperpolarizing shift of GABA activity is a result of developmental changes in the relative number of co-transporters and channels responsible for chloride ion transfer across the membrane (Rohrbough and Spitzer, 1996). In the adult brain, a higher extracellular concentration of $Cl^-$ ions causes its influx after opening of $GABA_A$ receptors. However, prior to complete neuronal maturation, intracellular $Cl^-$ concentrations are increased and the receptor's opening results in ion efflux and consequent membrane depolarization. Most importantly, this depolarization translates the action of GABA into trophic responses, such as synaptic patterning and changes in cell death (McCarthy et al., 2002). During development, increased intracellular levels of $Cl^-$ ions are established by ion accumulation via $Na^+$-$K^+$-$2Cl^-$ co-transporters (NKCC1), expressed from the mid-embryonic stages until the first week of postnatal life in rodents (Wang and Kriegsten, 2009). With neuronal maturation, the number of $K^+/Cl^-$ co-transporters (KCC2) that extrude $Cl^-$ from the cell and the number of $Cl^-$-permeable channels (ClC2) that prevent intracellular chloride accumulation increases, resulting in ontogenetic changes in $GABA_A$-mediated responses from depolarizing to hyperpolarizing (Rivera et al., 1999). The depolarizing effects of GABA on the postsynaptic membrane are frequently sufficient to open L-type voltage-gated $Ca^{2+}$ channels, thus increasing intracellular $Ca^{2+}$ concentration. In turn, this increase causes enhanced expression of KCC2 transporters that extrude $Cl^-$ from the neuron thus encouraging conversion of GABA effect to hyperpolarizing (Ganguly et al., 2001). In this manner, ambient GABA concentration is an important regulatory variable that tunes its output through a self-regulating feedback loop.

Since GABA is the first neurotransmitter active in the immature brain and provides the main excitatory drive, it has a crucial role in the early stages of brain development serving as an epigenetic factor that controls progenitor proliferation and survival, neuronal migration and circuits formation in the cortex (Wang and Kriegsten, 2009). GABA modulates early developmental processes acting on receptors in an extra-synaptic fashion. Patch-clamp recording has shown that immature neurons do not generate fast synaptic responses. In immature neurons electrical stimuli evoke giant currents, several orders of magnitude larger than synaptic currents. These very large currents are partially mediated by the activation of GABA receptors. Thus, at this early stage GABA acts as a paracrine factor. It is released tonically and diffusely activates receptors on distal neurons before synapse formation.

Blocking of GABA receptors in this early stage retards neuronal migration, indicating that GABA also acts as a morphogenetic factor (Ben-Ari, 2006). When primordial GABAergic cortical interneurons migrate to the embryonic cortical anlage, they display regionally specific pharmacological differences, as well as specific profiles of $GABA_A$ receptor subunit transcripts (Cuzon Carlson and Yeh, 2011). Thus, $GABA_A$ receptors constituted of diverse receptor subunits have different affinities for GABA and therefore various effects on neuronal migration. In slice cultures of embryonic rat cortex, it has been shown that $GABA_A$ and $GABA_C$ receptors participate in the migration of neurons from the proliferative to the intermediate zone, whereas $GABA_B$ receptors signal cell migration into the cortical plate (Behar et al., 2000). When neuronal migration was studied in the newborn rat parietal cortex (during the first postnatal days neocortical neurons in rodents are still migrating), local applications of a $GABA_A$ antagonist or agonist induce alterations in the cortical architecture when compared with control animals, indicating that they also may induce neuronal migration disorders. Additionally, electrophysiological recordings from migrating neurons revealed that prolonged application of muscimol in a dose-dependent manner reduces responsiveness of postsynaptic $GABA_A$ receptors due to pronounced receptor desensitization (Heck et al., 2007).

Normal neuronal migration requires calcium signalling, and GABA has a very important role in raising intracellular calcium levels. As explained earlier, due to the enhanced intracellular chloride concentration, following GABA receptor activation, chloride ions efflux from the cell, depolarize the cell membrane, generate action potentials and remove the voltage-dependent magnesium block from NMDA receptors that leads to calcium influx (Ben-Ari, 2006). Hence, in the early stages of brain development, GABA acts as a regulator of synaptogenesis because it can repeatedly excite neurons without producing long-term voltage-gated channel activation and excitotoxic effects of $Ca^{2+}$ influx.

During development the brain undergoes an enormous increase in the number of newly formed and refined synapses and neuronal circuits which causes changes in network activity. To become a functional unit of brain circuits, young neurons have to display mature morphology, be able to form synapses with other cells and refine those synapses. Following the migration process GABA acts in coordination with glutamate and stimulates developing networks intervening in the formation of cortical networks and exhibiting a wide range of trophic actions (Ben-Ari, 2006). These findings suggest that disturbances in the development of GABAergic interneurons and alterations of GABA synthesis and signaling, either because of genetic or environmental causes, can affect nearly all stages of cortical circuit formation leading to impaired brain functioning (Chattopadhyaya and Di Cristo, 2012). Indeed, aberrant development of GABAergic circuits has been implicated in various neurodevelopmental and psychiatric disorders such as schizophrenia, autism, mental retardation, and epilepsy (Ben-Ari, 2006; Di Cristo, 2007).

## GABA and Brain Masculinization

Sexually reproducing animals display differences between male and female reproductive behavior. These differences are a result of the developmental changes in the male and female nervous systems that can be observed without prior experience or training (Morris et al., 2004). Morphological brain sex differences can be observed in different collections of neurons in sex specific brain regions (e.g. hypothalamus), specific nuclei (e.g. the sexually dimorphic nucleus (SDN) of the preoptic area (POA) in rats) or in fiber tracts (e.g. corpus callosum). At the cellular level, hormonally induced sex differences are present in neuronal dendritic branching and synaptic patterning, and astrocyte differentiation in some hypothalamic nuclei (Mong et al., 1999; Todd et al., 2007). In addition, it appears that volumetric differences can also result from hormonally induced apoptosis in the developing POA (Arai et al., 1996).

It has also been established that GABA participates in the formation of brain sex differences. In specific brain regions, variations of three parameters can be observed: intrinsic timing of the depolarizing–hyperpolarizing GABA shift, the endogenous GABA concentration and the action of hormones, and these variations contribute to differential brain development between males and females.

Namely, during a critical period in development gonadal steroids act in a regionally specific manner and change neuronal architecture. Estradiol mediates many aspects of brain masculinization. Fetuses and newborns are exposed to estradiol derived from their mother, their own gonads, and synthesized locally in the brain. Although estradiol is found at high levels in the developing brain of both sexes, its expression is higher in some regions of the male rat brain, particularly in the hypothalamus (McCarthy, 2008). Estradiol enhances the effects of GABA and prolongs the developmental excitatory effects of GABA, resulting in divergence of signal transduction pathways activated in males versus females. In newborn male rats, the concentrations of GABA and glutamic acid decarboxylase (GAD), an enzyme that catalyzes the decarboxylation of glutamate to GABA, are higher in brain estrogen-receptor-expressing regions, than in those of females. In addition, treatment of females with testosterone propionate results in increased GABA levels. Thus, it has been assumed that hormonally mediated sex differences in GABA levels might contribute to the establishment of sexually dimorphic neuronal architecture in the adult brain (Davis et al., 1999). Studies on dissociated hypothalamic neurons have shown that estradiol pretreatment enhances $Ca^{2+}$ transients induced by $GABA_A$ receptor activation, further suggesting that estradiol, besides extending the developmental duration of depolarizing effects by GABA, may mediate sexual differentiation by increasing GABA-induced enhancement in intracellular $Ca^{2+}$ and influencing intracellular signaling (Perrot-Sinal et al., 2001). Inside the cell, $Ca^{2+}$ activates several kinases resulting in phosphorylation of cAMP-response-element-binding protein (CREB) at serine residues. Phosphorylated CREB (pCREB) is an important transcriptional factor that influences neuronal survival and plasticity (Murphy and Segal, 1997, Walton et al., 1999).

There is a sex difference in the number of cells expressing pCREB (McCarthy et al., 2002), and $GABA_A$-receptor activation has opposing effects on pCREB in steroid-concentrating regions of male and female brains. Depending on the sex, and the region in the developing brain, the response to GABA can be excitatory or inhibitory on signal transduction pathways that alter CREB phosphorylation (Auger et al., 2001). Thus, these pathways may play an important role in the modulation of sex specific differences during development (Tobet et al., 2009). A gene commonly regulated by pCREB encodes brain derived neurotrophic factor (BDNF) which is involved in both synaptic plasticity and cell survival.

It also appears that NKCC1 are also involved in estradiol-induced augmentation of depolarizing GABA action. The activity of these co-transporters, whose function is to move chloride ions into the cell, is controlled by phosphorylation of a cluster of threonine residues, and is counterbalanced by the activity of KCC2 co-transporters that extrude ions from the cell. Estradiol markedly increases phosphorylation of NKCC1 at two threonine residues indicating that estradiol-mediated enhancement of depolarizing GABA is regulated by the control of NKCC1 activity (Nugent et al., 2012).

## GABA and Adult Neurogenesis

Adult neurogenesis is an intensive ongoing process that necessitates tight homeostatic control mechanisms on neural stem cells and neuroblasts. During a lifetime, it is estimated that more than 10 000 immature neurons migrate to the olfactory bulb every day where they differentiate into interneurons. A postnatal subventricular zone contains the largest pool of dividing neuronal progenitors in the adult mammalian brain. The rate of neuroblast production and the number that ultimately integrate into the olfactory bulb is determined by the overall outcomes of cell proliferation, migration and survival that are regulated by diverse genetic and epigenetic mechanisms.

It has been proposed that cell number is determined by the concentration and supply of local GABA that provides a feedback control on cell proliferation through receptor activation (Platel et al., 2008). Similarly to developmental processes, tonic release of endogenous GABA regulates the rate of neurogenesis. In the subventricular zone nonsynaptically released GABA from neuroblasts activates $GABA_A$ receptors in glial fibrillary acidic protein (GFAP)-expressing cells thought to be stem cells. This tonic activation of $GABA_A$ receptors limits progression of GFAP-positive cells through the cell cycle. Thus, since a subset of GFAP-expressing cells is thought to generate neuroblasts, GABA released from neuroblasts provides a feedback mechanism to control the proliferation of GFAP-expressing progenitors and neuroblast production by activating $GABA_A$ receptors (Liu et al., 2005). Tonic $GABA_A$ receptor activation also reduces the speed of neuroblast migration (Bolteus and Bordey, 2004).

## GABA and Circadian Rhythms

Many aspects of mammalian physiology and behavior, including sleep, hormone levels, body temperature, physical activity, alertness and mood, follow regular circadian rhythms. An entrained circadian clock placed in the suprachiasmatic nuclei (SCN) ensures that endogenous rhythms are coordinated with the 24-h day-night cycle. SCN functions as an intrinsic self-sustaining oscillator and master circadian pacemaker of the mammalian circadian timing system (Antle and Silver, 2005). The nuclei are strategically positioned in the anterior hypothalamus, just above the optic chiasm, for receiving visual input for light-dark entrainment, primarily via the direct retinohypothalamic tract. Specialized retinal melanopsin-containing ganglion cells respond to light and send their axons to the SCN. The SCN are composed of multiple, autonomous, single-cell circadian oscillators - clock cells, that must be synchronized to generate a coordinated output signal and operate as a functional unit (Van den Pol and Dudek, 1993; Welsh et al., 1995; Aton and Herzog, 2005).

GABA plays a particularly important role in regulating this circadian clock. Although some results suggested that GABA could have an excitatory role during daytime and inhibitory role at night (Wagner et al., 1997), Gribkoff and colleagues (1999), using three independent electrophysiological approaches in hypothalamic slices, have reported only inhibitory responses to GABA in the SCN during subjective day. Most, if not all, SCN neurons express GABA and glutamic acid decarboxylase (Okamura et al., 1986). GABA is released in a daily rhythm in the SCN (Itri and Colwell, 2003), and is colocalized with one or more neuroactive peptides, predominantly with arginine vasopressin (AVP), vasoactive intestinal polypeptide (VIP), gastrin-releasing peptide (GRP) and calretinin (Moore et al., 2002). Since VIP meets most of the criteria to be a synchronizing factor of SCN cell populations by modulating frequency of GABA release (Itri and Colwell, 2003), GABA and VIP are considered the principal neurotransmitters of the SCN (Moore and Speh, 1993; Aton and Herzog, 2005). In addition, all SCN neurons also synthesize prokinecitin 2, a protein most probably involved in the transmission of circadian information to other brain regions (Zhang et al., 2009).

Both ionotropic $GABA_A$ and metabotropic $GABA_B$ receptors are involved in SCN function. Electrophysiological and pharmacological studies indicate that $GABA_A$ receptors predominantly function as postsynaptic somatodendritic receptors (Kim and Dudek, 1992), while $GABA_B$ receptor activation exerts a strong presynaptic inhibition of GABA release in SCN neurons, primarily by modulating P/Q-type calcium channels at axon terminals (Chen and van den Pol, 1998). However, SCN $GABA_A$ receptors are expressed not only in postsynaptic regions, but also in presynaptic terminals where they probably act as regulators of neurotransmitter release (Belenky et al., 2003).

GABA activity in the SCN can affect circadian phase and the ability of phase shifting stimuli to reset the clock. GABA, and both $GABA_A$ and $GABA_B$ receptor agonists phase shift circadian rhythms if applied to the SCN. Electrical activity rhythms of SCN clock cells in culture shows that GABA, acting through the $GABA_A$ receptor, can both synchronize and shift clock cells (Liu and Reppert, 2000). Although it was previously thought that GABA plays an important role in the synchronization of the individual clock-cells, recent studies indicate that GABA may be sufficient for synchronization, but not necessary. It seems that endogenous GABA controls the amplitude of SCN neuronal rhythms by reducing daytime firing since $GABA_A$ and $GABA_B$ antagonism increases circadian peak firing rates and rhythm precision of cultured SCN neurons, while G protein mediated signaling suppresses night time firing and synchronizes these rhythms (Aton et al., 2006). In addition, GABA also modulates the ability of light pulses to phase shift the circadian clock (Mintz et al., 2002). The in vivo effects of GABAergic drugs, such as competitive antagonist bicuculline, on light-induced phase shifts and c-Fos expression in the SCN are mediated by postsynaptic $GABA_A$ receptor mechanisms (Gillespie et al. 1999). However, inhibition alone was insufficient to cause a phase shift, indicating that other diffusible substances, such as neuropeptides, are also involved (Lall and Biello, 2003).

Furthermore, GABA accompanied by arginine vasopressin originating in the SCN mediates some output pathways of SCN. The daily synthesis of melatonin in the pineal gland, which occurs exclusively during the dark phase of the light/dark cycle, represents a stable and reliable output of the biological clock. Endogenous release of GABA from SCN is implicated in the further transmission of light information to the pineal gland. Retina-mediated photic activation of SCN neurons induces the release of GABA from efferent SCN nerve terminals, thus resulting in the inhibition of melatonin release (Kalsbeek et al., 1999).

## GABA and Sleep

The sleep-wake cycle is one of the most important processes regulated by the circadian clock. It results from the reciprocal functional switching between wakefulness promoting systems and sleep promoting systems. The ascending reticular activating system (ARAS), a functional unit involved in exchanging sleep-arousal behavior, gathers together neural systems with different neurotransmitters, mainly located in the brainstem reticular formation (Saper et al., 2010). However, the overall control of the sleep-wake cycle is attributed to the hypothalamic systems and their functional interactions (Hasan and Alóe, 2011). Orexinergic neurons from the lateral hypothalamus (LH) stimulate all the excitatory circuits responsible for wakefulness, while GABAergic neurons of the preoptic area of the anterior hypothalamus are mainly responsible for promoting sleep. Because of its crucial role in initiating and maintaining the sleep phase of the cycle, lack of the central inhibitory processes of GABA results in sleeping disorders, like insomnia. People suffering from insomnia have an average brain GABA level reduced by 30% (Winkelman et al. 2008), and three generations of commonly used hypnotics are based on $GABA_A$ receptor-mediated inhibitory processes (Gottesmann 2002).

Sleep can be defined as a behavior represented by a temporary change in the level of awareness and mobility, and a lack of responsiveness to external stimuli. At the beginning of sleep, consciousness fades but the brain remains active. It is considered that GABA plays an essential role in switching waking consciousness to the non-conscious state of sleep. Although spontaneous firing rates in the cortex remain relatively unchanged and sensory areas continue to respond to sounds and other stimuli, GABA limits neuronal activity thus causing unconsciousness. Enhanced GABA levels prevent axons from spreading stimulation to other areas leading to a reduction in effective connectivity from primary sensory areas to higher cortical areas (Massimini et al., 2005; Esser et al., 2009).

Normal sleep consists of an alternation between two distinct states: synchronized, slow-wave or non-rapid-eye-movement (non-REM) sleep, and desynchronized or rapid-eye-movement (REM) sleep. Sleep-active parts of the POA of the hypothalamus contain >75% GABAergic neurons that have elevated discharge rates during both non-REM and REM sleep compared to waking, i.e. sleep-active discharge pattern (Suntsova et al., 2002; Gong et al., 2004). Hence, the inhibitory effects of GABA are essential for the initiation and maintenance of sleep (Gottesmann, 2002). The GABA transporter that controls the duration and intensity of GABAergic activity at the synapse is also involved in the regulation of REM sleep and homeostasis of non-REM sleep (Xu et al., 2013).

During non-REM sleep, overall brain function declines. There is a significant reduction in energy consumption and cerebral blood flow in the thalamus and cortex, together with a reduction of sympathetic nervous system activity (Okada et al., 1991). Thus, non-REM sleep can be defined as a state of relative brain inactivity in a partially inactive neuromuscular system (Hasan and Alóe, 2011).

The preoptic area of the hypothalamus plays an important role in the regulation of non-REM sleep. By using different experimental approaches, the ventrolateral preoptic area (vlPOA) and median preoptic nucleus (MnPN) have been identified as critical structures involved in the occurrence of non-REM sleep. The activity of these neurons, as measured by their levels of c-Fos immunoreactivity, increases during sleep and the number of c-Fos-positive GABAergic cells is positively correlated with the amount of preceding sleep. Since sleep deprivation is associated with increased activation of GABAergic neurons in the MnPN and vlPOA, increased activation of these GABAergic neurons has been suggested as a potential mechanism by which a prior time of wakefulness causes increased sleep time and/or sleep depth (Gong et al., 2004). It seems that GABAergic MnPN neurons are most strongly activated in response to increasing sleep pressure (i.e. in response to sleep deprivation during the light/rest period), while GABAergic vlPOA neurons are most strongly activated in increasing sleep time during recovery sleep and spontaneous sleep in the light (Gvilia et al., 2006).

During wakefulness an organism is exposed to all kinds of sensory, somatic and visceral inputs that activate orexinergic and aminergic neurons. The absence of sunlight at the end of the photo-period that disables the SCN, the accumulation of adenosine combined with sensory reduction and overall calmness and resting posture of the organism potentiate the inhibitory activity of vlPOA and stimulate sleep. GABA released from neurons in the vlPOA inhibits neuronal circuits involved in wakefulness and arousal, while serotonergic, noradrenergic and histaminergic systems stimulated by orexinergic neurons inhibit these GABAergic neurons in the vlPOA. Based on a mutually inhibitory flip-flop switch mechanism, vlPOA neurons activate sleep by inhibitory modulatory control over multiple aminergic wakefulness promoting systems (Liu and Reppert, 2000; Hasan and Alóe, 2011). As well, released GABA also inhibits brain activity and promotes slow-wave sleep by reducing firing of the orexinergic neurons. Accordingly, microinjection of muscimol, a $GABA_A$ receptor agonist, increases time spent in slow-wave sleep (Nitz and Siegel, 1996).

On the other hand, REM sleep is characterized by rapid eye movements, muscle paralysis, desynchronized electroencephalogram as a result of cortical and hippocampal activation, and increased cerebral metabolism in brain regions involved in visual control (vivid dreams), but marked metabolic deactivation of cortical regions related to executive cognitive functions (Pace-Schott and Hobson, 2002; Lu et al., 2006).

Nevertheless, the occurrence of REM sleep also depends on GABAergic processes (Lu et al., 2006; Sapin et al. 2009). It has been considered that the main switching mechanism for REM sleep involves reciprocal interactions i.e. mutual inhibition between GABAergic REM-on and REM-off neurons (Dunmyre et al., 2014). REM-off neurons are placed in the ventrolateral division of the periaqueductal gray (vlPAG) and deep mesencephalic reticular nucleus in the pontine tegmentum. Inactivation of REM-off neurons by lesions or injection of the $GABA_A$ agonist muscimol into vlPAG and deep reticular nuclei provokes strong enhancement of REM sleep (Lu et al., 2006; Kaur et al., 2009). Similarly, GABAergic disinhibition of sublaterodorsal nucleus, where GABAergic REM-on neurons are predominantly localized, by using the $GABA_A$ receptor antagonists bicuculline and gabazine, induces a REM-like state (Boissard et al., 2002). Furthermore, muscimol applied in the nucleus reticularis pontis oralis and caudalis of rats suppresses REM (Sanford et al., 2003), whereas antagonizing GABA action by bicucculine and gabazine at $GABA_A$ receptors in the nucleus pontis oralis (PnO) induces dose-dependent increase in REM sleep (Marks et al., 2008). Methyl-6,7-dimethoxy-4-ethyl-β-carboline (DMCM), an inverse agonist of a benzodiazepine binding site at the $GABA_A$ receptor, injected into the PnO of rats was also capable of inducing a long-lasting increase in REM sleep. This effect was blocked by a preceding injection of the muscarinic antagonist atropine, suggesting that antagonizing GABA disinhibits acetylcholine release from cholinergic axons in the PnO and results in acetylcholine-mediated REM sleep induction (Nguyen et al., 2013).

During REM sleep GABA drive also triggers REM paralysis by switching off motoneuron activity. However, inactivation of both $GABA_A$ and $GABA_B$ receptors prevented and reversed REM paralysis of skeletal muscles, but neither ionotropic nor metabotropic receptors alone were sufficient to induce REM inhibition (Brooks and Peever, 2012).

In addition, it seems that the REM-off area is under GABAergic control of the extended part of vlPOA. It is proposed that GABAergic projections of sleep neurons from the preoptic hypothalamus inhibit vlPAG, allowing REM sleep generating neurons in the pontine reticular formation to become activated.

## GABA and Feeding

GABAergic transmission from the hypothalamus is essential for normal feeding regulation, and hyperphagia can be induced by local application of $GABA_A$-receptor agonists to different feeding-associated brain areas such as the ventral tegmental area (VTA), nucleus accumbens (NAc) shell, substantia nigra, median and dorsal raphe nuclei and ventromedial hypothalamus (Miner et al., 2010). Transgenic mice that overexpress the GABA transporter exhibit heritable obesity, indicating that an excessive level of GABA transporter may be an important part of the mechanism underlying certain types of obesity (Ma et al., 2000).

The role of GABA in feeding varies in different brain areas. The arcuate nucleus in the hypothalamus is considered an integrative site that receives satiety and hunger signals from the periphery reflecting energy status. Recent findings demonstrate that specific subpopulations of GABAergic neurons in the arcuate nucleus that are involved in the regulation of drive energy expenditure, contribute to the stimulatory effect of the hormone leptin on thermogenesis and protect against diet-induced obesity (Kong et al., 2011). It was also found that GABA regulates neuropeptide Y (NPY)-neurons in the arcuate nucleus via $GABA_A$ and $GABA_B$ receptors (Muroya et al., 2005). NPY is one of the most potent stimulants for food intake.

The paraventricular nucleus is exceptionally sensitive to the stimulatory effects elicited by GABA agonists and inhibitory effects of GABA antagonists. It has been proposed that a daily rise in plasma glucose concentration is caused by SCN-mediated withdrawal of GABAergic inputs to sympathetic preautonomic neurons in the paraventricular nucleus leading to an increase in hepatic glucose production (Kalsbeek et al., 2004).

GABAergic medium spiny neurons in the NAc shell are also implicated in the control of appetitive behavior. Acute inhibition of neuronal activity in NAc shell via administration of muscimol and baclofen elicit intense, dose-related feeding. Feeding elicited by muscimol, a selective $GABA_A$ receptor agonist, is specifically blocked by pretreatment with bicuculline, a selective $GABA_A$ receptor antagonist if administered at specific sites like VTA and NAc shells (Stratford and Kelley, 1997; Echo et al., 2002). Similarly, feeding elicited by the selective $GABA_B$ agonist baclofen is prevented with the selective $GABA_B$ antagonist saclofen. In addition to regional interactions aimed at identifying important relationships between GABAergic circuits, feeding behavior can be studied by administering an antagonist in one site of interest prior to administration of the feeding-active agonist in a second site of interest. Such studies have shown unidirectional $GABA_A$/$GABA_B$ receptor interactions between VTA and NAc shells, demonstrating that GABA employs a distributed brain network in mediating its ingestive action, and uses different receptor subtypes to underlie its regional effects (Miner et al., 2010).

Neurons within the lateral hypothalamus also play an important role in feeding behavior. In particular, GABA is involved in feeding inhibition. Agonists of $GABA_A$ receptors suppress feeding following injection into the LH and can reduce body weight, while $GABA_A$ receptor antagonists elicit eating when injected into the LH of satiated rats (Stanley et al., 2011). It is thought that stimulation of food intake is mediated by GABA projections from the NAc to LH. Inhibition of NAc-LH projections neurons leads to an arrest of GABA release, disinhibition of LH neurons and increase in food intake (Berhoud and Münzberg, 2011). In addition to LH, GABA injected into the ventromedial hypothalamus (VMH) also depresses food intake (Hansen and Ferreira, 1986).

## GABA and Aggressive Behavior

Aggression can be defined as a complex social behavior evolved primary for defending and obtaining resources. From a psychiatric perspective, it is thought to be motivated by hypothetical constructs such as anger, irritation, frustration and fear. There are many different brain areas and neurotransmitters involved in aggressive behavior. Different brain circuits characteristic for certain types of aggression are also part of social behavior networks that include the medial preoptic area, lateral septum, anterior hypothalamus, ventromedial hypothalamus, periaqueductal grey, medial amygdale and bed nucleus of the stria terminalis. In stress, aggressive behavior can be inhibited via inhibitory inputs from the orbital frontal cortex, hippocampus and paraventricular nucleus (Nelson and Trainor, 2007). Neurotransmitters involved in mammalian aggression include serotonin, dopamine, norepinephrine and GABA, as well as neuropeptides such as vasopressin and oxytocin (Yanowitch and Coccaro, 2011).

Different studies have shown that GABAergic neurons are present in brain structures involved in modulation of aggressive behavior (Shaikh and Siegel, 1990; Han et al., 1996; Cheu and Siegel, 1998). It seems that GABA exerts a critical role in the neurochemical control of aggressive behavior based on studies that directly modify GABAergic neurotransmission, and on neurochemical studies that correlate GABA measurements with aggressive behavioral responses (Miczek et al., 2002). Namely, GABA levels were found to be inversely correlated with some aspects of aggressiveness in human adults (Bjork et al., 2001). Brain levels of GABA and GAD activity are also lower in animals that exhibit aggressive behavior, particularly in regions such as the amygdala, striatum and olfactory bulbs (Clement et al., 1987; Guillot and Chapouthier, 1998). Similarly, blockade of GABA transaminase inhibits isolation-induced aggressive behavior in mice (Puglisi-Allegra and Mandel, 1980).

Shaikh and Siegel (1990) demonstrated that microinjection of muscimol into defensive rage sites within the PAG suppresses the affective defense response in a dose- and time-dependent manner, but does not have any effect upon predatory attack in a cat model. On the other hand, pretreatment with bicuculline blocked the suppressive effects of muscimol. These findings suggested that GABA selectively modulates defensive rage by serving as an inhibitory neurotransmitter within the PAG. Han and colleagues (1996) have microinjected bicuculline into sites within the lateral hypothalamus from which predatory attack is elicited. Bicuculline infusion produced a blockade of medial amygdaloid suppression of predatory attack in a time- and dose-dependent manner, while microinfusion of muscimol into the same attack site in LH in the absence of medial amygdaloid stimulation suppressed predatory attack. Thus, they confirmed the hypothesis that the medial amygdales mediate predatory attack inhibition through a GABAergic neurons that projects from the medial to lateral hypothalamus. It was also discovered that GABAergic neurons project in both directions and that their inhibition is reciprocal, so that signals that inhibit defensive rage (elicited from medial hypothalamus) will also facilitate predatory attack and vice versa (Cheu and Siegel, 1998). In particular, administration of bicuculline into medial hypothalamic sites from which defensive rage was elicited blocked the suppressive effects of lateral hypothalamic stimulation, while muscimol applied into the medial hypothalamus, suppressed defensive rage, and this suppression was blocked by bicuculline.

It was considered that GABA tonically inhibits aggressive behavior through the $GABA_A$ receptor complex, and that drugs that inhibit depolarization at the GABA receptor decrease aggression. It has also been shown that benzodiazepines, positive modulators of specific $GABA_A$ receptor subtypes reduce aggressive behavior (Skolnick et al., 1985), and psychiatric patients with violent outbursts are often treated with benzodiazepines (Dorevitch et al. 1999). However, current findings confirm the critical role of benzodiazepine binding sites at $GABA_A$ receptors in both reducing and heightening aggressive behavior. $GABA_A$ receptor agonists exhibit dual effects on aggression, i.e. at low doses increase aggression, while applied at high doses suppress aggressive behavior (Gourley et al., 2005). Other positive modulators of $GABA_A$ receptors such as ethanol and neurosteroid allopregnanolone also effectively increase aggressive behavior (Fish et al., 2001, 2005).

It is possible that the escalation of aggressive behavior involves increased activity of $GABA_A$ receptors that are modulated by serotonergic projections. Hence, modulation of

GABA and $GABA_A$ receptors by serotonin in corticolimbic neurons might be a promising approach for targeting selected forms of escalated aggressive behavior, in particular alcohol-heightened aggression. In addition, specific subunit combinations of the $GABA_A$ receptor complex might be particularly important for pharmacological interventions (de Almeida et al., 2005).

## GABA, Learning and Memory

The central GABAergic system also plays a role in cognitive processes, including learning, memory formation and consolidation. Learning is defined as a change in an organism's behavior as a result of experience, while memory refers to the ability to recall or recognize previous experiences. The processes that stabilize a trace of memory after its initial acquisition are known as memory consolidation. It is believed that memories are stored in the form of synaptic connections between neurons.

Numerous studies have shown that GABA receptor agonists and antagonists may modulate memory processing, although the results are not entirely consistent. In general, systemic administration of GABA inhibitors enhances memory in a variety of tests, while drugs that facilitate GABAergic function, slow memory acquisition. Thus, it has been shown that septal infusion of muscimol impairs memory. This effect probably involves the hippocampus since hippocampal bicuculline infusion blocks the memory–impairing effects produced by septal muscimol infusion (Krebs-Kraft et al., 2007). Accordingly, inactivation of GABA transaminase induces impairment of memory and lack of consolidation, presumably due to an increase in GABA concentration throughout the brain (Kalueff and Nutt, 1996-1997), while optogenic inhibition of GABAergic interneurons activity in the hilus of the hippocampus impairs spatial learning and memory retrieval up to 2 weeks after initial memory formation, without affecting spatial memory retention or short-term working memory (Andrews-Zwilling et al., 2012). Furthermore, clinical evidence suggests that inhibitors of GABA reuptake, in particular tiagabine, improve performance in verbal memory when used as an add-on anticonvulsant therapy (Shi et al., 2012), although another study on animals indicated that tiagabine impaired spatial learning in the Morris water maze (Schmitt and Hiemke, 2002).

Data in the literature also suggest that $GABA_A$ and $GABA_B$ receptor agonists, muscimol and baclofen respectively, may enhance memory (Sharma and Kulkarni, 1993). On the other hand, memory impairment was demonstrated in Balb/c mice lacking the $GABA_B(1)$ subunit (Schuler et al., 2001). Bianchi and Panerai (1993) studied the effects of CGP 35348, a centrally active blocker of $GABA_B$ receptors, on scopolamine-induced amnesia for a passive avoidance response in the mouse, and found that both pre- and post-training intraperitoneal administration of the $GABA_B$ antagonist exerts antiamnestic effects. In addition, Getova and Bowery (1998) showed that rats treated with different $GABA_B$ receptor antagonists show improved learning and memory retention.

Regarding fear memory, GABA is involved in acquisition, consolidation, reconsolidation and extinction. By using step-down typed passive avoidance and rapidly learned conditioned suppression tasks in mice it was shown that administration of the GABA antagonists, picrotoxin and bicuculline, and 3-mercaptopropionic acid, an inhibitor of GABA synthesis, just after the training, caused amnesia, while $GABA_A$ and $GABA_B$ receptor agonists, muscimol and baclofen respectively, and aminooxyacetic acid, an inhibitor of GABA transaminase, showed antiamnestic action (Nabeshima et al., 1988). As reviewed by Makkar and coauthors (2010), fear memory acquisition, consolidation, reconsolidation and extinction are dependent on a mechanism of reduced GABAergic neurotransmission, possibly within the amygdala and hippocampus. Pre- and post-training administrations of drugs that promote GABAergic transmission disturb formation of fear memories, while $GABA_A$ receptor antagonists applied before fear conditioning facilitate subsequent fear memory. It is also well known that administration of benzodiazepines alleviates symptoms of anxiety, while their infusion into the amygdale reduces learned fear responses in animals. GABAergic transmission is also important for the consolidation of fear memories. Thus, $GABA_A$ receptor agonists disturb reactivation of fear memories, while $GABA_A$ receptor antagonists facilitate fear memory retention.

Learning appears to involve an increase in inhibitory synaptic plasticity together with enhanced GABA release. Thus, in classical conditioning it was found that a simple form of learning involving mystacial vibrissae triggers a rapid increase in the density of inhibitory synapses on neuronal spines, while symmetrical synapses of cells located in barrels receiving the conditioned stimulus show enhanced concentration of GABA in their presynaptic terminals (Jasinska et al., 2010). Similarly, olfactory-discrimination learning was accompanied by long-lasting enhancement of synaptic inhibition onto excitatory pyramidal neurons in the piriform cortex, probably compensating for the increase of excitation in these neurons (Brosh and Barkai, 2009), while decreased GABA levels in the hippocampus due to overexpression of GABA transporter 1 impaired associative learning ability and new object recognition retention in mice (Hu et al., 2004).

Agonists and antagonists of $GABA_A$ and $GABA_B$ receptors also can modify spatial learning. Muscimol induced state-dependent learning in the Morris water maze task through $GABA_A$ receptors (Nakagawa et al., 1995). Baclofen, a $GABA_B$ receptor agonist, also dose-dependently impaired spatial learning in the water maze task (McNamara and Skelton, 1996), while the $GABA_B$ receptor antagonist CGP36742 attenuated the baclofen-induced deficit in the Morris water maze task in rats (Nakagawa and Takashima, 1997).

It seems that $GABA_A$ receptors containing the α5 subunit, expressed predominantly in the hippocampus, are particularly important for cognitive processes. A restricted distribution of the α5 subunit to the dendritic regions of CA1-CA3 fields of the hippocampus suggests that this subunit mainly contributes to the molecular processes underlying learning and memory. A mouse line with a disrupted α5 gene ($\alpha 5^{-/-}$ mice) showed enhanced performance in the Morris water maze model of spatial learning, while the performance of hippocampus-independent learning and anxiety tasks were not affected when compared with wild-type mice (Collinson et al., 2002). Furthermore, it has been shown that an α5 specific inverse agonist acting at benzodiazepine binding sites at $GABA_A$ receptor restores learning and memory performances in cognitively-impaired mouse model of Down syndrome (Braudeau et al., 2011).

$GABA_C$ receptors are also important for learning and memory. A drug named CGP36742, an antagonist of $GABA_B$ receptor sites that also antagonizes $GABA_C$ receptors, exerts memory-enhancing properties by acting on $GABA_C$ receptors. Another $GABA_C$ receptor antagonist that lacks $GABA_B$ receptor activity has been patented as a memory enhancer. In addition, resveratrol, a moderately potent $GABA_C$ receptor non-competitive antagonist from red wine, has been patented for the treatment of mild cognitive disorders (Chebib et al., 2004).

## REFERENCES

Antle MC, Silver R (2005) Orchestrating time: arrangements of the brain circadian clock. *Trends Neurosci.* 28(3):145-51.

Arai Y, Sekine Y, Murakami S (1996) Estrogen and apoptosis in the developing sexually dimorphic preoptic area in female rats. *Neurosci Res.* 25:403–7.

Aton SJ, Herzog ED (2005) Come together, right now: synchronization of rhythms in a mammalian circadian clock. *Neuron.* 48(4):531-4.

Aton SJ, Huettner JE, Straume M, Herzog ED (2006) GABA and Gi/o differentially control circadian rhythms and synchrony in clock neurons. *Proc Natl Acad Sci USA.* 103(50):19188-93.

Auger AP, Perrot-Sinal TS, McCarthy MM (2001) Excitatory versus inhibitory GABA as a divergence point in steroid-mediated sexual differentiation of the brain. *Proc Natl Acad Sci USA.* 98(14):8059-64

Behar TN, Schaffner AE, Scott CA, Greene CL, Barker JL (2000) GABA receptor antagonists modulate postmitotic cell migration in slice cultures of embryonic rat cortex. *Cereb Cortex.* 10(9):899-909.

Belenky MA, Sagiv N, Fritschy JM, Yarom Y (2003) Presynaptic and postsynaptic GABAA receptors in rat suprachiasmatic nucleus. *Neuroscience.* 118(4):909-23.

Ben-Ari Y (2006) Basic developmental rules and their implications for epilepsy in the immature brain. *Epileptic Disord.* 8:91–102.

Berthoud HR, Münzberg H (2011) The lateral hypothalamus as integrator of metabolic and environmental needs: from electrical self-stimulation to opto-genetics. *Physiol Behav.* 104(1):29-39.

Bianchi M, Panerai AE (1993) Reversal of scopolamine-induced amnesia by the GABAB receptor antagonist CGP 35348 in the mouse. *Brain Res Cogn Brain Res.* 1(2):135-6.

Bjork JM, Moeller FG, Kramer GL, Kram M, Suris A, Rush AJ, Petty F (2001) Plasma GABA levels correlate with aggressiveness in relatives of patients with unipolar depressive disorder. *Psychiatry Res.* 101(2):131-6.

Boissard R, Gervasoni D, Schmidt MH, Barbagli B, Fort P, Luppi PH (2002) The rat ponto-medullary network responsible for paradoxical sleep onset and maintenance: a combined microinjection and functional neuroanatomical study. *Eur J Neurosci.* 16(10):1959-73.

Bolteus AJ, Bordey A (2004) GABA release and uptake regulate neuronal precursor migration in the postnatal subventricular zone. *J Neurosci.* 24(35):7623-31.

Bowery NG, Bettler B, Froestl W, Gallagher JP, Marshall F, Raiteri M, Bonner TI, Enna SJ (2002) International Union of Pharmacology. XXXIII. Mammalian gamma-aminobutyric acid(B) receptors: structure and function. *Pharmacol Rev.* 54(2):247-64.

Braudeau J, Delatour B, Duchon A, Pereira PL, Dauphinot L, de Chaumont F, Olivo-Marin JC, Dodd RH, Hérault Y, Potier MC (2011) Specific targeting of the GABA-A receptor α5 subtype by a selective inverse agonist restores cognitive deficits in Down syndrome mice. *J Psychopharmacol.* 25(8):1030-42.

Brooks PL, Peever JH (2012) Identification of the transmitter and receptor mechanisms responsible for REM sleep paralysis. *J Neurosci.* 32(29):9785-95

Brosh I, Barkai E (2009) Learning-induced enhancement of feedback inhibitory synaptic transmission. *Learn Mem.* 16: 413–6.

Buzsaki G, Kaila K, Raichle M (2007) Inhibition and brain work. *Neuron.* 56:771–83.

Chattopadhyaya B, Cristo GD (2012) GABAergic circuit dysfunctions in neurodevelopmental disorders. *Front Psychiatry.* 3:51.

Chebib M, Hanrahan JR, Mewett N, Duke RK, Johnston GAR (2004) Ionotropic GABA receptors as therapeutic targets for memory and sleep disorders. *Annu Rep Med Chem.* 39:13-23.

Chen G, van den Pol AN (1998) Presynaptic GABAB autoreceptor modulation of P/Q-type calcium channels and GABA release in rat suprachiasmatic nucleus neurons. *J Neurosci.* 18(5):1913-22.

Clement J, Simler S, Ciesielski L, Mandel P, Cabib S, Puglisi-Allegra S (1987) Age-dependent changes of brain GABA levels, turnover rates and shock-induced aggressive behavior in inbred strains of mice. *Pharmacol Biochem Behav.* 26(1):83-8.

Collinson N, Kuenzi FM, Jarolimek W, Maubach KA, Cothliff R, Sur C, Smith A, Otu FM, Howell O, Atack JR, McKernan RM, Seabrook GR, Dawson GR, Whiting PJ, Rosahl TW (2002) Enhanced learning and memory and altered GABAergic synaptic transmission in mice lacking the alpha 5 subunit of the GABAA receptor. *J Neurosci.* 22(13):5572-80.

Cuzon Carlson VC, Yeh HH (2011) GABAA receptor subunit profiles of tangentially migrating neurons derived from the medial ganglionic eminence. *Cereb Cortex.* 21(8):1792-802.

Di Cristo G (2007) Development of cortical GABAergic circuits and its implications for neurodevelopmental disorders. *Clin Genet.* 72: 1–8.

de Almeida RM, Ferrari PF, Parmigiani S, Miczek KA (2005) Escalated aggressive behavior: dopamine, serotonin and GABA. *Eur J Pharmacol.* 526(1-3):51-64.

Davis AM, Ward SC, Selmanoff M, Herbison AE, McCarthy MM (1999) Developmental sex differences in amino acid neurotransmitter levels in hypothalamic and limbic areas of rat brain. *Neuroscience.* 90:1471–82.

Dorevitch A, Katz N, Zemishlany Z, Aizenberg D, Weizman A (1999) Intramuscular flunitrazepam versus intramuscular haloperidol in the emergency treatment of aggressive psychotic behavior. *Am J Psychiatry.* 156(1):142-4.

Dunmyre JR, Mashour GA, Booth V (2014) Coupled flip-flop model for REM sleep regulation in the rat. *PLoS One.* 9(4):e94481.

Echo JA, Lamonte N, Ackerman TF, Bodnar RJ (2002) Alterations in food intake elicited by GABA and opioid agonists and antagonists administered into the ventral tegmental area region of rats. *Physiol Behav.* 76(1):107-16.

Esser SK, Hill S, Tononi G (2009) Breakdown of effective connectivity during slow wave sleep: investigating the mechanism underlying a cortical gate using large-scale modeling. *J Neurophysiol.* 102(4):2096-111.

Fish EW, Faccidomo S, DeBold JF, Miczek KA (2001) Alcohol, allopregnanolone and aggression in mice. *Psychopharmacology* (Berl). 153(4):473-83.

Fish EW, DeBold JF, Miczek KA (2005) Escalated aggression as a reward: corticosterone and GABA(A) receptor positive modulators in mice. P*sychopharmacology* (Berl). 182(1):116-27.

Ganguly K, Schinder AF, Wong ST, Poo M (2001) GABA itself promotes the developmental switch of neuronal GABAergic responses from excitation to inhibition. *Cell.* 105:521–32.

Getova D, Bowery NG (1998) The modulatory effects of high affinity GABA(B) receptor antagonists in an active avoidance learning paradigm in rats. *Psychopharmacology* (Berl). 137(4):369-73

Gillespie CF, Van Der Beek EM, Mintz EM, Mickley NC, Jasnow AM, Huhman KL, Albers HE (1999) GABAergic regulation of light-induced c-Fos immunoreactivity within the suprachiasmatic nucleus. *J Comp Neurol*. 411(4):683-92.

Gong H, McGinty D, Guzman-Marin R, Chew KT, Stewart D, Szymusiak R (2004) Activation of c-fos in GABAergic neurones in the preoptic area during sleep and in response to sleep deprivation. *J Physiol.* 556:935-46.

Gourley SL, Debold JF, Yin W, Cook J, Miczek KA (2005) Benzodiazepines and heightened aggressive behavior in rats: reduction by GABA(A)/alpha(1) receptor antagonists. *Psychopharmacology* (Berl). 178(2-3):232-40.

Gottesmann C (2002) GABA mechanisms and sleep. *Neuroscience*. 111(2):231-9.

Gribkoff VK, Pieschl RL, Wisialowski TA, Park WK, Strecker GJ, de Jeu MT, Pennartz CM, Dudek FE (1999) A reexamination of the role of GABA in the mammalian suprachiasmatic nucleus. *J Biol Rhythms*. 14:126–30.

Guillot PV, Chapouthier G (1998) Intermale aggression, GAD activity in the olfactory bulbs and Y chromosome effect in seven inbred mouse strains. Behav Brain Res. 90(2):203-6.

Gvilia I, Turner A, McGinty D, Szymusiak R (2006) Preoptic area neurons and the homeostatic regulation of rapid eye movement sleep. *J Neurosci.* 26(11):3037-44.

Han Y, Shaikh MB, Siegel A. (1996) Medial amygdaloid suppression of predatory attack behavior in the cat: II. Role of a GABAergic pathway from the medial to the lateral hypothalamus. *Brain Res*. 716:72-83.

Hansen S, Ferreira A (1986) Effects of bicuculline infusions in the ventromedial hypothalamus and amygdaloid complex on food intake and affective behavior in mother rats. *Behav Neurosci*. 100(3):410-5.

Hasan R, Alóe F (2011) Updates on sleep-wake cycle. *Sleep Sci*. 4(2): 52-60.

Heck N, Kilb W, Reiprich P, Kubota H, Furukawa T, Fukuda A, Luhmann HJ (2007) GABA-A receptors regulate neocortical neuronal migration in vitro and in vivo. *Cereb Cortex* 17:138–48.

Hu JH, Ma YH, Jiang J, Yang N, Duan SH, Jiang ZH, Mei ZT, Fei J, Guo LH (2004) Cognitive impairment in mice over-expressing gamma-aminobutyric acid transporter 1 (GAT1). *Neuroreport.* 15(1):9-12.

Itri J, Colwell CS (2003) Regulation of inhibitory synaptic transmission by vasoactive intestinal peptide (VIP) in the mouse suprachiasmatic nucleus. *J Neurophysiol.* 90(3):1589-97.

Jasinska M, Siucinska E, Cybulska-Klosowicz A, Pyza E, Furness DN, et al. (2010) Rapid, learning-induced inhibitory synaptogenesis in murine barrel field. *J Neurosci* 30: 1176–84.

Kalueff A, Nutt DJ (1996) Role of GABA in memory and anxiety. *Depress Anxiety*. 4(3):100-10.

Kaur S, Thankachan S, Begum S, Liu M, Blanco-Centurion C, Shiromani PJ (2009) Hypocretin-2 saporin lesions of the ventrolateral periaquaductal gray (vlPAG) increase REM sleep in hypocretin knockout mice. *PLoS One*. 4(7):e6346.

Kalsbeek A, La Fleur S, Van Heijningen C, Buijs RM (2004) Suprachiasmatic GABAergic inputs to the paraventricular nucleus control plasma glucose concentrations in the rat via sympathetic innervation of the liver. *J Neurosci*. 24(35):7604-13.

Kilb W, Kirischuk S, Luhmann HJ (2013) Role of tonic GABAergic currents during pre- and early postnatal rodent development. *Front Neural Circuits*.7:139.

Kim YI, Dudek FE (1992) Intracellular electrophysiological study of suprachiasmatic nucleus neurons in rodents: inhibitory synaptic mechanisms. *J Physiol*. 458:247-60.

Kong D, Tong Q, Ye C, Koda S, Fuller PM, Krashes MJ, Vong L, Ray RS, Olson DP, Lowell BB (2012) GABAergic RIP-Cre neurons in the arcuate nucleus selectively regulate energy expenditure. *Cell*. 151(3):645-57

Korpi ER, Gründer G, Lüddens H (2002) Drug interactions at GABAA receptors. *Prog Neurobiol*. 67:113-59.

Krebs-Kraft DL, Wheeler MG, Parent MB (2007) The memory-impairing effects of septal GABA receptor activation involve GABAergic septo-hippocampal projection neurons. *Learn Mem*. 14(12):833-41.

Lall GS, Biello SM (2003) Neuropeptide Y, GABA and circadian phase shifts to photic stimuli. *Neuroscience*. 120(4):915-21.

Levitis DA, Lidicker WZ, Jr, Freund G (2009) Behavioural biologists do not agree on what constitutes behaviour. *Anim Behav*. 78:103-10.

Liu C, Reppert SM (2000) GABA synchronize clock cells within the suprachiasmatic circadian clock. *Neuron* 25:123–28.

Liu X,Wang Q, Haydar TF, Bordey A (2005) Nonsynaptic GABA signaling in postnatal subventricular zone controls proliferation of GFAP-expressing progenitors. *Nat Neurosci*. 8:1179–87.

Lu J, Sherman D, Devor M, Saper CB (2006) A putative flip-flop switch for control of REM sleep. *Nature*. 441(7093):589-94.

Ma YH, Hu JH, Zhou XG, Zeng RW, Mei ZT, Fei J, Guo LH (2000) Transgenic mice overexpressing gamma-aminobutyric acid transporter subtype I develop obesity. *Cell Res*. 10(4):303-10.

Makkar SR, Zhang SQ, Cranney J (2010) Behavioral and neural analysis of GABA in the acquisition, consolidation, reconsolidation, and extinction of fear memory. *Neuropsychopharmacology*. 35(8):1625-52.

Marks GA, Sachs OW, Birabil CG (2008) Blockade of GABA, type A, receptors in the rat pontine reticular formation induces rapid eye movement sleep that is dependent upon the cholinergic system. *Neuroscience*. 156(1):1-10.

Massimini M, Ferrarelli F, Huber R, Esser SK, Singh H, Tononi G (2005) Breakdown of cortical effective connectivity during sleep. *Science*. 309:2228–32.

McCarthy MM (2008) Estradiol and the developing brain. *Physiol Rev*. 88(1):91-124.

McNamara RK, Skelton RW (1996) Baclofen, a selective GABAB receptor agonist, dose-dependently impairs spatial learning in rats. *Pharmacol Biochem Behav*. 53(2):303-8.

Miczek KA, Fish EW, De Bold JF, De Almeida RM (2002) Social and neural determinants of aggressive behavior: pharmacotherapeutic targets at serotonin, dopamine and gamma-aminobutyric acid systems. *Psychopharmacology* (Berl). 163(3-4):434-58.

Miner P, Borkuhova Y, Shimonova L, Khaimov A, Bodnar RJ (2010) GABA-A and GABA-B receptors mediate feeding elicited by the GABA-B agonist baclofen in the ventral tegmental area and nucleus accumbens shell in rats: reciprocal and regional interactions. *Brain Res.* 1355:86-96.

Mintz EM, Jasnow AM, Gillespie CF, Huhman KL, Albers HE (2002) GABA interacts with photic signaling in the suprachiasmatic nucleus to regulate circadian phase shifts. *Neuroscience.* 109(4):773-8.

Mong JA, Glaser E, McCarthy MM (1999) Gonadal steroids promote glial differentiation and alter neuronal morphology in the developing hypothalamus in a regionally specific manner. *J Neurosci.* 19:1464–72.

Moore RY, Speh JC. (1993) GABA is the principal neurotransmitter of the circadian system. *Neurosci. Lett.* 150:112–6.

Moore RY, Speh JC, Leak RK (2002) Suprachiasmatic nucleus organization. *Cell Tissue Res.* 309:89–98.

Morris JA, Jordan CL, Breedlove SM (2004) Sexual differentiation of the vertebrate nervous system. *Nat Neurosci.* 7:1034–9.

Muroya S, Funahashi H, Uramura K, Shioda S, Yada T (2005) Gamma aminobutyric acid regulates glucosensitive neuropeptide Y neurons in arcuate nucleus via A/B receptors. *Neuroreport.* 16(9):897-901.

Murphy DD, Segal M (1997) Morphological plasticity of dendritic spines in central neurons is mediated by activation of cAMP response element binding protein. *Proc Natl Acad Sci USA.* 94:1482–7.

Nabeshima T, Noda Y, Kameyama T (1988) GABAergic modulation of memory with regard to passive avoidance and conditioned suppression task in mice. *Psychopharmacology* (Berl). 94(1):69-73.

Nakagawa Y, Ishibashi Y, Yoshii T, Tagashira E (1995) Muscimol induces state-dependent learning in Morris water maze task in rats. *Brain Res.* 681(1-2):126-30.

Nakagawa Y, Takashima T (1997) The GABA(B) receptor antagonist CGP36742 attenuates the baclofen- and scopolamine-induced deficit in Morris water maze task in rats. *Brain Res.* 766(1-2):101-6.

Nelson RJ, Trainor BC (2007) Neural mechanisms of aggression. *Nat Rev Neurosci.* 8(7):536-46.

Nguyen TQ, Liang CL, Marks GA (2013) GABA(A) receptors implicated in REM sleep control express a benzodiazepine binding site. *Brain Res.* 1527:131-40.

Nitz D, Siegel JM (1996) GABA release in posterior hypothalamus across sleep-wake cycle. *Am J Physiol.* 271:1707-12.

Nugent BM, Valenzuela CV, Simons TJ, McCarthy MM (2012) Kinases SPAK and OSR1 are upregulated by estradiol and activate NKCC1 in the developing hypothalamus. *J Neurosci.* 32(2):593-8.

Okada H, Iwase S, Mano T, Sugiyama Y, Watanabe T (1991) Changes in muscle sympathetic nerve activity during sleep in humans. *Neurology.* 41(12):1961-6.

Okamura H, Bérod A, Julien JF, Geffard M, Kitahama K, Mallet J, Bobillier P (1989) Demonstration of GABAergic cell bodies in the suprachiasmatic nucleus: in situ hybridization of glutamic acid decarboxylase (GAD) mRNA and immunocytochemistry of GAD and GABA. *Neurosci Lett.* 102(2-3):131-6.

Uusi-Oukari M, Korpi ER (2010) Regulation of GABA(A) receptor subunit expression by pharmacological agents. *Pharmacol Rev*. 62(1):97-135.

Pace-Schott EF, Hobson JA (2002) The neurobiology of sleep: genetics, cellular physiology and subcortical networks. *Nat Neurosci.* 3(8):591-605.

Perrot-Sinal TS, Davis AM, Gregerson KA, Kao JP, McCarthy MM (2001) Estradiol enhances excitatory gamma-aminobutyric acid-mediated calcium signaling in neonatal hypothalamic neurons. *Endocrinology.* 142:2238–43.

Platel JC, Dave KA, Bordey A (2008) Control of neuroblast production and migration by converging GABA and glutamate signals in the postnatal forebrain. *J Physiol*. 586:3739–43.

Puglisi-Allegra S, Mandel P (1980) Effects of sodium n-dipropylacetate, muscimol hydrobromide and (R,S) nipecotic acid amide on isolation-induced aggressive behavior in mice. *Psychopharmacology* (Berl). 70(3):287-90.

Rivera C, Voipio J, Payne JA, Ruusuvuori E, Lahtinen H, Lamsa K, Pirvola U, Saarma M, Kaila K (1999) The K+/Cl– co-transporter KCC2 renders GABA hyperpolarizing during neuronal maturation. *Nature.* 397:251–5.

Rohrbough J, Spitzer NC (1996) Regulation of intracellular Cl− levels by Na+-dependent Cl− cotransport distinguishes depolarizing from hyperpolarizing GABAA receptor-mediated responses in spinal neurons. *J Neurosci.* 16:82–91.

Sanford LD, Tang X, Xiao J, Ross RJ, Morrison AR (2003) GABAergic regulation of REM sleep in reticularis pontis oralis and caudalis in rats. *J Neurophysiol*. 90(2):938-45.

Sapin E, Lapray D, Bérod A, Goutagny R, Léger L, Ravassard P, Clément O, Hanriot L, Fort P, Luppi PH (2004) Localization of the brainstem GABAergic neurons controlling paradoxical (REM) sleep. *PLoS One*. 4(1):e4272.

Saper CB, Fuller PM, Pedersen NP, Lu J, Scammell TE (2010) Sleep state switching. *Neuron.* 68(6):1023-42.

Schmitt U, Hiemke C (2002) Tiagabine, a gamma-amino-butyric acid transporter inhibitor impairs spatial learning of rats in the Morris water-maze. *Behav Brain* Res. 133(2):391-4.

Schuler V, Lüscher C, Blanchet C, Klix N, Sansig G, Klebs K, Schmutz M, Heid J, Gentry C, Urban L, Fox A, Spooren W, Jaton AL, Vigouret J, Pozza M, Kelly PH, Mosbacher J, Froestl W, Käslin E, Korn R, Bischoff S, Kaupmann K, van der Putten H, Bettler B (2001) Epilepsy, hyperalgesia, impaired memory, and loss of pre- and postsynaptic GABA(B) responses in mice lacking GABA(B(1) *Neuron.* 31(1):47-58.

Shaikh MB, Siegel A (1990) GABA-mediated regulation of feline aggression elicited from midbrain periaqueductal gray upon affective defense behavior in the cat. *Brain Res.* 507:51-6.

Sharma AC, Kulkarni SK (1993) (+/-)Baclofen sensitive scopolamine-induced short-term memory deficits in mice. *Indian J Exp Biol*. 31(4):348-52.

Shi J, Cai Y, Liu G, Gong N, Liu Z, Xu T, Wang Z, Fei J (2012) Enhanced learning and memory in GAT1 heterozygous mice. *Acta Biochim Biophys Sin* (Shanghai). 44(4):359-66.

Sigel E, Steinmann ME (2012) Structure, function, and modulation of GABA(A) receptors. *J Biol Chem.* 287(48):40224-31

Skolnick P, Reed GF, Paul SM (1985) Benzodiazepine-receptor mediated inhibition of isolation-induced aggression in mice. *Pharmacol Biochem Behav*. 23(1):17-20.

Stanley BG, Urstadt KR, Charles JR, Kee T (2011) Glutamate and GABA in lateral hypothalamic mechanisms controlling food intake. *Physiol Behav*. 104(1):40-6.

Stratford TR, Kelley AE (1997) GABA in the nucleus accumbens shell participates in the central regulation of feeding behavior. *J Neurosci.* 17(11):4434-40.

Suntsova N, Szymusiak R, Alam MN, Guzman-Marin R, McGinty D (2002) Sleep-waking discharge patterns of median preoptic nucleus neurons in rats. *J Physiol*. 543:665-77.

Tobet S, Knoll JG, Hartshorn C, Aurand E, Stratton M, Kumar P, Searcy B, McClellan K (2009) Brain sex differences and hormone influences: a moving experience? *J Neuroendocrinol.* 21(4):387-92.

Todd BJ, Schwarz JM, Mong JA, McCarthy MM (2007) Glutamate AMPA/kainate receptors, not GABA(A) receptors, mediate estradiol-induced sex differences in the hypothalamus. *Dev Neurobiol.* 67(3):304-15.

Tyzio R, Represa A, Jorquera I, Ben-Ari Y, Gozlan H, Aniksztejn L (1999) The establishment of GABAergic and glutamatergic synapses on CA1 pyramidal neurons is sequential and correlates with the development of the apical dendrite. *J Neurosci.* 19(23):10372-82.

Van den Pol AN, Dudek FE (1993) Cellular communication in the circadian clock, the suprachiasmatic nucleus. *Neuroscience.* 56:793–811.

Xu XH, Qu WM, Bian MJ, Huang F, Fei J, Urade Y, Huang ZL (2013) Essential roles of GABA transporter-1 in controlling rapid eye movement sleep and in increased slow wave activity after sleep deprivation. *PLoS One.* 8(10):e75823.

Wagner S, Castel M, Gainer H, Yarom Y (1997) GABAin the mammalian suprachiasmatic nucleus and its role in diurnal rhythmicity. *Nature.* 387:598–603

Wang DD, Kriegstein AR (2009) Defining the role of GABA in cortical development. *J Physiol.* 587:1873-9.

Walton M, Woodgate AM, Muravlev A, Xu R, During MJ, Dragunow M (1999) CREB phosphorylation promotes nerve cell survival. *J. Neurochem.* 73:1836–42.

Welsh DK, Logothetis DE, Meister M, Reppert SM (19995) Individual neurons dissociated from rat suprachiasmatic nucleus express independently phased circadian firing rhythms. *Neuron.* 14(4):697-706.

Winkelman JW, Buxton OM, Jensen JE, Benson KL, O'Connor SP, Wang W, Renshaw PF (2008) Reduced brain GABA in primary insomnia: preliminary data from 4T proton magnetic resonance spectroscopy (1H-MRS). *Sleep*. 31(11):1499-506.

Yanowitch R, Coccaro EF (2011) The neurochemistry of human aggression. *Adv Genet.* 75:151-69.

Zhang C, Truong KK, Zhou QY (2009) Efferent projections of prokineticin 2 expressing neurons in the mouse suprachiasmatic nucleus. *PLoS One*. 4(9):e7151

Zhang D, Pan ZH, Awobuluyi M, Lipton SA (2001) Structure and function of GABA(C) receptors: a comparison of native versus recombinant receptors. *Trends Pharmacol Sci.* 22(3):121-32.

In: Gamma-Aminobutyric Acid (GABA) ISBN: 978-1-63321-838-3
Editors: Josipa Vlainić and Maja Jazvinšćak Jembrek 

*Chapter 5*

# THE EFFECTS OF GABA AND GABAERGIC DRUGS ON THE HPA AXIS ACTIVITY

***Dubravka Svob Strac**, Dorotea Muck-Seler and Nela Pivac***
Rudjer Boskovic Institute, Division of Molecular Medicine, Zagreb, Croatia

## ABSTRACT

Various studies have shown that γ-aminobutyric acid (GABA), the major inhibitory neurotransmitter in the brain, regulates neuroendocrine functions and affects the activity of hypothalamic-pituitary-adrenal (HPA) axis. Although most data suggest that GABA, as well as benzodiazepines, inhibit HPA axis function through central mechanisms involving the hypothalamic control, the reports regarding possible involvement of GABAergic drugs in the control of HPA axis are still contradictory. Namely, diverse effects of these drugs on corticosterone and adrenocorticotropic hormone (ACTH) levels have been demonstrated both in experimental animals and in humans. Besides being dependent on the dose, the effects of GABAergic drugs on the HPA axis activity appear to be influenced by the gender of the animals. Moreover, the reasons for the observed discrepancies might be sought in the complexity of neural circuits and neuroendocrine relations, the lack of specificity of drugs used in the studies, but also in different levels (central or peripheral) at which drugs affecting GABAergic neurotransmission primarily act. Our results demonstrating the stimulatory effect of GABA antagonists picrotoxin and bicuculline, administered intraperitoneally (i.p.), on the plasma corticosterone levels in rats, suggest that blockade of $GABA_A$ receptors stimulates the activity of the HPA axis. The observed inhibitory effect of a low dose (1 mg/kg) of diazepam (i.p.), the $GABA_A$ receptor enhancer, as well as of baclofen (i.p.), the $GABA_B$ receptor agonist, and GABA administered intracerebroventriculary (i.c.v.), on plasma corticosterone and ACTH levels, respectively, is also in agreement with the hypothesis suggesting GABAergic inhibition of the HPA axis. In contrast, the i.p. administration of GABA, the GABA agonist progabide and aminooxyacetic acid (AOAA), the inhibitor of GABA degradation,

* Corresponding author: Dubravka Svob Strac, Ph.D., Research Associate, Rudjer Boskovic Institute, Division of Molecular Medicine, Bijenicka cesta 54, 10 000 Zagreb, Croatia. Phone: 385 1 456 1126, Fax: + 385 1 456 1010. E-mail: dsvob@irb.hr.

increased corticosterone levels in plasma. While picrotoxin, bicuculline and progabide produced an increase of plasma corticosterone levels in both males and females (although more in female then in male rats), diazepam had a dual effect depending on the dose of the drug and on the sex of the animals. Namely, diazepam administered in lower dose (1 mg/kg) inhibited the activity of HPA axis only in female rats, while high dose of diazepam (10 mg/kg) stimulated the HPA axis activity of male and female rats. Hence, further studies are necessary to elucidate the complex mechanisms of GABAergic drugs on the activity of HPA axis and to consider the possible implications of these findings for the human therapy.

**Keywords**: GABA, GABAeric drugs, HPA axis, corticosterone, ACTH, sex differences, rats

## INTRODUCTION

Various studies suggested that γ-aminobutyric acid (GABA), besides its role as the major inhibitory neurotransmitter in the central nervous system (CNS) also regulates neuroendocrine function and affects the activity of hypothalamic-pituitary-adrenal (HPA) axis. A variety of findings provide an anatomical basis for a neuroendocrine role of GABA in the regulation of the HPA axis activity. The existence of intimate relationship between GABA and endocrine system is also obvious from the fact that GABA and hormones can even coexist in the same neurons (Lin et al., 1986). As many other neurotransmitters, GABA is present in the tissues which are parts of the endocrine system including hypothalamus, pituitary, as well as peripheral organs such as adrenal gland, pancreatic islets, thyroid, ovary, oviduct and uterus (Erdo, 1985). The hypothalamic control of many aspects of endocrine function involves the complex interplay of several neurotransmitters in which GABA exert a modulatory action on the secretion of hypothalamic releasing factors, pituitary hormones, as well as hormones in the target endocrine organs.

The hypothalamus has been reported to contain high levels of glutamate decarboxylase (GAD) and GABA transferase (GABA-T), enzymes involved in the GABA synthesis and catabolism, respectively (Okada et al., 1971; Tappaz et al., 1976, 1980). A dense plexus of GAD-like immunoreactivity, revealed in the median eminence and other hypothalamic nuclei, revealed the existence of tuberoinfundibular GABAergic system (Berod et al., 1984; Tappaz et al., 1983; Vincent et al., 1982). GABA represents the main neurotransmitter involved in the complex regulatory control in the hypothalamic function (Herman and Cullinan, 1997; Herman et al., 2002a). Namely, the HPA axis is controlled by a discrete set of neurosecretory neurons, located in the medial parvocellular region of hypothalamic paraventricular nucleus (mpPVN) (Antoni, 1986; Whitnall, 1993). These neurons integrate excitatory and inhibitory signals for appropriate release of corticotropin-releasing hormone (CRH) and arginine vasopressin (AVP), involved in the regulation of the magnitude and duration of the stress response. The prominent GABAergic modulation of CRH neurons has been established (Herman et al., 2004; Kovacs et al., 2004). Nearly half of all synapses in the mpPVN and majority of the local synaptic inputs to PVN neurons were identified as GABAergic (Decavel and van den Pol, 1990; Herman et al., 2003, 2004; Tasker and Dudek, 1993). However, substantial proportion of GABAergic innervations to the PVN neurons is also supplied by neighboring cell populations (Herman et al., 2002b). Moreover, the presence of GABA receptors has been determined in the hypothalamus (Beaumont et al., 1978), and the expression of both $GABA_A$ and $GABA_B$ receptors was found in the parvocellular region of PVN (Margeta-Mitrovic et al., 1999; Pirker et al., 2000). Anatomic studies have shown that CRH neurons express key $GABA_A$ receptor subunits (Cullinan, 2000; Roland and Sawchenko, 1993) as well as both splice variants of $GABA_B$ receptors (Pirker et al., 2000).

In addition to cells and axon terminals containing GABA and its receptors, located in the hypothalamus, GABA has been also found in the pituitary portal blood and its release from the median eminence can be increased following stimulation (Gudelsky et al., 1983; Nicoletti et al., 1982). GABA receptors were also observed in both the anterior and neurointermediate lobe of pituitary (Anderson and Mitchell, 1986; Berman et al., 1994). GABA has been reported to affect the release of several anterior pituitary hormones, such as prolactin, growth hormone, adrenocorticotropic hormone (ACTH), or thyroid-stimulating hormone (TSH) (De Feudis, 1983; Racagni et al., 1982). High concentrations of GABA and GAD found in the islet cells of the pancreas suggested that GABA may be involved in the regulation of pancreatic endocrine function (Gerber and Hare, 1979). In line with these findings, it has been reported that the administration of GABA might result in hyperinsulinemia and hyperglucagonemia (Cavagnini et al., 1982).

Although initial evidence for the importance of GABAergic neurotransmission in regulating the HPA axis activity dates back over four decades (Jones et al. 1976; Makara and Stark, 1974) and since then the influence of GABA and GABAergic drugs on the HPA axis has been extensively studied, the results are still contradictory. Besides being dependent on the dose, the effects of GABAergic drugs on the HPA axis activity appear to be influenced by the gender of the animals. The reasons for the discrepancies might be sought in the complexity of neural circuits and neuroendocrine relations, the lack of specificity of drugs used in the studies, but also in different levels (central or peripheral) at which drugs affecting GABAergic neurotransmission primarily act. However, most studies suggested the inhibitory effect of GABA on the CRH secretion (Calogero et al., 1988; Hillhouse and Milton, 1989; Plotsky et al., 1987; Tappaz et al., 1982), mediated via a local neurocircuitry involving limbic forebrain regions (Arvat et al., 2002; Herman et al., 2002a,b; Jones et al., 1984). Namely, GABA-mediated inhibition of the HPA axis activity at the level of the PVN originates from a series of local hypothalamic and adjacent forebrain regions which contain GABA, and which project to CRH-containing neurons (Cullinan et al., 2008). It has been shown that injection of GABA triggers inhibitory postsynaptic potentials in parvocellular neurons (Boudaba et al., 1996) indicating the direct physiologic actions on excitability. Activity of the HPA axis is also reduced after intracerebroventricular (i.c.v). injection of $GABA_A$ receptor agonists (Makara and Stark, 1974) or by peripheral injection of benzodiazepines (Imaki et al., 1995). Although GABA as well as benzodiazepines have been shown to suppress CRH secretion in the hypothalamus and locus coeruleus, these active substances did not modify basal or CRH-stimulated ACTH release in animals, as wells as in humans (Arvat et al., 2002; Grottoli et al., 2002; Kalogeras et al., 1990). Some authors demonstrated that microinjections of $GABA_A$ receptor agonist, muscimol, directly inhibit corticosterone responses to stress (Cullinan, 1998), whereas responses can be initiated by the $GABA_A$ antagonist bicuculline (Cole and Sawchenko, 2002), implying the existence of an inhibitory GABAergic tone. Moreover, in vitro studies demonstrated that GABA inhibits the release of CRH from the hypothalamic slices (Calogero et al., 1988; Hillhouse and Milton, 1989).

The role of GABA on the release of some other hormones such as prolactin is less clear, since both stimulatory (Lee and Pan, 2001; Mioduszewski et al., 1976; Ondo and Pass, 1976;

Pass and Ondo, 1977; Vijayan and Mccann, 1978) and inhibitory (Locatelli et al., 1978; Lux-Lantos et al., 1992; Schally et al., 1977; Vijayan and Mccann, 1978) effects have been described. It appears that the stimulating effect on the prolactin secretion is achieved by GABA action at a cerebral site, while the inhibiting effect on the prolactin secretion is presumably a result of its action on the anterior pituitary (Racagni et al., 1982). GABA also inhibits oxytocin secretion in response to osmotic stimuli (Bisset et al., 1990) or suckling (Voisin et al., 1995) via $GABA_A$ receptors. These results suggest a physiological role of GABA in regulating the activity of oxytocin neurons in the hypothalamus.

On the other hand, a vice versa relationship between endocrine function and GABA has been also suggested. Some studies demonstrated the involvement of GABA in the feedback action of estradiol on gonadotropin and prolactin release (Mansky et al., 1982). The changes in GABA concentration and synthesis have been observed due to actions of gonadal hormones (Earley and Leonard, 1978; Wuttke and Mansky, 1981). The activity of GAD in the medial basal hypothalamus and substantia nigra is affected under conditions of hyper- and hypo-prolactinemia (Nicoletti et al., 1982; 1983). Estrogen and progesteron have been demonstrated as potent inhibitors of GAD in several brain regions (McGinnis et al., 1980; Wallis and Luttge, 1980). The existence of GABAergic estrogen-receptive neurons in the preoptic/anterior hypothalamic area suggests that GABA release is directly regulated by estrogens (Flugge et al., 1986). It has been shown that estrogens and progesterone can regulate the number of GABA receptors as well (Maggi and Perez, 1984). The reported sex differences in GABA concentrations in discrete rat brain nuclei (Frankfurt et al., 1984) and sex-related differences in GABA and benzodiazepine receptor binding (Fiszer de Plazas et al., 1983; Shephard et al., 1982) also confirmed the influence of gonadal steroids on this neuronal system.

Hence, in order to find out whether the HPA axis in rats of both sexes responds equally to drugs affecting GABAergic neurotransmission, we studied the effects of GABA itself, as well as GABA agonist progabide, $GABA_A$ receptor enhancer diazepam, $GABA_B$ receptor agonist baclofen, inhibitor of GABA degradation aminooxyacetic acid (AOAA), or GABA antagonists picrotoxin and bicuculline, on the plasma corticosterone and ACTH levels.

## Materials and Methods

### Animals

Wistar rats (3 months old) bred in Rudjer Boskovic Institute were used. They were housed at a constant temperature (22° C) and under a light cycle of 12-h light/ 12-h darkness (lights on at 7:00 a.m.). They were caged in groups of 5. Food and water were freely available. The female rats weighting 180 g were primarily used in experiments with the intraperitoneal (i.p.) drug injections, while heavier animals (~ 250 g) of both sexes were used in the experiments with intracerebroventricular (i.c.v.) drug administration. For the later, animals were operated under i.p. administered pentobarbital anesthesia (30 mg/kg). A stainless still cannula (0.7 mm id, 12 mm length) was sterotaxically inserted into the 3rd ventricle and fixed with dental cement to the scull. Operated animals were housed individually in the cages and allowed to recover for 7 days. Before the experiments all animals were adapted to handling and injecting for 7 days. To minimize circadian variability of plasma ACTH and corticosterone levels, all experiments were performed between 8.00 and 11.00 am. All animal care and experimental procedures were carried out in accordance with the Directive 2010/63/EU of European Parliament and Council of the European Union on the protection of animals used for scientific purposes and with the Croatian law on animal welfare.

### Drugs

GABA, AOAA, baclofen and picrotoxin (all from Sigma) were dissolved in saline. Diazepam (Hoffman La Roche) and progabide (Synthelabo) were diluted with 0.1% solution of Tween 80 (Sigma) in saline. Bicuculline (Sigma) was dissolved in warm 0.1 N HCl followed by saline. All drugs and corresponding vehicles, including artificial cerebrospinal fluid (ACSF), were prepared fresh and their pH was adjusted. Drugs were injected to animals i.p. in a volume of 1 ml/100 g of body weight or i.c.v. in a volume of 1 μl.

### Experimental Procedure

Following administration of drugs or their vehicles, animals were sacrificed by decapitation with a guillotine. Trunk blood was collected in prechilled tubes containing EDTA (1 mg/ml of blood), centrifuged (4° C, 15 min, 1250 g) and plasma was separated and stored at -20° C. Corticosterone levels were determined in plasma samples of 500 μl by a slight modification of the fluorometric method (Pivac and Pericic, 1993). ACTH levels were measured directly, without prior extraction, in a 200 μl of plasma, by a radioimmunoassay (RIA) using commercially available ACTHK-PR kit (CIS bioindustries).

### Data Analysis

Results were expressed as mean ± SEM of the values. Statistical evaluation of the results was done using one-way analysis of variance (ANOVA) followed by Dunnett´s test, or using Student t-test, where appropriate. *P*-values of $<0.05$ were considered significant.

## RESULTS

### The Effects of Intraperitoneral Injection on the Plasma Corticosterone and ACTH Levels

Prior to experiments involving GABAergic drug administration the effects of i.p. injection itself on the plasma corticosterone levels of male and female rats were first examined. These effects were determined at different time points following i.p. saline injection. As shown in Figure 1, the corticosterone concentrations in plasma were significantly higher in male rats injected with saline 15, 30 and 60 min prior to sacrifice when compared to non-injected animals, while there were no differences 120 min following saline injection (Figure 1A). On the other hand, significantly elevated levels of plasma corticosterone were observed in female rats 15 and 30 min following injection and prior to sacrifice (Figure 1B).

Moreover, the significant sex-differences in plasma corticosterone levels were observed. As shown in Figure 1, in non-injected animals corticosterone leves were significantly higher in female then in male rats ($p < 0.02$, Student t-test). There were also significant sex differences in plasma corticosterone levels in animals injected with saline 15, 30 and 120 min prior to sacrifice ($p < 0.001$, $p < 0.02$ and $p < 0.02$, respectively, Student t-test), while 60 min following saline injection the corticosterone concentrations in plasma were not significantly different between male and female rats.

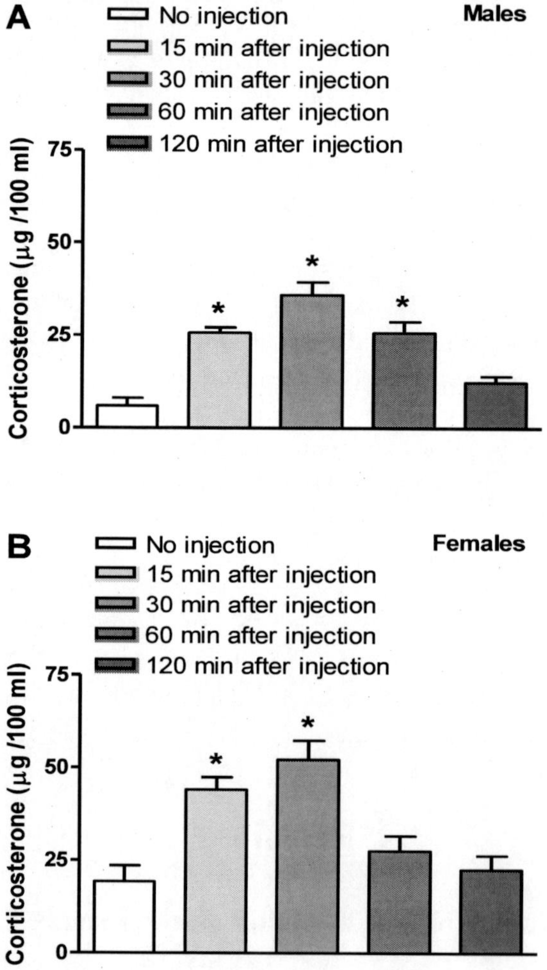


Figure 1. The effect of i.p. administered saline on plasma corticosterone concentrations in male (A) and female (B) rats. Saline was injected i.p. 15, 30, 60 and 120 min prior to sacrifice. The results are expressed as mean ± SEM of the values. The number of animals per group ranked from 5-15. *$p < 0.05$ or 0.01 vs. the control non-injected group (ANOVA followed by Dunnett's test).

Moreover, ACTH concentrations in the plasma of female rats were also significantly elevated 10 and 30 min following saline injection when compared to non-injected animals, while there were no differences in ACTH levels 60 min prior sacrifice (Figure 2).

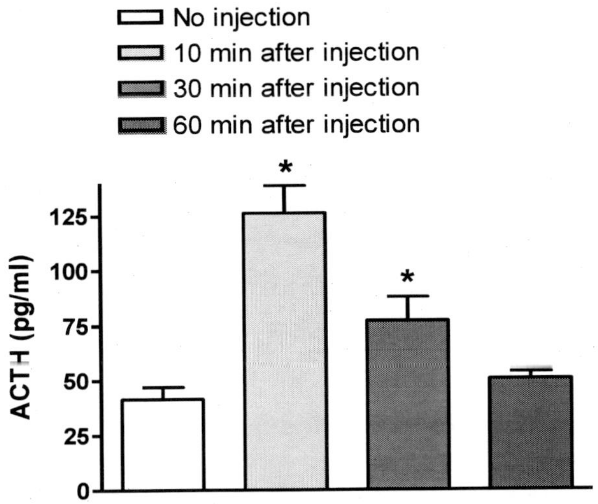


Figure 2. The effect of i.p. administered saline on plasma ACTH concentrations in female rats. Saline was injected i.p. 10, 30 and 60 min prior to sacrifice. The results are expressed as mean ± SEM of the values. The number of animals per group ranked from 6-13. **p*< 0.01 vs. the control non-injected group (ANOVA followed by Dunnett's test).

## The Effects of GABA on the Plasma Corticosterone and ACTH Levels

As in the case of i.p. injection, similar changes in plasma corticosterone, but also in ACTH levels were observed at different time points following i.c.v. administration of artificial cerebrospinal fluid (ACSF), Figure 3. Hence, plasma corticosterone as well as ACTH levels were significantly higher 30 min ($p < 0.01$, ANOVA followed by Dunnett's test or $p < 0.05$, ANOVA followed by Dunnett's test), but not 60 min following i.c.v. injection of ACSF in both female and male rats, in comparison to un-injected animals. GABA (8 μg/μl) administered i.c.v. 30 or 60 min prior to sacrifice induced no significant changes in the plasma corticosterone concentrations when compared to control group (injected i.c.v. with ACSF) in both male and female rats (Figure 3A and 3B). On the other hand, GABA decreased the levels of plasma ACTH in male rats when administered i.c.v. 30 min prior the sacrifice and in female rats when i.c.v. administered 60 min prior to sacrifice (Figure 3C and 3D).

Various concentrations of GABA (0.1, 1, 10 and 100 mg/kg) or its vehicle were also administered i.p. to female rats 60 min prior to sacrifice and plasma corticosterone was determined. As shown in Figure 4, GABA administered in the doses of 0.1, 1 and 10 mg/kg has not induced significant changes in the plasma corticosterone and ACTH levels. However, plasma corticosterone concentrations were significantly elevated following 100 mg/kg GABA (Figure 4A), while observed increase in ACTH levels was not significant (Figure 4B).

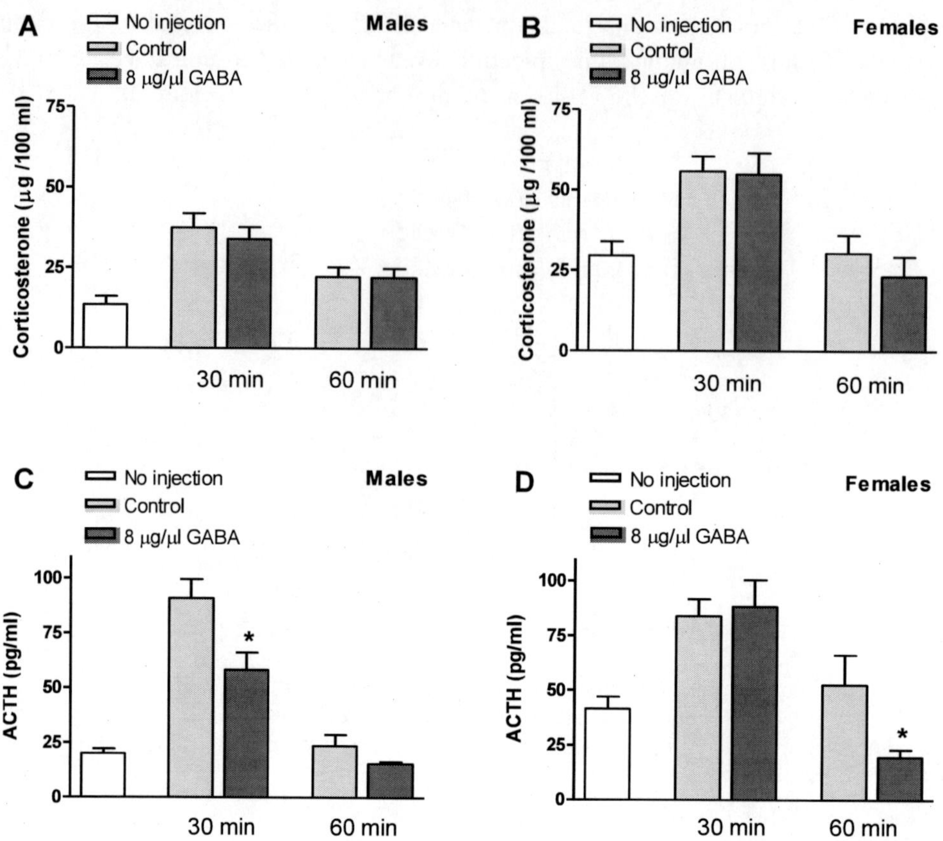


Figure 3. The effect of i.c.v. administered GABA on plasma corticosterone (A) and ACTH (B) concentrations in male and female rats. GABA (8 μg/ml) or ACSF were injected i.c.v. 30 or 60 min prior to sacrifice. The results are expressed as mean ± SEM of the values. The number of animals per group ranked from 5-12. *$p < 0.02$ or $p < 0.05$ vs. the control ACSF treated group (Student's t-test).

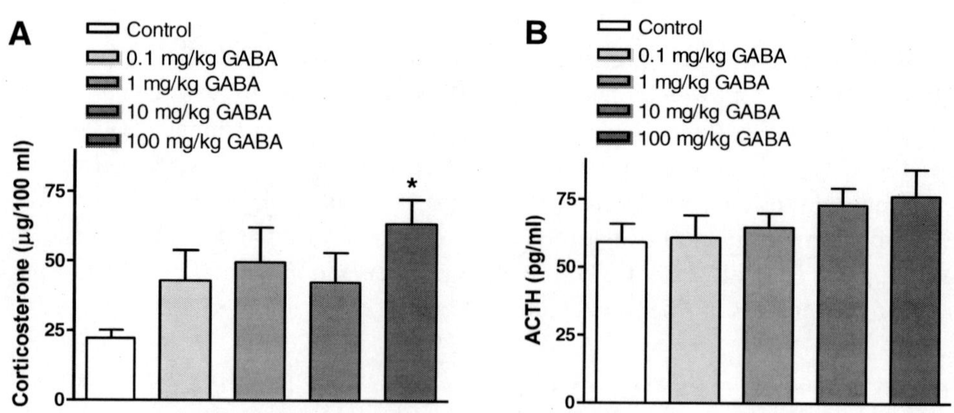


Figure 4. The effect of i.p. administered GABA on plasma corticosterone (A) and ACTH (B) concentrations in female rats. GABA (0.1, 1, 10 and 100 mg/kg) or its vehicle were injected i.p. 60 min prior to sacrifice. The results are expressed as mean ± SEM of the values. The number of animals per group ranked from 7-14. *$p < 0.01$ vs. the control vehicle treated group (ANOVA followed by Dunnett's test).

In addition to GABA treatment, the levels of GABA in the rat brain could be increased by administration of aminooxyacetic acid (AOAA), the inhibitor of GABA degradation. For that purpose various concentrations of AOAA (25, 50 and 75 mg/kg) or its vehicle were administered i.p. to female rats 60 min prior to sacrifice. The results demonstrated that all used doses of AOAA have significantly increased the levels of corticosterone in plasma of female rats (Figure 5).

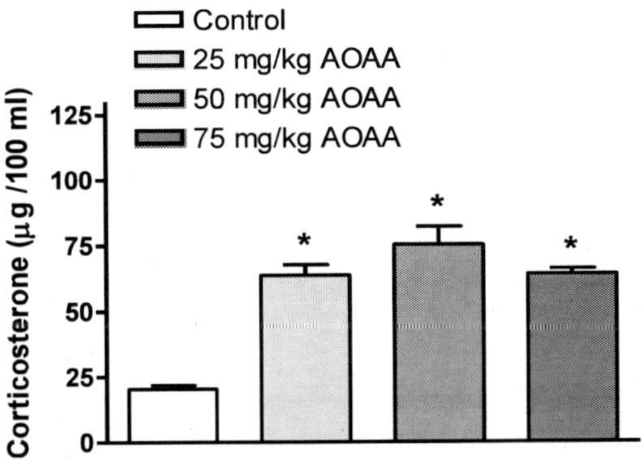


Figure 5. The effect of i.p. administered AOAA on plasma corticosterone concentrations in female rats. AOAA (25, 50 and 75 mg/kg) or its vehicle were injected i.p. 60 min prior to sacrifice. The results are expressed as mean ± SEM of the values. The number of animals per group ranked from 7-8. *$p < 0.01$ vs. the control vehicle treated group (ANOVA followed by Dunnett's test).

## The Effects of GABA Receptor Agonists Progabide and Baclofen on the Plasma Corticosterone Levels

As shown in Figure 6, GABA receptor agonist progabide administered i.p. to male and female rats in dose of 10 mg/kg, 60 min prior to sacrifice, induced no significant changes in the plasma corticosterone levels.

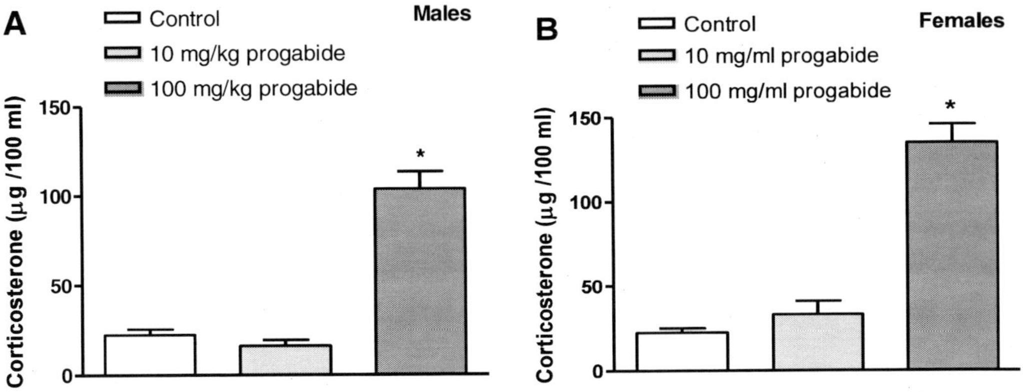


Figure 6. The effect of i.p. administered progabide on plasma corticosterone concentrations in male (A) and female (B) rats. Progabide (10 and 100 mg/kg) or its vehicle were injected i.p. 60 min prior to sacrifice. The results are expressed as mean ± SEM of the values. The number of animals per group ranked from 6-13. *$p < 0.01$ vs. the control vehicle treated group (ANOVA followed by Dunnett's test).

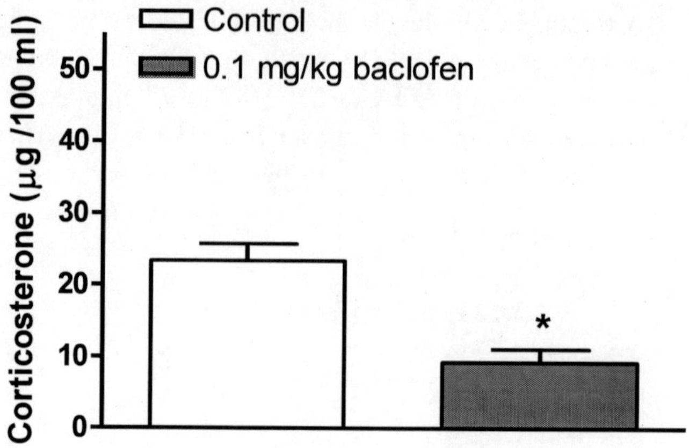


Figure 7. The effect of i.p. administered baclofen on plasma corticosterone concentrations in female rats. Baclofen (0.1 mg/kg) or its vehicle were injected i.p. 60 min prior to sacrifice. The results are expressed as mean ± SEM of the values. The number of animals per group was 10. *$p< 0.001$ vs. the control vehicle treated group (Student's t-test).

However, significantly increased concentrations of corticosterone in plasma were observed in male and female rats 60 min following administration of the higher dose of GABA mimetic drug progabide (100 mg/kg). On the other hand, 0.1 mg/kg baclofen, an agonist of $GABA_B$ receptor, injected i.p. 60 min prior to sacrifice, produced significant decrease in the plasma corticosterone levels in female rats (Figure 7).

## The Effects of GABA Antagonists Bicuculline and Picrotoxin on the Plasma Corticosterone and ACTH Levels

GABA antagonist bicuculline administered i.p. to female rats in the doses 0.5, 1.0 and 2.0 mg/kg, 10 min before sacrifice, demonstrated no significant effect on the plasma corticosterone levels (Figure 8A).

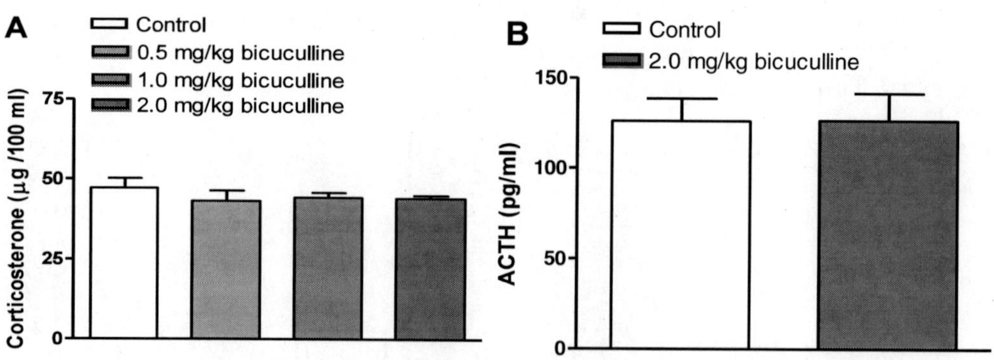


Figure 8. The effect of i.p. administered bicuculline on plasma corticosterone (A) and ACTH (B) concentrations in female rats. Bicuculline (0.5, 1 and 2 mg/kg) or its vehicle were injected i.p. 10 min prior to sacrifice. The results are expressed as mean ± SEM of the values. The number of animals per group ranked from 5-6.

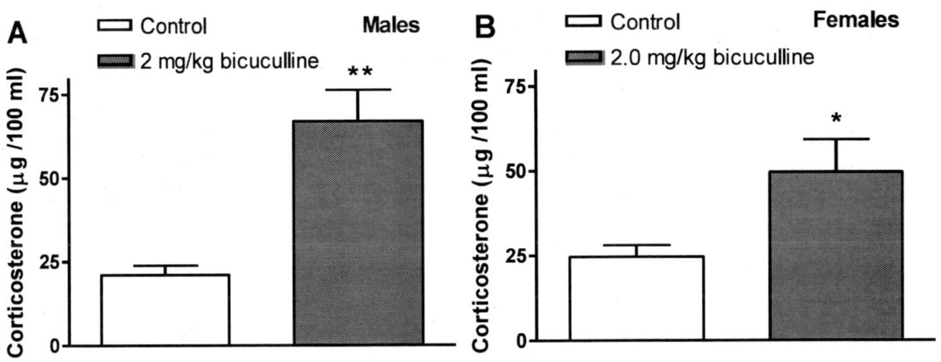


Figure 9. The effect of i.p. administered bicuculline on plasma corticosterone concentrations in male (A) and female (B) rats. Bicuculline (2 mg/kg) or its vehicle were injected i.p. 60 min prior to sacrifice. The results are expressed as mean ± SEM of the values. The number of animals per group ranked from 6-13. $^*p< 0.01$; $^{**}p< 0.001$ vs. the control vehicle treated group (Student's t-test).

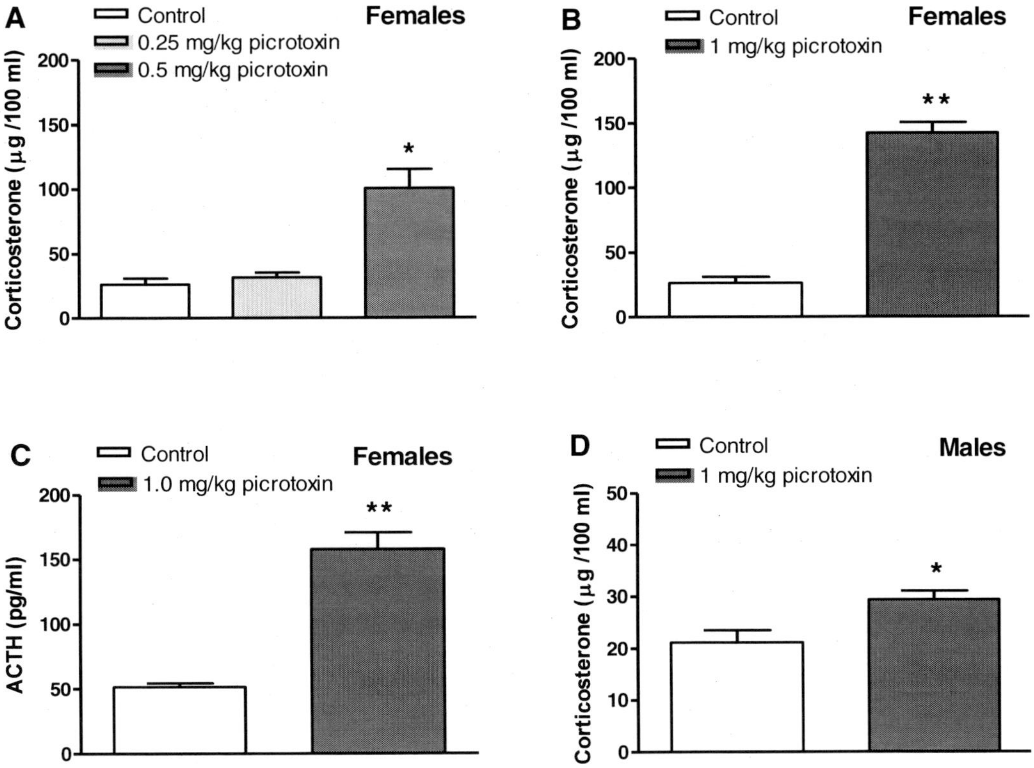


Figure 10. The effect of i.p. administered picrotoxin on plasma corticosterone (A, B and D) and ACTH (C) concentrations in male and female rats. Picrotoxin (0.25, 0.5 and 1 mg/kg) or its vehicle were injected i.p. 60 min prior to sacrifice. The results are expressed as mean ± SEM of the values. The number of animals per group ranked from 6-12. $^*p< 0.01$ or $p< 0.02$ vs. the control vehicle treated group (ANOVA followed by Dunnett's test or Student t-test, respectively); $^{**}$ $p< 0.0001$ vs. the control vehicle treated group (Student t-test).

Moreover, 2.0 mg/kg bicuculline demonstrated no significant changes in concentration of ACTH in plasma of female rats (Figure 8B). However, as shown in Figure 9, bicuculline (2 mg/kg) administered i.p. 60 min prior to sacrifice significantly increased the corticosterone levels in plasma of both male and female rats.

As shown in Figure 10, plasma corticosterone levels in female rats were not significantly different 60 min following i.p. administration of another GABA antagonist picrotoxin, given in the dose of 0.25 mg/kg. However, 0.5 and 1.0 mg/kg picrotoxin significantly elevated the levels of plasma corticosterone in female rats. Higher levels of corticosterone were also observed in male rats following administration of 1.0 mg/kg picrotoxin (Figure 10D) Moreover, 1.0 mg/kg picrotoxin administered 60 min prior to sacrifice induced significant increase in the plasma concentration of ACTH in female rats (Figure 10C).

Diazepam administered in the 0.1 mg/kg dose has not induced any changes in plasma corticosterone concentrations of male as well as female rats (Figure 11A). However, as shown in Figure 11B, 1 mg/kg diazepam significantly decreased plasma corticosterone levels only in female rats, while high dose of diazepam (10 mg/kg) significantly elevated corticosterone in rats of both sexes (Figure 11C). In addition, ACTH levels in plasma of female rats were also significantly lower following administration of 1 mg/kg diazepam, and significantly higher following treatment with diazepam in a dose of 10 mg/kg (Figure 11D).

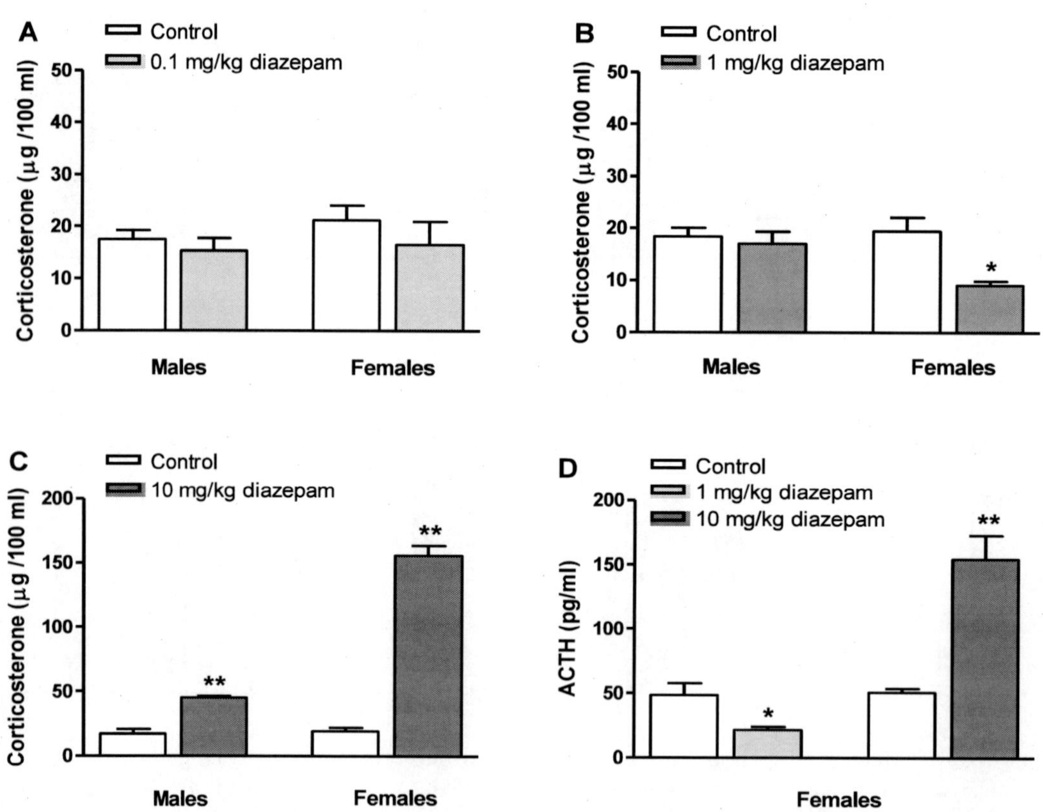


Figure 11. The effect of i.p. administered diazepam on plasma corticosterone (A, B and C) and ACTH (D) concentrations in male and female rats. Diazepam (0.1, 1 and 10 mg/kg) or its vehicle were injected i.p. 60 min prior to sacrifice. The results are expressed as mean ± SEM of the values. The number of animals per group ranked from 5-8. *$p< 0.004$ or $p<0.008$; **$p< 0.0001$ vs. the control vehicle treated group (Student t-test).

## DISCUSSION

It has been previously shown that intraperitoneal injection of saline or a vehicle itself results in the enhancement of plasma corticosterone levels in rats (Barett and Stockham, 1963; Pericic et al., 1984), indicating an induced activation of the HPA axis by a stressful stimulans, such as intraperitoneal injection and handling. In our study we also observed the injection-induced rise in plasma corticosterone and ACTH levels in both male and female rats, confirming previous data. However, this increase disappeared 60 min after injection in female and 120 min following injection in male rats. Moreover, we observed significant sex-related differences in plasma corticosterone levels in both non-injected and injected animals. Namely, higher levels of corticosterone in female than in male rats were detected following injection of saline 15, 30 and 120 min, but not 60 min prior to sacrifice, suggesting that female rats respond to stress induced by the injection and handling with higher corticosterone rise than male rats.

Our previous results (Manev and Pericic, 1983; Pericic et al., 1984) demonstrated that GABAergic drugs affect the activity of the HPA axis, and this conclusion was based on the determination of the plasma corticosterone levels. Other studies also reported the effect of GABA on the HPA axis activity (De Feudis, 1984; Elias et al., 1982; Imura et al., 1982; Racagni et al., 1982). In line with our findings demonstrating decreased levels of plasma corticosterone and/or ACTH, following administration of a low dose (1 mg/kg) of diazepam (i.p.), the $GABA_A$ receptor enhancer, baclofen (i.p.), the $GABA_B$ receptor agonist, and GABA itself (i.c.v.), most data show that GABA inhibits the activity of the HPA axis (Ixart et al., 1983; Jones et al., 1976; Makara and Stark, 1974). Some other studies also detected that GABA, when injected i.c.v. to animals, suppresses the HPA axis (Makara and Stark, 1974; Miguez and Aldegunde, 1990; Miguez et al., 1990; Plotsky et al., 1987). It has been reported that GABA itself also inhibits the stimulated release of CRH from the hypothalamus (Buckingham and Hodges, 1979; Hillhouse and Milton, 1988; Jones et al., 1976). This is not unexpected since the elements of GABA system were found in the hypothalamus (Meister et al., 1988; Vincent et al., 1982). Although GABA receptors are localized also in the pituitary (Grandison and Guidotti, 1979), the addition of GABA did not alter ACTH release from the dispersed pituitary cells in culture (Kalogeras et al., 1990) or from the hemipituitaries in vitro (Miguez and Aldegunde, 1990). These data suggest a central (hypotalamic) site of action of GABA on the HPA axis.

The results of our studies are supported also by "in vitro" experiments suggesting that both $GABA_A$ and $GABA_B$ receptors are involved in this inhibitory role of GABA in regulating the HPA function. Namely, Calogero and his group (Calogero et al., 1988; Kalogeras et al., 1990) reported that muscimol, a $GABA_A$ receptor agonist, and baclofen, a $GABA_B$ receptor agonist, both inhibit the stimulated secretion of CRH in hypothalamic organ culture. In line with the inhibitory role of GABA on the HPA axis activity, the results of our studies also demonstrated the stimulatory effect of administration of the $GABA_A$ receptor antagonists picrotoxin (i.p) and bicuculline (i.p.) on plasma corticosterone and/or ACTH levels. These resulst indicate that blockade of $GABA_A$ receptors stimulates the activity of the HPA axis (Lakic et al., 1985). In other studies bicuculline and picrotoxin have been also shown to stimulate the corticosterone secretion in vivo (Ixart et al., 1983; Lakic et al., 1986; Makara and Stark, 1974; Miguez and Aldegunde, 1990b; Pericic et al., 1985), and in vitro

(Buckingham and Hodges, 1979; Calogero et al., 1988; Jones et al., 1976; Hillhouse and Milton, 1988). In contrast, there are also some contradictory reports (Aldegunde et al., 1984; Garcy and Marotta, 1978). Namely, in the present study the i.p. administration of GABA, the GABA agonist progabide and aminooxyacetic acid (AOAA), the inhibitor of GABA degradation, increase corticosterone levels in plasma. In line with our findings, other authors also demonstrated that the intraperitoneal injection of GABA or GABA mimetic drugs elevates the release of corticosterone (Aldegunde et al., 1984).

The reason for these discrepancies (i.e. inhibitory as well as stimulatory effects of GABA-ergic drugs on the HPA axis) is at present unclear. These differences might be due to the differences in dose of GABA (since we have shown that GABAergic drugs affect the HPA axis in a dose-dependent fashion), or the differences at the level at which these drugs alter the HPA axis activity (i.e. central or peripheral level). The differences might be also due to the fact that GABA, progabide and AAOA act, besides via GABAergic, also via some other receptors, since it has been shown that drugs elevating GABAergic transmission stimulate the HPA axis by counteracting the noradrenergic inhibitory influence on CRH neurons (Aldegunde et al., 1984; Lakic et al., 1986).

While picrotoxin, bicuculline and progabide produced an increase of plasma corticosterone levels in both males and females (although more pronaunced increase was detected in female than in male rats), diazepam, positive allosteric modulator of $GABA_A$ receptor, administered in a lower dose (1 or 2 mg/kg) inhibited the activity of HPA axis only in female rats (Lakic et al., 1985; Pericic et al., 1984, 1985; Pivac and Pericic 1993), while high dose of diazepam (10 mg/kg) stimulated the HPA axis activity in rats of both sexes (Lakic et al., 1985,1986; Pericic et al., 1984). Whereas $GABA_A$ receptor complex seems to be involved in the suppressive effect of the lower dose of diazepam (2.0 mg/kg) on the HPA axis activity in female rats (Pivac and Pericic, 1993), mechanisms by which the higher dose of diazepam (10 mg/kg) increases corticosterone levels do not involve the stimulation of $GABA_A$ receptors, but rather the blockade of $\alpha_2$-adrenergic receptors (Lakic et al., 1986). Our results demonstrated that besides $GABA_A$ receptor complex (Pivac and Pericic, 1993), postsynaptic $\alpha_2$-adrenoreceptors activity and intact presynaptic noradrenergic function are required also for the suppressive effect of 2.0 mg/kg diazepam on the activity of the HPA axis in female rats (Svob Strac et al., 2012). Similar to GABA, administration of benzodiazepines, drugs which exert most pharmacological effects via $GABA_A$ receptors, has been also associated with alterations in neuroendocrine function both in experimental animals and in humans (Arvat et al., 2002; Heberlein et al., 2008; Mikkelsen et al., 2005). Most of the previous studies have demonstrated that classical benzodiazepines such as diazepam decrease the HPA axis activity in stressful conditions (Carrasco and Van de Kar, 2003; Fries et al., 2006; Kalman et al., 1997; Pericic and Pivac, 1995; Pomara et al., 2005). However, under basal conditions, stimulation (DeBoer et al., 1991; Kalman et al., 1997; Lakic et al., 1985, 1986; Mikkelsen et al., 2005; Vargas et al., 2001), inhibition (Kalogeras et al., 1990; Lakic et al., 1985; Pericic et al., 1985; Pivac and Pericic, 1993; Skelton et al., 2000; Svob Strac et al., 2012) and no alternation (Broadbear et al., 2005; DeBoer et al., 1991; Matheson et al., 1988; Olivier et al., 2003) of the HPA axis activity were observed following treatment with benzodiazepines.

Our results have also pointed out the differences in the regulatory mechanisms of the HPA axis activity between males and females (Kudielka and Kirschbaum, 2005; Pericic and

Pivac, 1995, 1996; Seeman et al., 2001; Wilson and Biscardi; 1994). These findings are in line with the studies demonstrating that the effects of benzodiazepine exposure on HPA axis activity, including CRH, ACTH and glucocorticoids, are influenced by the gender-related factors (Wilson et al., 1996; Wilson and Biscardi; 1994). Namely, gonadal steroid hormones including estrogens and androgens have been shown to modulate the GABA/BZ receptors or their responses, as well as the HPA axis activity implicated in the different stress responses between genders (Kageyama and Suda; 2009; Magiakou et al., 1997; Wilson et al., 1996; Wilson and Biscardi; 1994). Moreover, the basis for the different response of plasma corticosterone in male and female rats might be sought in sex differences in GABA concentration found in the pituitary (Manev et al., 1985) or hypothalamus (Frankurt et al., 1984). The inhibition of plasma corticosterone secretion observed in female but not in male rats following administration of 1 mg/kg diazepam might be due to its greater binding in the pituitary of females. Namely, the specific GABA binding could be detected in the pituitary of female but not male rats (Wuttke and Mansky, 1981). As GABA binding is also significantly higher in the hypothalamus of female rats (Fiszer de Plazas et al., 1983), and there are also sex differences in GABA and glutamate concentrations in several hypothalamic nuclei of the rat (Frankfurt et al., 1984), it is possible that the sex differences in diazepam binding, also at the hypothalamic level, might cause sex differences in the response of the HPA axis to diazepam. Sexually dimorphic alternations in CRH system and HPA responses to stress are suggested to play a role in the etiology of affective and anxiety-related disorders and may be affected by both estrogen and progesterone (Wilson et al., 1996).

## CONCLUSION

On the basis of our previous data (Lakic et al., 1985, 1986; Pericic et al., 1985; Pivac and Pericic, 1993) one might conclude that the blockade of $GABA_A$ receptors stimulates the activity of the HPA axis by acting at the pituitary and/or hypothalamic level. On the other hand, GABA and some drugs which enhance the GABAergic neurotransmission appear to achieve their stimulating effect on the HPA axis by decreasing the noradrenergic inhibitory activity on CRH neurons (Aldegunde et al., 1984; Lakic et al., 1986) The results of our studies summarized in this manuscript suggest that caution should be exercised in the interpretation of data regarding HPA axis activity which are obtained following administration of drugs affecting GABAergic neurotransmission. It is obvious that the response of the HPA axis may vary depending on the sex of the animals, the dose of the drug and even on the time and the route of drug administration. Hence, further studies are necessary to elucidate the complex mechanisms of GABAergic drugs on the activity of HPA axis and to consider the possible implications of these findings for the human therapy.

## REFERENCES

Aldegunde M, Miguez MI, Fernandez MP (1984) GABA administered intraperitoneally alters the release of corticosterone in male rats. *IRCS Med. Sci.* 12: 523-524.

Anderson RA, Mitchell R (1986) Distribution of GABA binding site subtypes in rat pituitary gland. *Brain Res.* 365: 78-84.

Antoni FA (1986) Hypothalamic control of adrenocorticotropin secretion: advances since the discovery of 41-residue corticotropin-releasing factor. *Endocr. Rev.* 7: 351-378.

Arvat E, Giordano R, Grottoli S, Ghigo E (2002) Benzodiazepines and anterior pituitary function. *J. Endocrinol. Invest.* 25: 735–747.

Barrett AM, Stockham MA (1963) The effect of housing conditions and simple experimental procedures upon the corticosterone level in the plasma of rats. *J. Endocrinol.* 26: 97-105.

Beaumont K, Chilton WS, Yamamura HI, Enna SJ (1978) Muscimol binding in rat brain: association with synaptic GABA receptors. *Brain Res.* 148: 153-162.

Berman JA, Roberts JL, Pritchett DB (1994) Molecular and pharmacological characterization of GABA-A receptors in the rat pituitary. *J. Neurochem.* 63: 1948–1954.

Berod A, Chat M, Paut L, Tappaz M (1984) Catecholaminergic and GABAergic anatomical relationship in the rat substantia nigra, locus coeruleus, and hypothalamic median eminence. *J. Histochem. Cytochem.* 32: 1331-1338.

Bisset GW, Chowdrey HS, Fairhall KM, Gunn LK (1990) Central inhibition by gamma-aminobutyric acid and muscimol of the release of vasopressin and oxytocin by an osmotic stimulus in the rat. *Br. J. Pharmacol.* 99: 529-535.

Boudaba C, Szabo K, Tasker JG (1996) Physiological mapping of local inhibitory inputs to the hypothalamic paraventricular nucleus. *J. Neurosci.* 16: 7151–7160.

Broadbear JH, Winger G, Woods JH (2005) Self-administration of methohexital, midazolam and ethanol: effects on the pituitary-adrenal axis in rhesus monkeys. *Psychopharmacology.* 178: 83-91.

Buckingham JC, Hodges JR (1979) The influence of some neurotransmitter substances and drugs on the secretion of corticotrophin releasing hormone by the rat hypothalamus in vitro. *J. Physiol.* 290: 40P-41P.

Calogero AE, Gallucci WT, Chrousos GP, Gold PW (1988) Interaction between GABAergic neurotransmission and rat hypothalamic corticotropin-releasing hormone secretion in vitro. *Brain Res.* 463: 28–36.

Carrasco GA, Van de Kar LD (2003) Neuroendocrine pharmacology of stress. *Eur. J. Pharmacol.* 463: 235-272.

Cavagnini F, Pinto M, Dubini A, Invitti C, Cappelletti G, Poli EE (1982) Effects of gamma-aminobutyric acid (GABA) and muscimol on endocrine pancreatic function in man. *Metabolism.* 31: 73-77.

Cole RL, Sawchenko PE (2002) Neurotransmitter regulation of cellular activation and neuropeptide gene expression in the paraventricular nucleus of the hypothalamus. *J. Neurosci.* 22: 959–969.

Cullinan WE (1998) Evidence for a PVN site of action of GABA in the regulatory control of the rat stress axis. *Physiologist.* 41: 353.

Cullinan WE (2000) GABA(A) receptor subunit expression within hypophysiotropic CRH neurons: a dual hybridization histochemical study. *J. Comp. Neurol.* 419: 344–351.

Cullinan WE, Ziegler DR, Herman JP (2008) Functional role of local GABAergic influences on the HPA axis. *Brain Struct. Funct.* 213: 63-72.

DeBoer SF, Van Der Gugten J, Slangen JL (1991) Effects of chlordiazepoxide, flumazenil and DMCM on plasma catecholamine and corticosterone concentrations in rats. *Pharm. Biochem. Behav.* 38: 13-19.

Decavel C, Van den Pol AN (1990) GABA: a dominant neurotransmitter in the hypothalamus. *J. Comp. Neurol.* 302: 1019-1037.

De Feudis FV (1984) GABA and hormonal secretion. Trends Pharmacol Sci. 5: 152-156.

Earley CJ, Leonard BE (1978) GABA and gonadal hormones. *Brain Res.* 155: 27-34.

Elias AN, Valenta LJ, Szekeres AV, Grossman MK (1982) Regulatory role of gamma-aminobutyric acid in pituitary hormone secretion. Psychoneuroendocrinology. 7: 15-30.

Erdo SL (1985) Peripheral GABAergic mechanisms. *Trends Pharmacol. Sci.* 6: 205-208.

Fiszer de Plazas S, Seilicovich A, Duvilanski B, Gonzales NN, Rettori V (1983) Sex related differences in GABA binding sites of rat anterior pituitary and hypothalamus. *IRCS Med. Sci.* 11: 976.

Flugge G, Oertel WH, Wuttke W (1986) Evidence for estrogen-receptive GABAergic neurons in the preoptic/anterior hypothalamic area of rat brain. *Neuroendocrinology.* 43: 1-5.

Frankfurt M, Fuchs E, Wuttke W (1984) Sex differences in γ-amino-butyric acid and glutamate concentrations in discrete rat brain nuclei. *Neurosci. Lett.* 50: 245-250.

Fries E, Hellhammer DH, Hellhammer J (2006) Attenuation of the hypothalamic-pituitary-adrenal axis responsivity to the Trier Social Stress Test by the benzodiazepine alprazolam. *Psychoneuroendocrinology.* 31: 1278-1288.

Garcy AM, Marotta SF (1978) Plasma cortisol of conscious cats during cerebroventricular perfusion with adrenergic, cholinergic and GABAergic antagonists. *Neuroendocrinology.* 25: 343-353.

Gerber JC, Hare TA (1979) Gamma-aminobutyric acid in peripheral tissue, with emphasis on the endocrine pancreas. Presence in two species and reduction by streptozotocin. *Diabetes.* 28: 1073-1076.

Grandison L, Guidotti A (1979) Gamma-aminobutyric acid receptor function in rat anterior pituitary: evidence for control of prolactin release. *Endocrinology.* 105: 754-759.

Grottoli S, Maccagno B, Ramunni J, Di Vito L, Giordano R, Gianotti L, DeStefanis S, Camanni F, Ghigo E, Arvat E (2002) Alprazolam, a benzodiazepine, does not modify the ACTH and cortisol response to hCRH and AVP, but blunts the cortisol response to ACTH in humans. *J. Endocrinol. Invest.* 25: 420–425.

Gudelsky GA, Apud JA, Masotto C, Locatelli V, Cocchi D, Racagni G, Muller EE (1983) Ethanolamine-O-sulphate enhance γ-aminobutyric acid secretion into hypophysial portal blood and lowers serum prolactin concentrations. *Neuroendocrionology.* 37: 397-399.

Heberlein A, Bleich S, Kornhuber J, Hillemacher T (2008) Neuroendocrine pathways in benzodiazepine dependence: new targets for research and therapy. *Hum. Psychopharmacol.* 23: 171-181.

Herman JP, Cullinan WE (1997) Neurocircuitry of stress: central control of the hypothalamo-pituitary-adrenocortical axis. *Trends Neurosci.* 20: 78-84.

Herman JP, Cullinan WE, Ziegler DR, Tasker JG (2002a) Role of the paraventricular nucleus microenvironment in stress integration. *Eur. J. Neurosci.* 16: 381–385.

Herman JP, Mueller NK, Figueiredo H (2004) Role of GABA and Glutamate Circuitry in Hypothalamo-Pituitary-Adrenocortical Stress Integration. *Ann. N Y Acad. Sci.* 1018: 35–45.

Herman JP, Renda A, Bodie B (2003) Norepinephrine-gamma-aminobutyric acid (GABA) interaction in limbic stress circuits: effects of reboxetine on GABAergic neurons. *Biol. Psychiatry.* 53: 166-174.

Herman JP, Tasker JG, Ziegler DR, Cullinan WE (2002b) Local circuit regulation of paraventricular nucleus stress integration: glutamate-GABA connections. *Pharmacol Biochem. Behav.* 71: 457-468.

Hillhouse EW, Milton NG (1989) Effect of noradrenaline and gamma-aminobutyric acid on the secretion of corticotrophin-releasing factor-41 and arginine vasopressin from the rat hypothalamus in vitro. *J. Endocrinol.*. 122: 719-723.

Imaki T, Wang XQ, Shibasaki T, Harada S, Chikada N, Takahashi C, Naruse M, Demura H (1995) Chlordiazepoxide attenuates stress-induced activation of neurons, corticotropin-releasing factor (CRF) gene transcription and CRF biosynthesis in the paraventricular nucleus (PVN). *Brain Res. Mol. Brain Res.* 32: 261–270.

Imura H, Nakai Y, Nakao K, Oki S, Tanaka I (1982) Control of biosynthesis and secretion of ACTH, endorphins and related peptides. In. Muller EE, MacLeod RM (eds) Neuroendocrine Perspectives, Vol 1, Elsevier Biomedical Press, New York, p 137.

Ixart G, Cryssogelou H, Szafarczyk A, Malaval F, Assenmacher I (1983) Acute and delayed effects of picrotoxin on the adrenocorticotropic system of rats. *Neurosci. Lett.* 43: 235-240.

Jones MT, Gillham B, Altaher AR, Nicholson SA, Campbell EA, Watts SM, Thody A (1984) Clinical and experimental studies on the role of GABA in the regulation of ACTH secretion: a review. *Psychoneuroendocrinology.* 9: 107–123.

Jones MT, Hillhouse EW, Burden J (1976) Effect of various putative neurotransmitters on the secretion of corticotrophin-releasing hormone from the rat hypothalamus in vitro- a model of the neurotransmitters involved. *J. Endocr.* 69: 1-10.

Kageyama K, Suda T (2009) Regulatory mechanisms underlying corticotropin-releasing factor gene expression in the hypothalamus. *Endocr. J.* 56: 335-344.

Kalman BA, Kim PJ, Cole MA, Chi MS, Spencer RL (1997) Diazepam attenuation of restraint stress-induced corticosterone levels is enhanced by prior exposure to repeated restraint. *Psychoneuroendocrinolog*y. 22: 349-360.

Kalogeras KT, Calogero AE, Kuribayashi T, Khan I, Gallucci WT, Kling MA, Chrousos GP, Gold PW (1990) In vitro and in vivo effects of the triazolobenzodiazepine alprazolam on hypothalamic-pituitary-adrenal function: pharmacological and clinical implications. *J. Clin. Endocrinol. Metab* 70: 1462–1471.

Kovács KJ, Miklós IH, Bali B (2004) GABAergic mechanisms constraining the activity of the hypothalamo-pituitary-adrenocortical axis. *Ann. N Y Acad. Sci.* 1018: 466-476.

Kudielka BM, Kirschbaum C (2005) Sex differences in HPA axis responses to stress: a review. *Biol. Psychol.* 69: 113-132.

Lakic N, Pericic D, Manev H (1985) The influence of GABA system on the activity of the hypothalamo-hypophysial-adrenal (HHA) axis. *Iugoslav Physiol. Pharmacol. Acta.* 21: 161-162.

Lakic N, Pericic D, Manev H (1986) Mechanisms by which picrotoxin and high dose of diazepam elevate plasma corticosterone level. *Neuroendocrinology.* 43: 331-335.

Lee TY, Pan JT (2001) Involvement of central GABAergic neurons in basal and diurnal changes of tuberoinfundibular dopaminergic neuronal activity and prolactin secretion. *Life Sci.* 68: 1965-1975.

Lin CS, Lu SM, Schmechel DE (1986) Glutamic acid decarboxylase and somatostatin immunoreactivities in rat visual cortex. *J. Comp. Neurol.* 244: 369-383.

Locatelli V, Cocchi D, Racagni G, Cattabeni F, Maggi A, Krogsgaard-Larsen P, Müller EE (1978) Prolactin-inhibiting activity of gamma-aminobutyric acid-mimetic drugs in the male rat. *Brain Res.* 145: 173-179.

Lux-Lantos V, Rey E, Libertun C (1992) Activation of $GABA_B$ receptors in the anterior pituitary inhibits prolactin and luteinizing hormone secretion. *Neuroendocrinology.* 56: 687-693.

Maggi A, Perez J (1984) Progesterone and estrogens in rat brain: modulation of GABA (γ-aminobutyric acid) receptor activity. *Eur. J. Pharmacol.* 103: 165-168.

Magiakou MA, Mastorakos G, Webster E, Chrousos GP (1997) The hypothalamic-pituitary-adrenal axis and the female reproductive system. *Ann. N Y Acad. Sci.* 816: 42-56.

Margeta-Mitrovic M, Mitrovic I, Riley RC, Jan LY, Basbaum AI (1999) Immunohistochemical localization of GABA(B) receptors in the rat central nervous system. *J. Comp. Neurol.* 405: 299-321.

Makara GB, Stark E (1974) Effect of gamma-aminobutyric acid (GABA) and GABA antagonist drugs on ACTH release. *Neuroendocrinology.* 16: 178–190.

Manev H, Pericic D (1985) Hypophysial GABA after ether stress, dexamethasone or inhibition of GABA catabolism. *Pharmacol. Biochem. Behav.* 23: 697-700.

Manev H, Pericic D (1983) Hypothalamic GABA system and plasma corticosterone in ether stressed rats. *Pharmacol. Biochem. Behav.* 18: 847-850.

Mansky T, Mestres-Ventura P, Wutke W (1982) Involvement of GABA in the feedback action of estradiol on gonadotropin and prolactin release: Hypothalamic GABA and catecholamine turnover rates. *Brain Res.* 231: 353-364.

Matheson GK, Gage D, White G, Dixon V, Gipson D (1988) A comparison of the effects of buspirone and diazepam on plasma corticosterone levels in rat. *Neuropharmacology.* 27: 823-830.

McGinnis MY, Gordon JH, Gorski RA (1980) Time course and localization of the effects of estrogen on glutamic acid decarboxylase activity. *J. Neurochem.* 34: 785-792.

Meister B, Hökfelt T, Geffard M, Oertel W (1988) Glutamic acid decarboxylase- and gamma-aminobutyric acid-like immunoreactivities in corticotropin-releasing factor-containing parvocellular neurons of the hypothalamic paraventricular nucleus. *Neuroendocrinology.* 48: 516-526.

Miguez I, Aldegunde MA (1990) Effect of gamma-aminobutyric acid on corticosterone secretion: Involvement of the noradrenergic system. *Life Sci.* 46: 875-880.

Miguez MI, Aldegunde M (1990) Effect of naloxone on the secretion of corticosterone induced by gamma-hydroxybutyric acid in male rats. *J. Neuroendocrinol.* 2: 501-503.

Mikkelsen JD, Soderman A, Kiss A, Mirza N (2005) Effects of benzodiazepines receptor agonists on the hypothalamic-pituitary-adrenocortical axis. *Eur. J. Pharmacol.* 519: 223-230.

Mioduszewski R, Grandison L, Meites J (1976) Stimulation of prolactin release in rats by GABA. *Proc. Soc. Exp. Biol. Med.* 151: 44-46.

Nicoletti F, Clementi G, Prato A, Canonico PL, Rampello L, Patti F, Di Giorgio RM, Scapagnini U (1983) Effects of hyper- and hypoprolactinemia on glutamate decarboxylase activity in medial basal hypothalamus of male rat. *Neuroendocrinology.* 36: 13-16.

Nicoletti F, Patti F, Ferrara N, Canonico PL, Giammona G, Condorelli DF, Scapagnini U (1982) Comparative effects of estrogens and prolactin on nigral and striatal GAD activity. *Brain Res.* 232: 238-241.

Okada Y, Nitsch-Hasser C, Kim JS, Bak IJ, Hassler R (1971) Role of γ –aminobutyric acid (GABA) in the extrapyramidal motor system. Regional distribution of GABA in rabbit, rat, guinea pig and baboon CNS. *Exp. Brain Res.* 13: 514-518.

Olivier B, Zethof T, Pattij T, van Boogaert M, van Oorschot R, Leahy C, Oosting R, Bouwknecht A, Veening J, van der Gugten J, Groenink L (2003) Stress-induced hyperthermia and anxiety: pharmacological validation. *Eur. J. Pharmacol.* 463: 117-132.

Ondo JG, Pass KA (1976) The effects of neurally active amino acids on prolactin secretion. *Endocrinology.* 98: 1248-1252.

Pass KA, Ondo JG (1977) The effects of gamma-aminobutyric acid on prolactin and gonadotropin secretion in the unanesthetized rat. *Endocrinology.* 100: 1437-1442.

Pericic D, Lakic N, Manev H (1984) Effect of diazepam on plasma corticosterone levels. *Psychopharmacology.* 83: 79-81.

Pericic D, Manev H, Lakic N (1985) Sex differences in the response of rats to drugs affecting GABAergic transmission. *Life Sci.* 36: 541-547.

Pericic D, Pivac N (1995) Sex differences in conflict behaviour and in plasma corticosterone levels. *J. Neural Transm. Gen. Sect.* 101: 213-21.

Pericic D, Pivac N (1996) Effect of diazepam on conflict behavior and on plasma corticosterone levels in male and female rats. *Naunyn Schmiedeberg's Arch Pharmacol.* 323: 369-376.

Pirker S, Schwarzer C, Wieselthaler A, Sieghart W, Sperk G (2000) GABA(A) receptors: immunocytochemical distribution of 13 subunits in the adult rat brain. *Neuroscience.* 101: 815-850.

Pivac N, Pericic D (1993) Inhibitory effect of diazepam on the activity of the hypothalamo-pituitary-adrenal axis in female rats. *J. Neural Transm.* 92: 173-186.

Plotsky PM, Otto S, Sutton S (1987) Neurotransmitter modulation of corticotropin releasing factor secretion into the hypophysial-portal circulation. *Life Sci.* 41:1311-1317.

Pomara N, Willoughby LM, Sidtis JJ, Cooper TB, Greenblatt DJ (2005) Cortisol response to diazepam: its relationship to age, dose, duration of treatment, and presence of generalized anxiety disorder. *Psychopharmacology.* 178: 1-8.

Racagni G, Apud JA, Cocchi D, Locatelli V, Muller EE (1982) GABAergic control of anterior pituitary hormone secretion. *Life Sci.* 31: 823-838.

Roland BL, Sawchenko PE (1993) Local origins of some GABAergic projections to the paraventricular and supraoptic nuclei of the hypothalamus in the rat. *J. Comp. Neurol.* 332: 123-143.

Schally AV, Redding TW, Arimura A, Dupont A, Linthicum GL (1977) Isolation of gamma-amino butyric acid from pig hypothalami and demonstration of its prolactin release-inhibiting (PIF) activity in vivo and in vitro. *Endocrinology.* 100: 681-691.

Seeman TE, Singer B, Wilkinson CW, McEwen B (2001) Gender differences in age-related changes in HPA axis reactivity. *Psychoneuroendocrinology.* 26: 225-240.

Shephard RA, Nielson EB, Broadhurst PL (1982) Sex and strain differences in benzodiazepine receptor binding in roman rat strains. *Eur. J. Pharmacol.* 77: 327-330.

Skelton KH, Nemeroff CB, Knight DL, Owens MJ (2000) Chronic administration of the triazolobenzodiazepine alprazolam produces opposite effects on corticotropin-releasing factor and urocortin neuronal systems. *J. Neurosci.* 20: 1240-1248.

Svob Strac D, Muck-Seler D, Pivac N (2012) The involvement of noradrenergic mechanisms in the suppressive effects of diazepam on the hypothalamic-pituitary-adrenal axis activity in female rats. *Croat Med. J.* 53: 214-223.

Tappaz M, Aguera M, Beliu MF, Pujol JF (1980) Autoradiography of GABA in the rat hypothalamic median eminence. *Brain Res.* 186: 379-391.

Tappaz ML, Brownstein MJ, Palkovits M (1976) Distribution of glutamate decarboxylase in discrete brain nuclei. *Brain Res.* 108: 317-379.

Tappaz ML, Oertel WH, Wassef M, Mugnaini E (1982) Central GABAergic neuroendocrine regulations: pharmacological and morphological evidence. *Prog. Brain Res.* 55: 77-96.

Tappaz M, Wassef M, Oertel WH, Paut L, Pujol JF (1983) Light- and electron-microscopic immunocytochemistry of glutamic acid decarboxylase (GAD) in the basal hypothalamus: morphological evidence for neuroendocrine γ-aminobutyrate (GABA). *Neuroscience* 9: 271-287.

Tasker JG, Dudek FE (1993) Local inhibitory synaptic inputs to neurones of the paraventricular nucleus in slices of rat hypothalamus. *J. Physiol.* 469: 179-192.

Vargas ML, Abella C, Hernandez J (2001) Diazepam increases the hypothalamic-pituitary-adrenocortical (HPA) axis activity by a cyclic AMP-dependent mechanism. *Br. J. Pharmacol.* 133: 1355-1361.

Vijayan E, McCann SM (1978) The effects of intraventricular injection of gamma-aminobutyric acid (GABA) on prolactin and gonadotropin release in conscious female rats. *Brain Res.* 155: 35-43.

Vincent JR, Hokfelt T, Wu JY (1982) GABA neuron systems in hypothalamus and pituitary gland. Immunohistochemical demonstration using antibodies against glutamate decarboxylase. *Neuroendocrinology.* 34: 117-125.

Voisin DL, Herbison AE, Poulain DA (1995) Central inhibitory effects of muscimol and bicuculline on the milk ejection reflex in the anaesthetized rat. *J. Physiol.* 483:211-224.

Wallis CJ, Luttge WG (1980) Influence of estrogen and progesterone on glutamic acid decarboxylase activity in discrete regions of rat brain. *J. Neurochem.* 34: 609-613.

Whitnall MH (1993) Regulation of the hypothalamic corticotropin-releasing hormone neurosecretory system. *Prog. Neurobiol.* 40: 573-629.

Wilson MA, Biscardi R (1994) Sex differences in GABA/benzodiazepine receptor changes and corticosterone release after acute stress in rats. *Exp. Brain Res.* 101: 297-306.

Wilson MA, Biscardi R, Smith MD, Wilson SP (1996) Effects of benzodiazepine agonist exposure on corticotropin-releasing factor content and hormonal stress responses: divergent responses in male and ovariectomized female rats. *J. Pharmacol. Exp. Ther.* 278: 1073-1082.

Wuttke W, Mansky T (1981) Gonadal steroids and brain monoamines: How do they interact? In Wutke W, Horowski R (eds) Gonadal steroids and brain function. Springer Verlag, Berlin, p 130.

In: Gamma-Aminobutyric Acid (GABA)
Editors: Josipa Vlainić and Maja Jazvinšćak Jembrek
ISBN: 978-1-63321-838-3


*Chapter 6*

# GABAergic Drugs in the Treatment of Cerebellar Ataxia and Other Motor Disorders of the Central Nervous System

***José Gazulla[1*], Carlota Ruiz-Gazulla[2] and María Tintoré[3]***
[1]Department of Neurology, Hospital Universitario Miguel Servet, Zaragoza, Spain
[2]Faculty of Science, University of Zaragoza, Zaragoza, Spain
[3]Nucleic Acid Chemistry, Institute for Advanced Chemistry of Catalonia, Barcelona CSIC, Spain

## Abstract

GABAergic drugs are mostly used in the treatment of epilepsy, spasticity and neuropathic pain. However, gamma-aminobutyric acid (GABA) is the main inhibitory neurotrasnmitter in the central nervous system, and other diseases that associate a deficiency in GABA, might benefit from its use. The cerebellar cortex is very rich in GABA, and Purkinje cells are the main cell type to employ it as a neurotransmitter. In consequence, diseases of the cerebellar cortex of any aetiology, could have their clinical manifestations improved by GABAergic drugs. Cortical cerebellar atrophy is a disease that meets the referred to characteristics, and the ataxia caused by this disease was alleviated by the drugs gabapentin and pregabalin. This disease is proposed as a model of selective deficiency in GABA content in the central nervous system, which may benefit clinically from administration of GABAergic drugs, in a manner similar in which motor manifestations in Parkinson's disease are improved by levodopa.

Other diseases of the cerebellum, in which a loss of Purkinje cells constitutes a prominent finding, and ataxia their main clinical expression, could also benefit from administration of GABAergic drugs. This was the case in adult-onset GM2 gangliosidosis, olivopontocerebellar atrophy, cerebellar ataxia with hypogonadotropic hypogonadism, spinocerebellar ataxias type 1, 2 and 6, and adult-onset ataxia-telangiectasia. On the other hand, in complex cerebellar diseases, such as multisystem atrophy, ataxia was worsened by administration of GABAergic drugs. Some disorders of

* Corresponding author: Department of Neurology, Hospital Universitario Miguel Servet. Zaragoza, Spain. C/ Luis Vives 6, esc dcha, 7° B, 50006 Zaragoza, Spain. Tel: +34976563649. josegazulla@wanadoo.es.

the central nervous system that associate a deficiency in GABA content, had their clinical manifestations relieved or suppressed by admistration of GABAergic drugs. This was the case in a patient with progressive encephalomyelitis with rigidity, who had painful muscular spasms suppressed by a combination of gabapentin and tizanidine, and in another with diaphragmatic myoclonus, who required a combination of gabapentin and tiagabine to control myoclonus. On the contrary, administration of GABAergic drugs was not successful in cervical dystonia, amyotrophic lateral sclerosis and Parkinson's disease, presumably because a tissue deficiency in GABA is not an essential neurochemical abnormality in these diseases. Research aimed at identifying effective therapies to treat cerebellar ataxias and other motor disorders of the central nervous system is warranted. Meanwhile, therapeutic tests with GABAergic drugs might yield clinical improvement in these diseases.

**Keywords**: GABAergic drugs; cortical cerebellar atrophy; olivopontocerebellar atrophy; spinocerebellar atrophy; progressive encephalomyelitis with rigidiy; diaphragmatic myoclonus

## INTRODUCTION

The objective of this work has been to review some therapeutic trials undertaken by the authors with GABAergic drugs, such as gabapentin, pregabalin, tiagabine and baclofen, in the treatment of various types of cerebellar ataxia and other motor disorders of the central nervous system, such as progressive encephalomyelitis with rigidity, diaphragmatic myoclonus, cervical dystonia, Parkinson's disease and amyotrophic lateral sclerosis.

## NEUROTRANSMISSION IN THE CEREBELLUM

The cerebellum is made up of four pairs of nuclei located in the deep white matter that covers the fourth ventricle, and is surrounded by a superficial layer of grey matter. The cerebellar cortex has a very uniform cellular structure and great cell density. In the cortex of the cerebellum, several types of inhibitory interneurons utilize $\gamma$-aminobutyric acid (GABA) as neurotransmitter. These are Golgi cells (that coexpress GABA and glycine), stellate cells, basket cells and Lugaro cells. Purkinje cells are the main GABAergic cells in the cerebellum, and their axons are the only efferent fibres to leave the cerebellar cortex and project to the cerebellar and vestibular nuclei. They also use taurine as an osmotic regulator.

The excitatory amino acid glutamate is used by granule cells and unipolar brush cells in the cerebellar cortex. The axons of granule cells constitute the parallel fibres in the molecular layer. Most of the afferent fibres to the cerebellum are excitatory, and use glutamate as neurotransmitter. Climbing fibres that leave the contralateral inferior olive and synapse with Purkinje cell dendrites are mostly glutamatergic, as well as using aspartate and homocysteic acid. Mossy fibres are more numerous and originate in a number of areas, such as the pontine nuclei, reticular formation, spinal cord, deep cerebellar nuclei (as collaterals to nuclear axons) and unipolar brush cells. They reach granule cell dendrites in the so called glomerular structures. The great majority of mossy fibres use glutamate, and a small proportion use acetylcholine (afferents from the vestibular nuclei and others from the cerebellar nuclei) and peptides such as enkephalins, cholecystokinin, corticotrophin, or calcitonin gene related peptide (CGRP). Some of the fibres that originate in precerebellar structures emit collateral ramifications that reach the deep cerebellar nuclei on their trajectory towards the cortex. The efferent nuclear fibres are excitatory, with the exception of those destined for the inferior olives, which have an inhibitory function.

In addition to mossy and climbing fibres, there is a group of beaded fibres that use monoamines as neurotransmitters, and reach the three layers of the cerebellar cortex.

A contingent of noradrenergic fibres stems from the locus coeruleus, and there also seems to be a group of dopaminergic afferents of indeterminate origin. Serotonergic fibres originate at the paramedian and lateral reticular nuclei, the periolivary reticular formation and the lateral tegmental region; it has not been possible to demonstrate connections between the raphe nuclei and the cerebellar cortex. Some histaminergic fibres reach the cerebellar cortex from the hypothalamus.

Nitric oxide (NO) is a non-synaptic neurotransmitter present in the cerebellar cortex, mostly generated in the soma and parallel fibres of granule cells. This substance spreads through membranes and acts on glial cells and neurons, stimulating the synthesis of cyclic guanosine-monophosphate. Basket and unipolar brush cells also synthesise NO, although Purkinje cells do not (Table 1).

In conclusion, neurotransmission in the cerebellum essentially implicates the amino acids GABA and glutamate, which establish an equilibrium between inhibitory and excitatory phenomena (Bastian and Thach 2002; Colin et al. 2002; Kwong et al. 2000; Mugnaini 1993; Ottersen 1993; Ottersen and Walberg 2002; Trouillas 1993).

**Table 1. Neurotransmitters in the cerebellum**

| | |
|---|---|
| Glutamate | Mossy fibres<br>Climbing fibres<br>Granule cells<br>Parallel fibres<br>Unipolar brush cells |
| GABA | Golgi cells<br>Stellate cells<br>Basket cells<br>Lugaro cells<br>Purkinje cells |
| Glycine | Golgi cells (coexpressed with GABA) |
| Noradrenaline | Origin in locus ceruleus |
| Serotonin | Origin in reticular formation |
| Acetylcholine | Origin in vestibular nuclei |
| Histamine | Origin in hipothalamus |

## GABAergic Drugs

The drugs referred to in this chapter are gabapentin, pregabalin, tiagabine and baclofen, which are mostly used in the treatment of epilepsy, anxiety disorder, neuropathic pain and spasticity. Their mechanisms of action are briefly described below.

Gabapentin and pregabalin target the $\alpha 2\delta$ subunit of the P/Q-type voltage-dependent calcium channels (VDCC), which are located on the presynaptic membrane, and mediate their effect on neurotransmission at the terminal axon (Belliotti et al. 2005). Gabapentin has been shown to increase brain GABA concentration in healthy volunteers (Kuzniecky et al. 2002). Gabapentin binds preferentially to the $\alpha 2\delta$-1 subunit, while pregabalin does so to $\alpha 2\delta$-2 (a subtype of $\alpha 2$-$\delta$ subunit predominantly represented in the Purkinje cell layer) (Gong et al., 2001). Pregabalin has exhibited more delayed VDCC inactivation, a larger capacity to let calcium into the neuron and greater antiepileptic power than gabapentin, under experimental conditions (Belliotti et al. 2005; Gong et al., 2001).

In addition, gabapentin inhibited L-type calcium currents in isolated rat hippocampal neurons, and AMPA-evoked excitatory responses in rat spinal dorsal horn neurons (Belliotti et al. 2005; Kang et al., 2002; Stefani et al., 1998).

Tiagabine inhibits GABA reuptake, the result being an increased content of this neurotransmitter at the synaptic fissure (Ostergaard et al. 1995).

Baclofen selectively activates GABA-B presynaptic receptors, which are linked to calcium channels through GTP-sensitive proteins. It reduces neuronal calcium inflow and inhibits the release of excitatory neurotransmitters; its main therapeutic role is in the treatment of spasticity (Cooper et al. 2003; Pazos and Pascual 2008).

## Treatment of Cerebellar Ataxia with GABAergic Drugs

A deficiency in GABA in the cerebellum may lead to cerebellar ataxia, as suggested by coexistence of ataxia with antibodies directed against the enzyme glutamic decarboxylase (GAD) (Honnorat et al. 2001; Saiz et al., 1997; Vulliemoz et al. 2007), and the finding of abnormal GABAergic neurotransmission in the presence of the aforementioned antibodies (Ishida et al. 1999). Anti-GAD antibodies are present in juvenile neuronal ceroid-lipofuscinosis, a disorder that may associate ataxia (Chattopadhyay et al. 2002), and a selective vulnerability of GABAergic neurons has been found in other lysosomal disorders (Walkley et al. 1991).

### 1. Cortical Cerebellar Atrophy

Cortical cerebellar atrophy (CCA) of idiopathic etiology may constitute a relatively uncomplicated neurochemical model: a loss of Purkinje cells in the anterior vermis (Oppenheimer 1982) causes a selective decrease in the concentration of GABA in the dentate nuclei (Kanazawa et al. 1985) and cerebrospinal fluid (CSF) (Kuroda et al. 1982; Manyam et al. 1990; Ogawa et al. 1982; Toghi et al. 1991), with no reduction in glutamate (Kanazawa et al. 1985), homovanillic acid (HVA), 5-hydroxiindolacetic acid (5-HIAA), or the noradrenergic metabolite 3-methoxy-4-hydroxyphenylglycol (MHPG) levels (Aldo et al. 2006).

Ten patients (five males and five females) diagnosed with cortical cerebellar atrophy, aged 72.7 ± 7.2 years, with duration of disease of 5.6 ± 2.71 years, were recruited. Clinical examinations were performed on baseline conditions, three hours after administration of single doses of 400 mg of gabapentin (time to peak plasma level of this drug) on alternate days, over a five day period (amounting to three doses of gabapentin); and four weeks later, receiving doses between 900 and 1600 mg of gabapentin per day. A substantial clinical improvement, and statistically significant differences in the scores of intermalleolar distance, spread of feet, walking capacities, knee-tibia test and finger-to-nose items, selected from the International Cerebellar Ataxia Rating Scale (ICARS) (Trouillas et al. 1997), were obtained. Furthermore, gait became normal in three of them (Gazulla et al. 2004).

Pregabalin, a molecule closely related to gabapentin, improved ataxia in a single blind, placebo controlled trial that included two patients with CCA. A 73-year-old woman and a 42-year-old man with progressive ataxia caused by cortical cerebellar atrophy, scored 19 and 15 points on the Scale for the Assessment and Rating of Ataxia (SARA) (Schmitz-Hübsch et al. 2006), respectively, while receiving placebo. Pregabalin, administered at a dose of 225 mg/day during 15 days, induced an amelioration of ataxic signs and a reduction of SARA scores to 11 and 8, respectively. The drug was well tolerated and the alleviation of ataxia was maintained after 6 months of treatment (Gazulla et al. 2007). On follow-up, the first patient is still on pregabalin at a dose of 150 mg/day (peripheral oedema being the reason for the decreased dose) after seven years of follow-up, while the second patient suffered a cranioencephalic traumatism that caused spastic tetraparesis, pregabalin being then withdrawn.

## 2. Adult-Onset GM2 Gangliosidosis

A 32 year-old man was diagnosed with adult GM2 gangliosidosis, after finding compound heterozygous mutations (F4343L/R510X) in the gene that codifies for the α chain of the β-hexosaminidase enzyme. The main clinical features were proximal lower limb weakness, myokymia in upper and lower limb muscles, dysmetria in the finger-to-nose and heel-to-shin manoeuvres, stance with an intermalleolar distance of 16 cm, wide based gait, and impossible tandem gait. Cerebellar hemispheric and vermian atrophy was observed on a cranial MR, without brainstem or cerebral anomalies. An electrophysiological study showed a continuous spontaneous activity integrated by myokymia and neuromyotonic discharges, in addition to signs of acute and chronic denervation in upper and lower limb muscles.

Administration of gabapentin, 2.000 mg/day, induced disappearance of myokymia; stance was then attained with an intermalleolar distance of 4 cm, and independent tandem gait became possible. Tiagabine, at a dose of 40 mg/day, brought about a similar improvement at the cost of a severe and transient encephalopathy integrated by amnesia, delirium and agitation. Phenytoin, 300 mg/day, acetazolamide, 750 mg/day, and a placebo did not modify ataxia, and proximal lower-limb weakness was not diminished by any drug (Gazulla and Benavente 2002). After fourteen years of treatment with gabapentin, 2400 mg/day, lower-limb muscle weakness has worsened, but ataxic signs remain stationary.

## 3. Cerebellar Ataxia with Hypogonadotropic Hypogonadism

The pathological substrate of ataxia with hypogonadotropic hypogonadism (Holmes' cerebello-olivary atrophy) is an almost selective loss of Purkinje cells in the cerebellar cortex (Eadie 1991), quite similar to that in CCA (Oppenheimer 1982). Recently, it was found that recessive mutations in *PNPLA6* caused Holmes' ataxia and Boucher-Neuhäuser syndrome (Synofzik et al. 2014). The authors considered it likely that cerebellar ataxia caused by Holmes' disease could be improved by administration of GABAergic drugs; the following observation has not yet been published.

A 25-year-old female with primary amenorrhea was diagnosed with hypogonadotropic hypogonadism, for which she received hormonal replacement; a slowly progressive unsteadiness of gait had been present since childhood. On examination, wide-based stance, independent ataxic gait of moderate intensity, impossible tandem gait, and dysmetria of limb movements were observed. A cranial MR revealed atrophy of the cerebellar vermis and normal tractography of corticospinal tracts.

Pregabalin, 25 mg twice a day, was started in March 2013, as gabapentin was not tolerated because of somnolence. Stance became possible with feet close together, gait ataxia became slighter, and dysmetria was not present on the finger-to-nose manoeuvre; the amelioration of ataxia persists after a fourteen-month follow-up.

## 4. Spinocerebellar Ataxia Type 6

SCA 6 is an autosomal dominant cerebellar degeneration associated with the expansion of a trinucleotide CAG repeat in the last exon of *CACNA1A*, the gene that codes for the $\alpha$1A subunit of the P/Q type VDCC, on chromosome 19p13.1-p13.2. Pathological findings in SCA 6 include diffuse loss of Purkinje cells, predominant in the cerebellar vermis; thus, it shares neuropathological findings with CCA (Frontali and Jodice 2002). No etiologic treatment is available for SCA 6 yet. In spite of this, these authors proposed that the P/Q-type VDCC might represent an accessible, potentially important therapeutic target in SCA 6, especially as the pore-forming region is preserved in this disease (Gazulla and Tintoré 2007a; Gazulla and Tintoré 2007b).

The use of gabapentin and pregabalin could hold promise in SCA 6, because stimulation of the ancillary $\alpha2\delta$ subunit (Gong et al. 2001) might offset an increased VDCC inactivation demonstrated by mutated $\alpha$1A subunits (Imbrici et al. 2004; Matsuyama et al. 1999). Moreover, pregabalin might prove particularly favourable in SCA 6, because expression of $\alpha$2-$\delta$2 is maximal in Purkinje cells (Toru et al. 2000). Ideally, improved adjustments in calcium homeostasis provided by gabapentin and pregabalin could give way to an amelioration of ataxia in SCA 6, even if other cell disturbances were not dealt with.

Following this line of thought, Nakamura et al. performed an open-label study and found that treatment with gabapentin, 1.200 mg/day during four weeks, decreased mean ICARS scores by more than 10% in 11 patients with SCA 6, compared to baseline. Although the comparative analysis of ICARS scores did not reach statistical significance, these results indicated that gabapentin was beneficial in SCA 6 (Nakamura et al. 2009).

## 4. Olivopontocerebellar Atrophies

The olivopontocerebellar atrophies comprise a heterogeneous group of disorders whose histological substrate is: 1) loss of neurons in the inferior olive and ventral portion of the pons; 2) loss of mossy and climbing fibres, and 3) atrophy of the cerebellar cortex (Berciano 1982). There is depletion of Purkinje and granule cells in the cerebellar cortex, especially in the hemispheres (Kanazawa et al. 1985). The clinical expression is a global cerebellar syndrome, usually accompanied by additional neurological signs. It may be sporadic or familial, familial cases being associated more frequently with spinal signs (with the exception of spasticity), dystonia and oculomotor abnormalities (Berciano 1982).

A quarter of sporadic olivopontocerebellar atrophy (OPCA) patients eventually develop multisystem atrophy (which associates parkinsonism and/or cerebellar ataxia with autonomic failure) (Berciano et al. 2006; Gilman et al. 2000). Analysis of pathological material has shown immunoreactive inclusions to alpha-synuclein in oligodendrocytes and neurons, in this disease (Berciano 1981; Berciano 2002; Tu et al. 1998). However, this is not the case with SCA1 or SCA2 (disorders caused by expansion of CAG triplets in 6p22.3 and 12q24.13, respectively), in which atrophy of olivopontocerebellar structures constitutes their pathological basis (Berciano et al. 2006). Possible atrophy of the locus coeruleus, red nucleus, substantia nigra, dentate, hypoglossal and dorsal motor nuclei, nucleus ambiguus, etc, in addition to the core pathological changes described above, may blur the nosological limits of OPCA (Perry et al. 1981).

Neurochemical studies in OPCA have demonstrated an important decrease in GABA content in the dentate nuclei (Albin and Gilman 1990; Kish et al. 1981; Ogawa et al. 1982) and cerebellar cortex (Kish et al. 1981).

The content of glutamate in the cerebellum varied between an important reduction, and normality (Albin and Gilman 1990; Kish et al. 1981; Ogawa et al. 1982); this discordance might be justified by the extensive distribution of glutamate in the brain. Kanazawa and colleagues (Kanazawa et al. 1985) found positive correlations in brains with OPCA, between: 1) content of glutamate in the anterior vermis, and density of granule cells; 2) concentration of glutamate in the posterior vermis and cerebellar hemispheres, and cellular density of the inferior olive; and, 3) content of GABA in the dentate nuclei, and density of Purkinje cells.

In an autoradiographic receptor study, Albin and Gilman found a statistically significant reduction in the density of GABA and glutamate receptors in the cerebellar cortex of OPCA brains, compatible with loss of granule and Purkinje cells (Albin and Gilman 1990). A PET study found diminished flumazenil binding in the brainstem and cerebellum in OPCA, thus confirming a deficiency in GABA (Gilman et al. 1995).

PET studies have shown decreases in dopamine and HVA levels in the striatum, in familial and sporadic OPCA (Rinne et al. 1995; Whitehouse et al. 1986). In CSF, a low content of GABA was found in sporadic OPCA (Kuroda et al. 1982; Ogawa et al. 1982; Toghi et al. 1991), in addition to low levels of glutamate, HVA and MHPG (Botez and Young 2001; Higgins et al. 1995; Orozco et al. 1989; Toghi et al. 1991). To summarise, deficiencies in GABA, glutamate, dopamine and probably noradrenaline, are present in OPCA.

In the experience of these authors, two patients with OPCA experienced improvement in cerebellar signs during treatment with gabapentin.

A 60-year-old woman with sporadic OPCA exhibited stance with a 16-centimetre intermalleolar distance, and slow, wide-based gait with ample trunk oscillations. Three hours after receiving a single dose of 400 mg of gabapentin, stance was possible with feet close together, gait was faster, with minimal body sway, and ataxia had become slight. In spite of significant improvement, the patient rejected treatment with gabapentin for fear of somnolence.

A 55-year-old female with sporadic OPCA of fourteen-year duration complained of dysarthria and oscillopsia which prevented her from focusing her eyes properly. On examination, it was found that severe ataxia made gait impossible, and she exhibited severe nystagmus evoked by horizontal and vertical gaze, together with a very elaborate and explosive dysarthria that made her speech almost unintelligible. Gabapentin, 2.000 mg/day, decreased the oscillopsia and reduced the amplitude of gaze-evoked nystagmus. Word articulation became faster and easier, so that her speech was easily understandable. The amelioration described was maintained during a twelve-month follow-up.

The authors hypothesized from these observations, that OPCA expressing a relatively pure cerebellar syndrome probably associates a comparatively isolated deficiency in GABA in the cerebellum; this could imply a possible benefit from treatment with GABAergic drugs, as described in the first patient. A persistent amelioration of dysarthria and oscillopsia brought about by gabapentin, as in the second case, has not been reported in the medical literature, and probably corresponds with the presence of a steady gabapentin plasma level (Gazulla and Benavente 2005).

## 5. Adult-Onset Ataxia-Telangiectasia

In an ataxia-telangiectasia (AT) brain with cerebellar, inferior olive and dentate nuclei atrophy, the contents of GABA and glutamate in the cerebellar cortex, and of GABA in the dentate nuclei, were lower than those in controls (Perry et al. 1984). These neurochemical findings were attributed to a loss of Purkinje and granule cells in the cerebellar cortex, and were similar to those described in OPCA (Perry et al. 1981).

A 34-year-old male patient was diagnosed with adult-onset AT. On examination, distal weakness and hypopalesthesia in the lower limbs, oculomotor apraxia, dysarthria, and conjunctival telangiectasiae were found. Independent stance required an intermalleolar distance of 28 cm, and gait was slow and severely ataxic, requiring episodic support to walk 10 metres. Carcinoembrionic antigen levels were raised in plasma, and those of alphafetoprotein were normal. MR imaging showed atrophy of the cerebellar vermis and thinning of the spinal cord.

Administration of gabapentin, 1200 mg/day, acetazolamide, 500 mg/day and placebo did not improve the patient's ataxia. Pregabalin, 225 mg/day, reduced intermalleolar distance to 8 cm while standing, and allowed him to walk 20 metres without support. The addition of tiagabine, 7.5 mg/day, increased his independent walking distance to over 20 metres (Gazulla et al. 2006). This treatment regime was well tolerated during seven years, but was abandoned when AT progressed and the patient became wheelchair-bound.

The authors suggested that the beneficial effect on ataxia might have been related either to a higher affinity of pregabalin towards $\alpha 2$-$\delta 2$ than that of gabapentin, or to its larger capacity to let calcium into the neuron (Gong et al. 2001; Imbrici et al. 2004; Matsuyama et al. 1999), or to a combination of these two factors. These differences might justify a greater effectiveness of pregabalin in the stimulation of cerebellar structures, and account for the amelioration of ataxia seen in this case. A synergistic effect with pregabalin was proposed as the cause of the supplementary benefit obtained from the addition of tiagabine (Gazulla et al. 2006).

### 6. Spinocerebellar Ataxia Types 1 and 2

It was mentioned above that atrophy of olivopontocerebellar structures constitutes the pathological basis of SCA 1 and 2 (Berciano et al. 2006), and that neurochemical studies in OPCA demonstrated a significant decrease in GABA content in the dentate nuclei and cerebellar cortex (Albin and Gilman 1990; Kish et al. 1984; Ogawa et al. 1982). Therefore, cerebellar ataxia caused by these diseases might be improved by administration of GABAergic drugs. The following observations have not previously been published.

A 39-year-old woman with a molecular diagnosis of SCA 1 (47 repeat CAG triplets; normal range, between 6 and 36) suffered from progressively unsteady gait during 5 years. On examination, enhanced tendon reflexes and severe dysmetria in the heel-to-shin manoeuvre were found. Unaided stance required a 22-centimetre intermalleolar distance, and wide-based ataxospastic gait and gaze-evoked nystagmus were also observed. Cranial MR showed cerebellar and brainstem atrophy. Pregabalin induced drowsiness, but gabapentin, at a dose of 400 mg/day, improved stance and gait.

A 56 year-old male with a molecular diagnosis of SCA 2 underwent a trial of GABAergic drugs in an attempt to improve ataxic symptoms. Gabapentin (600 mg/day), pregabalin (150 mg/day) and placebo did not ameliorate ataxia. However, baclofen at a dose of 20 mg/day, and tiagabine, 10 mg/day, improved the scores of the SARA items of stance, gait, finger-to nose, heel-to-shin and dysdiadocokinesia, without adverse side effects.

### 7. Multisystem Atrophy

Three male patients with the cerebellar variety of multisystem atrophy experienced orthostatic hypotension, together with trunk and limb cerebellar ataxia; all three were treated with gabapentin or pregabalin. No improvement in ataxia was noticed; instead, worsening of gait or dysarthria, or generalized weakness, were noticed, which forced withdrawal of the drugs (unpublished observations).

## TREATMENT OF OTHER MOTOR DISORDERS WITH GABAERGIC DRUGS

### 1. Progressive Encephalomyelitis with Rigidity

Progressive encephalomyelitis with rigidity (PER) is an inflammatory disease of the central nervous system that associates brain and spinal clinical signs with muscle rigidity (Whiteley et al. 1976). Muscle rigidity in PER has been attributed to a loss of spinal inhibitory interneurones, which might bring about a deficiency in GABA and glycine in the spinal cord (Howell et al. 1979).

PER may appear in association with GAD-autoantibodies, as a paraneoplastic syndrome, or as an essential disease (Brown and Marsden 1999).

A 72-year-old man presented with left hand amyotrophy and extensor plantar responses in 1992. In 1998, painful spasms and muscle rigidity affecting upper and lower limbs, trunk and neck, either spontaneous or triggered by stimuli, were added to previous manifestations, together with spastic paraparesis, bilateral hand amyotrophy, trismus and a pseudobulbar syndrome; no fasciculations were seen. Muscle rigidity disappeared during sleep.

An electrophysiological study showed continuous and spontaneous muscle activity integrated by normal motor unit potentials in the limbs, trunk and face, which could not be suppressed voluntarily.

Extensive blood and CSF analysis, and cranial and spinal MR were normal; these results pointed to a diagnosis of idiopathic PER.

Intravenous diazepam, at a dose of 100 mg/day, suppressed muscle spasms at the cost of severe lethargy, while baclofen, tramadol and codeine failed to decrease them. Gabapentin, 1.200 mg/day, reduced pain and muscle rigidity, while a dose of 2.000 mg/day suppresed electromyographic continuous motor unit activity and muscle spasms, and brought about an amelioration in dysarthria and gait; muscle weakness was not changed (Gazulla et al. 2001). Four years later, tiagabine 7.5 mg/day and intravenous immunoglobulin were added to gabapentin, when the muscle spasms relapsed (Gazulla et al. 2004). After six years of follow-up, muscle rigidity remained slight.

## 2. Diaphragmatic Myoclonus

The case of a 35-year-old woman with diaphragmatic myoclonus of four year duration is presented. Myoclonus occurred in clusters triggered by menstruation, and caused abdominal pain, dyspnea and blood oxygen desaturation; it was frequently accompanied by urinary retention or incontinence. During these episodes, myoclonus was severe enough to warrant hospital admission on over 20 occasions, and intravenous diazepam was repeatedly required to suppress it.

Many drugs (carbamazepine, phenytoin, baclofen, tramadol, clonazepam, bromazepam, alprazolam, trihexiphenidyl, cinitapride and otilonium) failed to prevent the appearance of myoclonus. Gabapentin, 2.100 mg/day, reduced the frequency and severity of myoclonus, although larger doses caused lethargy and were rejected. The addition of tiagabine, 10 mg/day, and an increase in dose of gabapentin to 2.400 mg/day during menstruation, finally suppressed myoclonus.

The respiratory centre was proposed as an originary location for diaphragmatic myoclonus; a deficiency in GABA in brainstem structures, as its neurochemical substrate; and GABAergic enhancement, as an effective therapeutic measure.

Experimental evidence suggested that lesions in the brainstem structures in charge of initiation of inspiratory movements, could originate diaphragmatic myoclonus. Gabapentin and tiagabine exhibited a synergistic action in this case, and these drugs were recommended as valuable means to treat diseases with increased inspiratory drive (Gazulla et al. 2003).

### 3. Dystonia

Three female patients with cervical dystonia received up to 450 mg/day of pregabalin, as adjunctive therapy to intramuscular infiltration of botulinum neurotoxin type A. No additional improvement in dystonia was observed, and pregabalin was withdrawn (unpublished observations).

### 4. Parkinson's Disease

Gabapentin was shown to improve rigidity, bradykinesia and tremor induced by Parkinson's disease and parkinsonian syndromes in a double blind, placebo-controlled, crossover trial (Olson et al. 1997). Three male patients with Parkinson's disease received 1200 mg/day of gabapentin as additional therapy to levodopa and selegiline, without alleviation of rigidity or bradykinesia; accordingly, gabapentin was discontinued for lack of efficacy (unpublished observations).

### 5. Amyotrophic Lateral Sclerosis

A phase II trial evaluated the efficacy of gabapentin in slowing the rate of decline in muscle strength of patients with amyotrophic lateral sclerosis (ALS). Gabapentin (800 mg) or placebo was administered t.i.d. in a randomized, double-blind, placebo-controlled trial for 6 months. A nonstatistically significant trend towards slower decline of arm strength in patients taking gabapentin compared with those taking placebo was observed (Miller et al. 1996). However, another group of patients with ALS was randomly assigned in a double-blinded fashion, to receive oral gabapentin 3,600 mg or placebo daily for 9 months. The primary outcome measure was the average rate of decline in isometric arm muscle strength, and no evidence of a beneficial effect of gabapentin on disease progression was found (Miller et al. 2001).

The authors treated two female patients with ALS with gabapentin, 2.000 mg/day, during four weeks, without apparent benefit in muscle strength or dysphagia. Consequently, gabapentin was discontinued (unpublished observations).

## Summary and Conclusion

GABAergic drugs have been shown to alleviate ataxia caused by CCA. As an essential neurochemical anomaly in CCA consists of an isolated deficiency in GABA in the cerebellar nuclei, related to loss of Purkinje cells, this could be considered a comparatively straightforward neurochemical model of cerebellar disease. It shares obvious similarities with Parkinson's disease, in which administration of dopamine agonists is able to reverse motor symptoms caused by depletion of dopamine in the substantia nigra. Presumably, the more selective the deficiency in GABA in the cerebellum, the more effective GABAergic substitution might become. Interestingly, single doses of 400 mg of gabapentin, or of 75 mg of pregabalin, proved useful in identifying cerebellar ataxias that might benefit from treatment with these drugs.

In addition, other ataxias with a loss of Purkinje cells as a major component of their pathology, in which a deficiency in GABA in the cerebellum may constitute an essential neurochemical anomaly, might benefit as well from treatment with GABAergic drugs, as referred to in OPCA, ataxia-telangiectasia, SCA 1 and SCA 2. Their aetiologies need not be necessarily degenerative, as metabolic disorders, such as adult-onset GM2 gangliosidosis, also benefited from these drugs.

On the other hand, ataxia caused by complex diseases of the central nervous system, such as multisystem atrophy, which inevitably combine various neurotransmitter deficiencies, has proved resistant to GABAergic drugs.

Other hyperkinetic disorders with a presumed deficiency in GABA in the central nervous system, such as PER and diaphragmatic myoclonus, were improved by GABAergic drugs in this series. However, cervical dystonia, Parkinson's disease and ALS patients did not benefit from GABAergic drugs, presumably because a tissue deficiency in GABA **is** not an essential neurochemical abnormality in these diseases.

Research aimed at identifying effective therapies to treat cerebellar ataxias and other motor disorders of the central nervous system is warranted. Meanwhile, therapeutic tests with GABAergic drugs might yield unexpected and welcome improvements in these diseases.

## REFERENCES

Albin RL, Gilman S. (1990) Autoradiographic localization of inhibitory and excitatory amino acid neurotransmitter receptors in human normal and olivopontocerebellar atrophy cerebellar cortex. *Brain Res.* 522: 37-45.

Aldo WF, van de Warrenburg BPC, Munneke M, van Geel WJA, Bloem BR, et al. (2006) CSF analysis differentiates multiple-system atrophy from idiopathic late-onset cerebellar ataxia. *Neurology* 67: 474-479.

Bastian AJ, Thach WT. (2002) Structure and function of the cerebellum. In: Manto MU, Pandolfo M, editors. The cerebellum and its disorders. Cambridge: *Cambridge University Press*. 49-66.

Belliotti TR, Capiris T, Ekhato IV, Kinsora JJ, Field MJ, Heffner TG, et al. (2005) Structure-activity relationships of pregabalin and analogues that target the $\alpha_2$-$\delta$ protein. *J. Med. Chem.* 48: 2294-2307.

Berciano J, Boesch S, Pérez-Ramos JM, Wenning GK (2006) Olivopontocerebellar atrophy: toward a better nosological definition. *Mov. Disord.* 10: 1607-1613.

Berciano J (1981) La nosología de la atrofia olivopontocerebelosa. Revisión crítica. *Arch. Neurobiol.* 44: 163-181.

Berciano J (2002) Multiple system atrophy and idiopathic late-onset cerebellar ataxia. In: Manto MU, Pandolfo M, editors. The cerebellum and its disorders. Cambridge: *Cambridge University Press.* 178-197.

Berciano J (1982) Olivopontocerebellar atrophy. A review of 117 cases. *J. Neurol. Sci.* 53: 253-272.

Botez MI, Young SN (2001) Biogenic amine metabolites and thiamine in cerebrospinal fluid in heredo-degenerative ataxias. *Can. J. Neurol. Sci*. 28: 134-140.

Brown P, Marsden CD (1999) The stiff man and stiff man plus syndromes. *J. Neurol*. 246: 648- 652.

Chattopadhyay S, Kriscenski-Perry E, Wenger DA, Pearce DA (2002) An autoantibody to GAD65 in sera of patients with juvenile neuronal ceroid lipofuscinosis. *Neurology*. 59: 1816-1817.

Colin F, Ris L, Godaux E (2002) Neuroanatomy of the cerebellum. In: Manto MU, Pandolfo M, editors. The cerebellum and its disorders. Cambridge: *Cambridge University Press*. 6-27.

Cooper JR, Bloom FE, Roth RH (2003) The biochemical basis of neuropharmacology. Oxford: *Oxford University Press*.

Eadie MJ (1991) Cerebello-olivary atrophy. In: Vinken PJ, Bruyn GW, Klawans HL, editors. Handbook of Clinical Neurology, volume 60. Amsterdam: Elsevier Science Publishers B.V. 569-573.

Frontali M, Jodice C (2002) Spinocerebellar ataxia type 6. In: Manto MU, Pandolfo M, editors. The cerebellum and its disorders. Cambridge: *Cambridge University Press*. 451-458.

Gazulla J, Benavente I, Capablo JL (2001) Encefalomielitis progresiva con rigidez. Aspectos clínicos, electrofisiológicos y tratamiento con gabapentina. *Neurología* 16: 85-88.

Gazulla J, Benavente I. (2002) Gangliosidosis GM2 del adulto: mejoría de la ataxia con fármacos GABAérgicos. *Neurología*. 17: 157-161.

Gazulla Abío J, Feijóo de Freixo M, Val Adán P, Benavente Aguilar I (2003) Aspectos clínicos y terapéuticos de las mioclonias diafragmáticas. *Neurología*. 18: 473-477.

Gazulla J, Errea JM, Benavente I, Tordesillas C (2004a) Treatment of ataxia in cortical cerebellar atrophy with the GABAergic drug gabapentin. A preliminary study. *Eur. Neurol*. 52: 7-11.

Gazulla J, Benavente I, Capablo JL (2004b) Actualización farmacológica de un caso de encefalomielitis progresiva con rigidez, con respuesta favorable a gabapentina. *Neurología*. 19 (8): 460-461.

Gazulla J, Benavente I (2005) Mejoría sintomática de la atrofia olivopontocerebelosa con gabapentina. *Rev. Neurol*. 40: 285-288

Gazulla J, Benavente I, Sarasa M (2006) Ataxia-telangiectasia del adulto. Observación clínica y terapéutica. *Neurología*. 21: 447-451.

Gazulla J, Benavente I (2007) Single-blind, placebo-controlled pilot study of pregabalin for ataxia in cortical cerebellar atrophy. Acta. Neurol. Scand. 116: 235-8.

Gazulla J, Tintoré M (2007a) The P/Q-Type Voltage-Dependent Calcium Channel as Pharmacological Target in Spinocerebellar Ataxia Type 6: Gabapentin and Pregabalin may be of Therapeutic Benefit. *Medical Hypotheses*. 687: 131-136.

Gazulla J, Tintoré M (2007b) The P/Q-Type Voltage-Dependent Calcium Channel: a Therapeutic Target in Spinocerebellar Ataxia type 6. *Acta. Neurologica Scand*. 115 (5): 356-363.

Gilman S, Koeppe RA, Junck L, Kluin KJ, Lohman M, St Laurent RT (1995) Benzodiazepine receptor binding in cerebellar degenerations studied with positron emission tomography. *Ann Neurol*. 38: 176-185.

Gilman S, Little R, Johanns J, Heumann M, Kluin KJ, Junck L, et al. (2000) Evolution of sporadic olivopontocerebellar atrophy into multiple system atrophy. *Neurology*. 55: 527-532.

Gong HC, Hang J, Kobler L, Li L, Su TZ (2001) Tissue-specific expression and gabapentin-binding properties of calcium channel α2δ subunit subtypes. *J. Membrane Biol.* 184: 35-43.

Gong HC, Hang J, Kobler L, Li L, Su TZ (2001) Tissue-specific expression and gabapentin-binding properties of calcium channel α2- δ subunit subtypes- *J. Membrane Biol.* 184: 35-43.

Higgins JJ, Harley-White J, Kopin IJ (1995) Low lumbar CSF concentrations of homovanilic acid in the autosomal dominant ataxias. *J. Neurol. Neurosurg. Psychiatry*. 58: 760.

Honnorat J, Saiz A, Giometto B, Vincent A, Brieva L, de Andrés C, et al. (2001) Cerebellar ataxia with anti-glutamic acid decarboxylase antibodies. *Arch. Neurol.* 58: 225-230.

Howell DA, Lees AJ, Toghill PJ (1979) Spinal internuncial neurones in progressive encephalomyelitis with rigidity. *J. Neurol. Neurosurg. Psychiatry*. 42: 773-785.

Imbrici P, Jaffe S, Eunson LH, Davies NP, Herd C, Robertson R, et al. (2004) Dysfunction of the brain calcium channel $Ca_v2.1$ in absence epilepsy and episodic ataxia. *Brain*. 127: 2682-2692.

Ishida K, Mitoma H, Song S, Uchihara T, Inaba K, Eguchi S, et al. (1999) Selective suppression of cerebellar GABAergic transmission by an autoantibody to glutamic acid decarboxylase. *Ann. Neurol.* 46: 263-267.

Kanazawa I, Kwak S, Sasaki H, Mizusawa H, Muramoto O, Yoshizawa K, et al. (1985) Studies on neurotransmitter markers and neuronal cell density in the cerebellar system in olivopontocerebellar atrophy and cortical cerebellar atrophy. *J. Neurol. Sci.* 71: 193-208.

Kang MG, Felix R, Campbell KP (2002) Long-term regulation of voltage-gated $Ca^{2+}$ channels by gabapentin. *FEBS Lett.* 528: 177-182.

Kish SJ, Perry TL, Hornykiewicz O (1984) Benzodiazepine receptor binding in cerebellar cortex: observations in olivopontocerebellar atrophy. *J. Neurochem.* 42: 466-469.

Kuroda H, Ogawa N, Yamawaki Y, Nukina I, Ofuji T, Yamamoto M, et al. (1982) Cerebrospinal fluid GABA levels in various neurological and psychiatric diseases. *J. Neurol. Neurosurg. Psychiatry*. 45: 257-260.

Kuzniecky R, Ho S, Pan J, Martin R, Gilliam F, Faught E, et al. (2002) Modulation of cerebral GABA by topiramate, lamotrigine, and gabapentin in healthy adults. *Neurology*. 58: 368-372.

Kwong WH, Chan WY, Lee KKH, Fan M, Yew DT (2000) Neurotransmitters, neuropeptides and calcium binding proteins in developing human cerebellum: a review. *J. Histochem.* 32: 521-534.

Manyam BV, Giacobini E, Ferraro TN, Hare TA (1990) Cerebrospinal fluid as a reflector of central cholinergic and amino acid neurotransmitter activity in cerebellar ataxia. *Arch. Neurol.* 47: 1194-1199.

Matsuyama Z, Wakamori M, Mori Y, Kawakami H, Nakamura S (1999) Direct alteration of the P/Q-type Ca 2+ channel property by polyglutamine expansion in spinocerebellar ataxia 6. *J. Neurosci.* 19 RC 14:1-5.

Miller RG, Moore D, Young LA, Armon C, Barohn RJ, Bromberg MB, Bryan WW, Gelinas DF, Mendoza MC, Neville HE, Parry GJ, Petajan JH, Ravits JM, Ringel SP, Ross MA (1996) Placebo-controlled trial of gabapentin in patients with amyotrophic lateral sclerosis. WALS Study Group. Western Amyotrophic Lateral Sclerosis Study Group. Neurology. 47: 1383-8.

Miller RG, Moore DH 2nd, Gelinas DF, Dronsky V, Mendoza M, Barohn RJ, Bryan W, Ravits J, Yuen E, Neville H, Ringel S, Bromberg M, Petajan J, Amato AA, Jackson C, Johnson W, Mandler R, Bosch P, Smith B, Graves M, Ross M, Sorenson EJ, Kelkar P, Parry G, Olney R (2001) Western ALS Study Group. Phase III randomized trial of gabapentin in patients with amyotrophic lateral sclerosis. Neurology. 56: 843-8.

Mugnaini E (2000) GABAergic inhibition in the cerebellar system. In: Martin DL, Olsen RW, editors. GABA in the Nervous System: the view at fifty years. Philadelphia: *Lippincott, Williams & Wilkins*. 383-407.

Nakamura K, Yoshida K, Miyakazi D, Morita H, Ikeda S (2009) Spinocerebellar ataxia type 6 (SCA 6): clinical pilot trial with gabapentin. *J. Neurol. Sci.* 278: 107-111.

Ogawa N, Kuroda H, Ota Z, Yamamoto M, Otsuki S (1982) Cerebrospinal fluid gamma-aminobutiric acid variations in cerebellar ataxia. *Lancet.* 2:215.

Olson WL, Gruenthal M, Mueller ME, Olson WH (1997) Gabapentin for parkinsonism: a double-blind, placebo-controlled, crossover trial. *Am. J. Med.* 102: 60-66.

Oppenheimer DR (1982) Diseases of the basal ganglia, cerebellum and motor neurons. In: Adams JH, Corsellis JAN, Duchen LW, editors. Greenfield´s Neuropathology. London: Edward Arnold. 699-747.

Orozco G, Estrada R, Perry TL, Araña J, Fernández R, González-Quevedo A, et al. (1989) Dominantly inherited olivopontocerebellar atrophy from Eastern Cuba. Clinical, neuropathological, and biochemical findings. *J. Neurol. Sci.* 93: 37-50.

Ostergaard LH, Gram L, Dam M (1995) Potential antiepileptic drugs. In: Levy RH, Mattson RH, Meldrum BS, editors. Antiepileptic drugs. New York: *Raven Press Ltd.* 1057-1061.

Ottersen OP, Walberg F (2002) Neurotransmitters in the cerebellum. In: Manto MU, Pandolfo M, editors. The cerebellum and its disorders. Cambridge: *Cambridge University Press.* 38-48.

Ottersen OP (1993) Neurotransmitters in the cerebellum. *Rev Neurol* (Paris). 149: 629-636.

Pazos A, Pascual J (2008) Farmacología de los movimientos anormales. Fármacos antiespásticos. In: Flórez J, Armijo JA, Mediavilla A, editors. Farmacología Humana. Barcelona: *Elsevier Masson*. 607-627.

Perry TL, Kish SJ, Hansen S, Currier RD (1981) Neurotransmitter amino acids in dominantly inherited cerebellar disorders. *Neurology.* 31: 237-242.

Perry TL, Kish SJ, Hinton D, Hansen S, Becker LE, Gelfand EW (1984) Neurochemical abnormalities in a patient with ataxia-telangiectasia. *Neurology.* 34: 187-191.

Rinne JO, Burn DJ, Mathias CJ, Quinn NP, Marsden CD, Brooks DJ (1995) Positron emission tomography studies on the dopaminergic system and striatal opioid binding in the olivopontocerebellar atrophy variant of multiple system atrophy. *Ann. Neurol.* 37: 568-573.

Saiz A, Arpa J, Sagasta A, Casamitjana R, Zarranz JJ, Tolosa E, et al. (1997) Autoantibodics to glutamic acid decarboxylase in three patients with cerebellar ataxia, late-onset diabetes mellitus, and polyendocrine autoimmunity. *Neurology.* 49: 1026-1030.

Schmitz-Hübsch T, du Montcel ST, Baliko L, Berciano J, Boesch S, Depondt C, et al. (2006) Scale for the assessment and rating of ataxia: development of a new clinical scale. *Neurology.* 66: 1717-1720.

Stefani A, Spadoni F, Bernardi G (1998) Gabapentin inhibits calcium currents in isolated rat brain neurons. *Neuropharmacol.* 37: 83-91.

Synofzik M, Gonzalez MA, Lourenco CM, Coutelier M, Haack TB, Rebelo A, Hannequin D, Strom TM, Prokisch H, Kernstock C, Durr A, Schöls L, Lima-Martínez MM, Farooq A, Schüle R, Stevanin G, Marques W Jr, Züchner S (2014) PNPLA6 mutations cause Boucher-Neuhäuser and Gordon Holmes syndromes as part of a broad neurodegenerative spectrum. Brain. 137: 69-77.

Tohgi H, Abe T, Hashiguchi K, Takahashi S, Nozaki Y, Kikuchi T (1991) A significant reduction of putative transmitter amino acids in cerebrospinal fluid of patients with Parkinson´s disease and spinocerebellar degeneraton. *Neurosci. Letter.* 126: 155-158.

Toru S, Murakoshi T, Ishikawa K, Saegusa H, Fujigasaki H, Uchihara T, et al. (2000) Spinocerebellar ataxia type 6 mutation alters P-type calcium channel function. *J. Biol. Chem.* 275: 10893-10898.

Trouillas P, Takayanagi T, Currier RD, Subramony SH, Wessel K, Bryer A, et al. (1997) International Cooperative Ataxia Rating Scale for pharmacological assessment of the cerebellar syndrome. *J. Neurol. Sci.* 145: 205-211.

Trouillas P (1993) Bases théoriques et propositions pour une neuropharmacologie de l´ataxie cérébelleuse. *Rev. Neurol.* (Paris). 149: 637-646.

Tu P, Galvin JE, Baba M, Giasson B, Tomita T, Leight S, et al. (1998) Glial cytoplasmatic inclusions in white matter oligodendrocytes of multiple system atrophy brains contain insoluble α-sinuclein. *Ann. Neurol.* 44: 415-422.

Vulliemoz S, Vanini G, Truffert A, Chizzolini C, Seeck M (2007) Epilepsy and cerebellar ataxia associated anti-glutamic acid decarboxylase antibodies. *J. Neurol. Neurosurg Psychiatry.* 78 : 187-189.

Walkley SU, Baker HJ, Rattazzi MC, Haskins ME, Wu JY (1991) Neuroaxonal dystrophy in neuronal storage disorders: evidence for major GABAergic neuron involvement. *J. Neurol. Sci.* 104: 1-8.

Whitehouse PJ, Muramoto O, Troncoso JC, Kanazawa I (1986) Neurotransmitter receptors in olivopontocerebellar atrophy: an autoradiographic study. *Neurology.* 36: 193-197.

Whiteley AM, Swash M, Urich H (1976) Progressive encephalomyelitis with rigidity: its relation to subacute myoclonic spinal neuronitis and to the stiff man syndrome. *Brain.* 99: 27- 42.

In: Gamma-Aminobutyric Acid (GABA)
Editors: Josipa Vlainić and Maja Jazvinšćak Jembrek ISBN: 978-1-63321-838-3


*Chapter 7*

# GABA-MEDIATED OVER-INHIBITION IN DOWN SYNDROME: IMPLICATIONS FOR COGNITIVE AND NEUROMORPHOLOGICAL PHENOTYPES

***Paula Martínez and Carmen Martínez-Cué[1*]***
Department of Physiology and Pharmacology, Faculty of Medicine, University of Cantabria, Santander, Spain

## ABSTRACT

Down syndrome (DS) is the most common cause of cognitive disability of a genetic origin. In the last few years, different murine models of DS have been developed, but the most commonly used and best characterized is the Ts65Dn mouse. Two main mechanisms have been proposed to underlie the cognitive alterations of DS individuals and Ts65Dn mice: excessive inhibition and the hypocellularity found in different brain areas due to altered neurogenesis. Evidence for enhanced inhibition in the trisomic brain comes from studies demonstrating that long-term potentiation (LTP), the electrophysiological substrate of learning, results from unbalanced excitatory and inhibitory neurotransmission. In addition, an increased number of GABAergic interneurons and alterations in GABA receptor subunit composition and in GABAergic synapse morphology and/or function have been reported in Ts65Dn brains. Moreover, both $GABA_A$ and $GABA_B$ receptor-mediated inhibition have been demonstrated in this mouse model of DS. Different pharmacological approaches that reduce GABAergic activity have been demonstrated to enhance cognitive abilities and LTP and to increase adult hippocampal neurogenesis and neuronal density in Ts65Dn mice. Because several other drugs targeting different transmitter systems have also been shown to have these beneficial effects on functional and neuromorphological abilities in Ts65Dn mice, we analyze here the relation between alterations in GABA transmission and neurogenesis and the putative role of their interaction on other transmitter systems leading to the pro-cognitive effects of the different therapeutic strategies.

* Corresponding autor: Carmen Martinez Cue, Department of Physiology and Pharmacology, Faculty of Medicine, University of Cantabria, Santander, Spain, Email: martinec@unican.es.

**Keywords:** Down syndrome, hippocampus, GABAergic system, over-inhibition, therapy

# 1. Introduction

Down syndrome (DS) is the most common cause of intellectual disability of a genetic origin. It affects 1 in 850-1000 infants (Shin et al., 2009) and is characterized by a number of phenotypes, including cardiovascular, skeletal and motor alterations. However, the most prominent feature of DS is an intellectual disability that affects 100% of the individuals with this condition. DS individuals show an array of altered cognitive and behavioral phenotypes, including impairments in learning and memory (Carlesimo et al., 1997; Chapman and Hesketh, 2000; Nadel, 2003; Vicari, 2006).

Based on the homology of human chromosome 21 (Hsa21) and the three mouse chromosomes: Mmu16, Mmu17 and Mmu10, in the last few years, several murine models of DS that are trisomic for different sets of Hsa21 orthologous genes have been developed. Studies on these models have provided important insight into the neurobiological mechanisms underlying the cognitive deficits in DS (Bartesaghi et al., 2011; Rueda et al., 2012a).

The Ts65Dn mouse, which is the most commonly used and best characterized model of DS, bears a partial trisomy of a segment of Mmu16, extending from the *Mrp139* gene to the *Znf295*, and contains approximately 92 genes orthologous to Hsa21 genes (Sturgeon and Gardiner, 2011). This murine model recapitulates several fundamental features of DS including cognitive deficits and alterations in brain morphology and function (Bartesaghi et al., 2011; Haydar and Reeves, 2012; Rueda et al., 2012a). Ts65Dn mice show alterations in different processes involved in learning and memory such as spatial reference and working memory and reduced attention (Driscoll et al., 2004; Escorihuela et al., 1998; Martinez-Cue et al., 2013; Martinez-Cue et al., 2006; Rueda et al., 2012a).

Different neuromorphological alterations present in the Ts65Dn mouse are likely to be partially responsible for their cognitive deficits including changes in the size, morphology and cellular density of different brain areas, alterations in pre- and post-natal neurogenesis, in dendritic structure and in the morphology of synapses and spines (Bartesaghi et al., 2011; Rueda et al., 2012a).

In addition, abnormal synaptic plasticity, as shown by the reduction in long-term potentiation (LTP), considered to be the electrophysiological substrate of learning, in the hippocampal CA1 and dentate gyrus (DG) areas have also been demonstrated to compromise cognitive abilities in Ts65Dn mice (Kleschevnikov et al., 2004; Siarey et al., 1999).

Among these morphological and functional alterations, two mechanisms have been proposed to underlie the cognitive alterations in DS individuals and Ts65Dn mice, namely over-inhibition and the hypocellularity found in different brain areas due to alterations in pre- and post-natal neurogenesis. In this review, we will summarize the evidence supporting the role of both altered processes and the putative relation between them. We will focus on the alterations in GABA transmission and neurogenesis and their interactions, and we will discuss the possibility that the interplay between both processes can lead to the cognitive deficits found in DS individuals and in the Ts65Dn mouse.

# 2. The over-Inhibition Hypothesis in Down Syndrome

Excess of inhibition in the adult brain could be responsible for the synaptic plasticity deficits that may be a major mechanism underlying cognitive impairments. Several studies have demonstrated that the functional defects in the DS and in the Ts65Dn brain may be due to an imbalance between excitatory and inhibitory neurotransmission (Martínez-Cué et al., 2014). The cognitive impairment displayed by Ts65Dn mice has been consistently related to excessive levels of neuronal inhibition in the medial temporal lobe circuitry. Accordingly, this excessive inhibition has been proposed as one of the underlying causes of the cognitive deficits in DS.

Increased inhibition in the trisomic condition is caused by alterations in both excitatory and inhibitory transmission, although this review will mainly focus on the latter.

## 2.1. Excitatory Transmitters

Although similar levels of glutamate (Pollonini et al., 2008) are found in fetuses with and without DS, decreased levels of aspartate and glutamate have been found in several areas of the adult DS brain (Godridge et al., 1987; Risser et al., 1997; Yates et al., 1986), therefore leading to enhanced inhibition.

Reduced activation of NMDA receptors is also thought to interfere with normal LTP induction in Ts65Dn mice (Belichenko et al., 2009a; Belichenko et al., 2007; Hanson et al., 2007; O'Doherty et al., 2005).

In addition, Ts65Dn mice show a reduction of the GluR1 subunit of the AMPA receptor (Belichenko et al., 2009b) and of the NR2A and NR2B subunits of the NMDA receptor (Sairanen et al., 2005). However, other studies failed to find changes in the GluR1 subunit in brain homogenates or changes in the NR2A and NR2B subunits in synaptosomes of these mice (Fernandez et al., 2009).

Alterations in the signaling mechanisms downstream of the NMDA receptor have also been reported; the hippocampi of Ts65Dn mice show disturbances in the calcium/calmodulin-dependent protein kinase II (CaMKII), phosphatidylinositol 3-kinase (PIP3K)/Akt, extracellular signal-regulated kinase (ERK), protein kinase A (PKA) and protein kinase C (PKC), all of which have been shown to be involved in synaptic plasticity (Siddiqui et al., 2008).

Altogether, these results provide evidence implicating altered excitatory transmission in the over-inhibition found in DS and in Ts65Dn mice.

## 2.2. GABA

The first evidence for the role of the GABAergic system in the over-inhibition displayed by Ts65Dn mice came from studies demonstrating that their reduced LTP results from an unbalanced excitatory and inhibitory neurotransmission (Hanson et al., 2007; Popov et al., 2011; Scott-McKean and Costa, 2011). The involvement of the $GABA_A$ receptor in the altered synaptic plasticity of Ts65Dn mice was demonstrated by a study showing that administering the $GABA_A$ receptor antagonist picrotoxin rescued LTP in Ts65Dn mice (Belichenko et al., 2004). These results were confirmed by Fernandez et al. (2007), who demonstrated that picrotoxin and other $GABA_A$ receptor antagonists such as bilobalide or pentilenetetrazol also rescued LTP and the cognitive alterations of Ts65Dn mice. More recently, Kleschevnikov et al. (2012b) have shown that both $GABA_A$ and $GABA_B$ receptor-mediated components of evoked inhibitory postsynaptic currents (IPSCs) were significantly higher in Ts65Dn mice, suggesting an increase in presynaptic release of GABA. Therefore, both $GABA_A$ and $GABA_B$ receptors are implicated in the reduced synaptic efficiency found in the hippocampal dentate gyrus (DG) of Ts65Dn mice.

However, while GABA-mediated overinhibition has been observed in some brain areas, this might not be true for all brain areas and it may vary between synapses within a brain area and with age. The increase in $GABA_A$ receptor-mediated synaptic transmission is cell and age specific because it does not occur in all subtypes of CA1 neurons or at all ages (Mitra et al., 2012). In addition, hippocampal CA3 pyramidal neurons of newborn Ts65Dn mice show a reduction in inhibitory $GABA_A$ receptor-mediated synaptic input and no impairment in LTP (Hanson et al., 2007). Finally, in contrast to the augmented GABAergic inhibition in dentate granule cells and CA1 pyramidal neurons of Ts65Dn hippocampi, the cerebellar granule cells of Ts65Dn mice show smaller tonic $GABA_A$ receptor currents (Szemes et al., 2013).

The enhanced GABA-mediated over-inhibition in the trisomic brain may be due to changes in GABA neurotransmitter levels, the number of GABAergic interneurons, alterations in receptor subunit composition and in GABAergic synapses morphology and/or function.

#### *2.2.1. GABA Levels*

Over-inhibition in the DS brain might be due to an increased concentration of GABA; however, different studies have shown a decrease or lack of changes in the concentration of this neurotransmitter. In the frontal cortex of fetuses with DS, GABA levels are reduced by 60 % (Whittle et al., 2007). In addition, *in vivo* magnetic resonance spectroscopy (MRS) studies in children between 3 and 17 years of age also demonstrated a decrease of GABA in the temporal lobes, while no change could be identified in the frontal lobes (Smigielska-Kuzia et al., 2010; Smigielska-Kuzia and Sobaniec, 2007).

However, during prenatal and early postnatal phases, GABAergic responses are depolarizing and turn to inhibitory responses during the first postnatal weeks. Therefore, the lower GABA levels found in DS fetuses could lead to a reduced depolarization (i.e., enhanced inhibition). Moreover, most cells in the rodent central nervous system (CNS) achieve a $Cl^-$ concentration low enough for inhibitory responses at approximately the end of the second postnatal week (Owens and Kriegstein, 2002), which corresponds approximately with early childhood in humans. However, several studies provide evidence that demonstrate that the maturation of membrane and synaptic properties of interneurons are not completed with puberty (Doischer et al., 2008; Okaty et al., 2009), and the postnatal maturation of the GABAergic system lasts until late adolescence (Kilb, 2012). Therefore, once again, the reduced GABA levels found in children and adolescence with DS could also be indicative of enhanced inhibition.

In adult DS patients with AD neuropathology, GABA levels are reduced in the hippocampus and temporal cortex (Reynolds and Warner, 1988); although these investigators also found a significant deficit of glutamate in the hippocampus. These results could be due to the loss of neurons containing these neurotransmitters.

Regarding GABA levels in the Ts65Dn brain, in the only MRS study published the resonance peak corresponding to GABA was not identified from the spectrum (Huang et al., 2000).

### *2.2.2. Gabaergic Neuron Density*

DS individuals present a reduction in the number of small, granular, presumably GABAergic neurons in layer II and layer IV of the cortex (Ross et al., 1984). In addition, microarray studies of DS human neural progenitor cells (hNPCs) revealed gene changes indicative of defects in interneuron progenitor development that may lead to decreased GABAergic interneuron neurogenesis (Bhattacharyya et al., 2009).

In contrast to what has been reported in the DS brain, in the Ts65Dn mouse, an increased number of GABAergic interneurons in the somatosensory cortex has been reported (Perez-Cremades et al., 2010), which implies an enhancement of inhibitory drive. In addition, an increased number of inhibitory neurons in the forebrains of newborn Ts65Dn mice that was paralleled by an increase in spontaneous inhibitory postsynaptic currents in the pyramidal neurons of the CA1 region has been reported (Chakrabarti et al., 2010).

In summary, while most of the studies performed in the Ts65Dn mouse support an increased density of GABAergic interneurons presumably enhancing inhibition, there is no evidence of the same alteration in the DS brain.

### *2.2.3. Alterations in Synapses*

DS and mouse models of DS display a reduced number of synaptic contacts and alterations in synaptic plasticity. Ts65Dn mice show a reduction in synaptic density in the neocortex and CA1 at P9 (Chakrabarti et al., 2007) and in the hippocampal DG, CA1 and CA3 regions in adulthood (Kurt et al., 2004). Not only the number of synapses but also the characteristics and the relative distribution of different types of synapses are altered in Ts65Dn mice, leaving the balance between excitatory and inhibitory synapses shifted toward increased inhibition in the trisomic brain. Ts65Dn mice have less excitatory (asymmetric) synapses in the temporal cortex, DG, CA1 and CA3 (Kurt et al., 2004; Perez-Cremades et al., 2010), and glutamatergic synapse markers are reduced in the hippocampus of Ts65Dn mice (Rueda et al., 2010). Ts65Dn brains also show a redistribution of inhibitory synapses, with a relative decrease in inputs to the dendritic shafts and an increase in inputs to the spine necks (Belichenko et al., 2007; Popov et al., 2011).

Moreover, the efficacy of individual inhibitory synaptic connections is decreased in Ts65Dn animals, leading to reduced intrinsic activity of interneurons (Hanson et al., 2007).

In addition, an increased expression of different inhibitory synapse markers has been reported in the brains of trisomic mice. Although gene expression profiles from the hippocampus of Ts65Dn mice or from the adult brain of DS individuals revealed that GABA synthesis enzymes glutamate decarboxylase (GAD), GAD65 and GAD67 were unchanged compared to euploids (Lockstone et al., 2007), increased levels of these synaptic proteins at hippocampal and cortical inhibitory synapses have been found in mice. GAD65, GAD67 and the vesicular GABA transporter (VGAT) were increased in the brain of Ts65Dn mice (Martinez-Cue et al., 2013; Perez-Cremades et al., 2010). Moreover, a significant increase in co-localization of GAD65 and VGAT was reported in the fascia dentata of Ts65Dn mice (Belichenko et al., 2009b).

### *2.2.4. Receptors*

In the CNS, GABA acts on two main classes of membrane-bound receptors: the ionotropic chloride permeable $GABA_A$ receptors (ligand-gated $Cl^-$ channels) and the metabotropic (G protein-coupled) $GABA_B$ receptors. A wide array of studies has shown that the Ts65Dn mouse presents both enhanced $GABA_A$ and $GABA_B$ mediated transmission.

The $GABA_A$ receptor contains an intrinsic ligand-gated $Cl^-$ channel formed by the pentameric assembly of different subunits (α1-6, β1-4, γ1-3, δ, ε, θ and π subunits) (Bonnert et al., 1999; Macdonald and Olsen, 1994; Mohler et al., 1996; Olsen et al., 1990; Rabow et al., 1995; Whiting et al., 1999).

A number of alterations have been reported in the expression of various GABA receptor subunits in DS and in the Ts65Dn mouse. In neurospheres from fetuses with DS, up-regulation of the α2 and down-regulation of the α5 and ß3 subunits of the $GABA_A$ receptor have been reported (Bhattacharyya et al., 2009). In the hippocampus of Ts65Dn mice, reductions in the number of ß2 and ß3 subunits of the $GABA_A$ receptor were found (Belichenko et al., 2009b). Brain synaptosomes of Ts65Dn mice show a reduction in $GABA_A$ α1 receptor expression (Fernandez et al., 2009). Changes in the R1 subunit of the $GABA_B$ receptor have also been reported in Ts65Dn mice (Belichenko et al., 2009b), and the levels of $GABA_B$ receptors R2 were 19% less. This decrease was attributed to a compensatory mechanism in response to the increase of G protein-coupled inward rectifier potassium channel 2 (GIRK2) levels, an inwardly rectifying potassium channel mapping to the trisomic region (Best et al., 2012). However, other studies (Kleschevnikov et al., 2012b) did not find changes in the levels of $GABA_A$ or $GABA_B$ receptor subunits using western blot analysis. Finally, no changes in the binding of RO0154513, a selective $GABA_A$ α5-selective NAM, were found *in vivo* in Ts65Dn mice (Martinez-Cue et al., 2013).

#### 2.2.4.1. $GABA_B$

The *Girk2* gene is overexpressed throughout the brain in DS individuals and in Ts65Dn mice, especially in the hippocampus. Girk channels generate a $GABA_B$ receptor-dependent slow inhibitory postsynaptic potential in hippocampal neurons (Lüscher et al., 1997). Synaptically evoked $GABA_B$/GIRK currents may serve as a primary inhibitory modulator of the direct, perforant path inputs onto CA1 pyramidal neurons (Pham et al., 1998). This pathway is likely to play a role in learning/memory, because it is strongly activated during cognitive tasks and is a principal mediator of hippocampal place field memory (Brun et al., 2002; Sybirska et al., 2000). It has been proposed that an increase in *Girk2* gene expression may produce overinhibition in hippocampal neurons and contribute to LTP failure in the trisomic condition (Best et al., 2007). In the Ts65Dn mouse, the overexpression of the *Girk2* gene leads to a significant increase in $GABA_B$-mediated Girk currents in hippocampal neuron cultures, which affects the balance between excitatory and inhibitory transmission (Best et al., 2012; Best et al., 2007). *Girk2* overexpression in the Ts65Dn hippocampus functionally alters the integration of synaptic inputs in CA1 pyramidal neurons in a pathway-specific manner. In addition to this impact on signal transmission through its coupling to $GABA_B$ receptors, GIRK2 channel expression levels can alter neuronal resting potentials and consequently impact LTP and cognitive processes (Cramer et al., 2010).

In addition, *Girk* channel overexpression may be involved in the reduced neuronal density found in Ts65Dn mice, because chronic treatment with a *Girk* channel antagonist increased neurogenesis of hippocampal neurons (Kobayashi et al., 2003). Interestingly, the serotonin reuptake inhibitor fluoxetine, which is also a *Girk* channel antagonist, rescues cognitive performance and neurogenesis in Ts65Dn mice (Kobayashi et al., 2003). However, chronic administration of ethosuximide, another inhibitor of *Girk* channels, was not able to rescue the cognitive alterations of Ts65Dn mice (Vidal et al., 2012). Therefore, the cognitive enhancing effects of fluoxetine may be secondary to other mechanisms (see below).

Recent studies demonstrated that signaling through postsynaptic $GABA_B$ receptors is significantly enhanced in the Ts65Dn DG (Kleschevnikov et al., 2012b).

In addition, antagonizing the activity of $GABA_B$ receptors reduced the cognitive alterations of Ts65Dn mice. Treatment with the $GABA_B$ receptor antagonist CGP55845 restored memory of Ts65Dn mice, increased hippocampal levels of BDNF and enhanced LTP in the DG. These findings demonstrate the contribution of $GABA_B$ receptors to the impaired cognitive abilities of Ts65Dnmice (Kleschevnikov et al., 2012a; Kleschevnikov et al., 2012b).

#### 2.2.4.2. $GABA_A$

It is firmly established that the $GABA_A$ receptor system plays an important role in cognition. Non-selective positive allosteric modulators (PAMs) of the $GABA_A$ receptor disrupt learning and memory processes (Cole, 1986; Ghoneim and Mewaldt, 1990; Lister, 1985), whereas non-selective negative allosteric modulators (NAMs) improve cognitive processes (Jensen et al., 1987; Sarter et al., 2001; Venault and Chapouthier, 2007; Venault et al., 1987). In addition, non-selective $GABA_A$ NAMs, such as DMCM, increase LTP (Seabrook et al., 1997), whereas nonselective $GABA_A$ agonists (e.g., diazepam) impair LTP (del Cerro et al., 1992).

## 2.3. Pharmacological Approaches to Reduce $GABA_A$-Mediated Inhibition

As previously mentioned, chronic administration of non-selective $GABA_A$ receptor antagonists picrotoxin, bilobalide or pentylenetetrazole (PTZ) reverses the deficits in LTP, produces power normalization of the EEG anomalies and enhances hippocampal-mediated memory of Ts65Dn mice (Fernandez et al., 2007). In spite of their pro-cognitive effects, these compounds cannot be safely used to improve cognition due to their anxiogenic and proconvulsant effects (Dorow et al., 1983). The ongoing clinical trial (http://compose21.com/study.htm) that assesses the safety and potential efficacy of PTZ in individuals with DS will clarify this point.

The identification of different functions of $GABA_A$ receptor subtypes has led to the hypothesis that receptor subtype-selective compounds could avoid the limitations of classical non-selective modulators of the $GABA_A$ receptor.

Among the different $GABA_A$ receptor subtypes, α5 subunit-containing $GABA_A$ receptors are predominantly expressed in the hippocampus, both in rodents and humans (Fritschy and Mohler, 1995; Klausberger, 2009; Laurie et al., 1992; Lingford-Hughes et al., 2002; Olsen and Sieghart, 2009). They are concentrated in the dendrites of hippocampal CA1 pyramidal neurons and play a role in regulating tonic inhibition through extrasynaptic receptors (Caraiscos et al., 2004). However, they have also been detected at GABAergic synapses on the dendrites of hippocampal pyramidal neurons and could modulate phasic GABAergic inhibition (Serwanski et al., 2006). $GABA_A$ α5-subunit-containing receptors are known to facilitate cognition in hippocampal-dependent tasks (Collinson et al., 2002; Crestani et al., 2002). Based on these results it was hypothesized that α5 subunit -containing $GABA_A$ receptors may represent a valuable target for memory-enhancing drugs.

Recently, the efficacy of two NAMs selective for α5-containing receptors to reduce the cognitive impairments of Ts65Dn mice has been assessed (Martínez-Cué et al., 2014). The first molecule tested was α5IA (3-(5-Methyllisoxazol-3-yl)6[(1-methyl-1,2,3-triazol-yl)methyl-oxy]-1,2,4-triazolo[3,4,-α]phthalazine), a NAM that has a higher binding selectivity for the α5 subunit compared to the α1 subunit and is a weak positive allosteric modulator of the α2 and the α3 subunit-containing receptors; the functional selectivities are similar for all subunits (Sternfeld et al., 2004).

The second NAM recently tested was RO4938581 (3-bromo-10-(difluoromethyl)-9H-benzo[f]imidazo[1,5-a][1,2,4]triazolo[1,5-d][1,4]diazepine), a molecule that has a higher affinity for the α5-containing $GABA_A$ receptors than for the α1, α2 and α3 containing $GABA_A$ receptors and is a NAM of α5-containing $GABA_A$ receptors only (Ballard et al., 2009).

In normal animals, both selective $GABA_A$ α5 NAMs have cognitive-enhancing effects and enhance LTP without inducing anxiogenic or proconvulsant side effects associated with the activity of other subtypes of $GABA_A$ receptors (Atack et al., 2006; Ballard et al., 2009; Braudeau et al., 2011; Chambers et al., 2004; Collinson et al., 2006; Dawson et al., 2006; Nutt et al., 2007; Rudolph and Mohler, 2006; Sternfeld et al., 2004).

In T65Dn mice, chronic administration of α5IA (Braudeau et al., 2011) or RO4938581 (Martinez-Cue et al., 2013) had cognitive enhancing effects. In addition, chronic treatment with RO4938581 completely rescued the LTP deficit of trisomic mice.

Because α5 subunit-containing $GABA_A$ receptors are predominantly localized extrasynaptically, mediate tonic inhibition (Glykys and Mody, 2006) and regulate the excitability of hippocampal pyramidal neurons by influencing the strength of depolarization required to generate an action potential (Bonin et al., 2007), $GABA_A$ α5-containing receptors are likely to modulate long-term synaptic plasticity and may be a mechanism whereby RO4938581 treatment rescues cognitive deficits in Ts65Dn mice.

In addition, the increased density of the GABAergic synapse markers GAD65, GAD67 and VGAT in the molecular layer of the hippocampus of Ts65Dn mice was normalized by chronic RO4938581 administration (Martinez-Cue et al., 2013). Because numerous studies have shown that TS mice display morphological and functional alterations in inhibitory circuitries in the hippocampus and cerebral cortex (Begenisic et al., 2011; Belichenko et al., 2009b; Belichenko et al., 2004; Chakrabarti et al., 2010; Perez-Cremades et al., 2010), it is possible that RO4938581 rescued cognitive deficits in TS mice by normalizing the number and/or function of inhibitory synapses and, therefore, re-established circuit inhibitory/excitatory balance and neuroplasticity.

Finally, the normalization of adult cell proliferation and survival in the hippocampal Ts65Dn dentate gyrus achieved after chronic treatment with RO4938581 could also be a mechanism underlying the pro-cognitive effects of this NAM (see below).

In the next sections, we will review the evidence that suggests a common mechanism underlying the cognitive enhancing-effects of drugs acting upon the GABA neurotransmitter system and drugs acting upon other targets. We propose here an enhancement of hippocampal neurogenesis as a putative common mechanism in many of the cases.

## 3. NEUROGENESIS

### 3.1. Neurogenesis and Down Syndrome

Neurogenesis is severely compromised in DS from early developmental stages due to impaired neuronal precursor proliferation, slowing of the cell cycle and altered differentiation (Contestabile et al., 2007; Guidi et al., 2008). In Ts65Dn mice, reduced neural precursor proliferation is also found in the neocortical ventricular zone (VZ) and in CA3 during embryonic stages (Chakrabarti et al., 2007) and in early postnatal life in the DG (Contestabile et al., 2007). In addition, alterations in neural differentiation are also a hallmark in the developing Ts65Dn mouse brain (Bartesaghi et al., 2011; Rueda et al., 2012b).

Adult hippocampal neurogenesis has been demonstrated in many species, including humans and rodents (Kempermann et al., 2002; Kempermann et al., 1997; van Praag et al., 1999b; van Praag et al., 2002). During the entire life span, cell proliferation takes place in the subventricular zone (SVZ) and in the subgranular zone (SGZ) of the DG where a pool of multipotent progenitor cells is located. In the SGZ, newborn neurons migrate into the granular cell layer and establish functional connections in the dentate molecular region where they receive excitatory synaptic input from perforant path afferents (van Praag et al., 2002). Increasing evidence indicates that adult hippocampal neurogenesis is implicated in the establishment of LTP and has a role in hippocampal-dependent learning and memory (Bianchi et al., 2010a; Malberg et al., 2000; Shors et al., 2002). Therefore, the neurogenesis impairment found in DS and in brains of Ts65Dn mice is likely to be one of the mechanisms responsible for their widespread hypocellularity leading to altered synaptogenesis, connectivity, synaptic plasticity and cognitive disabilities.

Consistent with the notion of the role of adult hippocampal neurogenesis in cognitive processes, in the last few years several drugs have been demonstrated to rescue neurogenesis and cognitive abilities in adult Ts65Dn mice.

### 3.2. GABA and Neurogenesis

It is well established that, in addition to its classical inhibitory role, GABA is an important signal modulating the development of the CNS. The high equilibrium potential for $Cl^-$ in neuroblasts causes GABA, acting through $GABA_A$ receptors, to depolarize, rather than hyperpolarize, young neurons (Pathania et al., 2010). The GABAergic depolarization mediates essential functions during the development of the nervous system (Ben-Ari, 2002; Wang and Kriegstein, 2009). During prenatal stages, GABA regulates different steps of adult neurogenesis, including proliferation of neural progenitors (Represa and Ben-Ari, 2005), migration (Manent et al., 2005), differentiation of neuroblasts (Markwardt and Overstreet-Wadiche, 2008; Marty and Llano, 2005) and synaptic integration of newborn neurons (Cancedda et al., 2007; Wang and Kriegstein, 2008).

Therefore, it is possible that the reduced levels of GABA found in DS brains during pre- and early post-natal stages might be implicated in the altered neurogenesis and neuromorphological anomalies that they display (Bartesaghi et al., 2011).

Adult-born neurons go through the same sequence of developmental milestones as those in the developing CNS (Ge et al., 2006). In the adult hippocampus, neural progenitors and newborn neurons initially receive exclusively GABAergic synaptic input, and the depolarizing actions of GABA contribute to activity-dependent regulation (Gaiarsa and Porcher, 2013; Markwardt and Overstreet-Wadiche, 2008). In adult mice, treatment with a $GABA_A$ receptor antagonist increases proliferation of neuronal progenitors in the hippocampal subgranular zone (SGZ), while treatment with a $GABA_A$ receptor agonist decreases proliferation and promotes neuronal differentiation via its GABA-mediated excitation (Tozuka et al., 2005). Therefore, GABAergic inputs to hippocampal progenitor cells promote activity-dependent neuronal differentiation. In addition, GABA regulates the synaptic integration of newly generated neurons in the adult brain (Ge et al., 2006).

Although most of the trophic actions of GABA have been attributed to the activation of $GABA_A$ receptors, $GABA_B$ receptors also play an important role regulating network development, including cell migration, differentiation and synaptogenesis (Gaiarsa and Porcher, 2013).

Therefore, GABA transmission acting through both $GABA_A$ and $GABA_B$ receptors modulates neuronal network formation by modifying cell survival and migration, neuritic growth and guidance, synapse formation and maturation.

## 3.3. Is Neurogenesis the Common Mechanism Responsible for the Cognitive-Enhancing Effects of Therapeutic Strategies Targeting Different Neurotransmitter Systems?

In the last few years, several pharmacological, genetic and behavioral therapeutic strategies targeting different neurotransmitter systems have proven to have cognitive-enhancing effects that correlate with the normalization of neurogenesis and LTP in Ts65Dn mice. Here, we summarize the data that suggest that the enhancement of neurogenesis, possibly through the direct or indirect action upon the GABAergic system, could be a common mechanism underlying the pro-cognitive effects of the different treatments.

### *3.3.1. GABA*

As discussed in the previous section, because GABA activity is known to regulate neuronal proliferation, migration, differentiation and integration of newly generated neurons (Earnheart et al., 2007; Ge et al., 2006; Tozuka et al., 2005), the alterations in GABA transmission in the Ts65Dn mouse could be partially responsible for the neurogenesis deficits in this mouse model of DS.

The first evidence of the implication of over-inhibition on the alterations in neurogenesis found in the Ts65Dn mouse was reported by Chakrabarti et al. (2010). These investigators demonstrated the involvement of the *Olig1* and *Olig2* genes, which encode transcription factors that play a role in neurogenesis and oligodendrogenesis (Lu et al., 2002; Takebayashi et al., 2000; Zhou and Anderson, 2002) in the regulation of the number of inhibitory neurons during embryonic development of the Ts65Dn mouse. These genes are overexpressed in DS and in the Ts65Dn mouse, and normalization of *Olig1* and *Olig2* expression in Ts65Dn mice rescued the abnormal interneuron production and the balance between excitatory and inhibitory transmission (Chakrabarti et al., 2010).

In addition, pharmacologically reducing GABA-mediated over-inhibition by chronically administering the α5-selective NAM RO4938581 fully restored the density of proliferating cells and of mature granule cells in the DG of Ts65Dn mice. Because both newborn and mature neurons are implicated in hippocampal-dependent learning and memory, the restoration of proliferation and of the density of mature neurons is likely to be involved in the cognitive-enhancing effects of RO4938581 in TS mice (Martinez-Cue et al., 2013).

In addition, *GIRK* channel overexpression may also be involved in the altered neurogenesis found in Ts65Dn mice, because chronic treatment with a GIRK channel antagonist increased neurogenesis of hippocampal neurons to levels comparable to those of euploid mice (Kobayashi et al., 2003).

### *3.3.2. Serotonin*

The $5\text{-}HT_{1A}$ receptor has also been implicated in the regulation of neurogenesis (Encinas et al., 2006; Malberg et al., 2000; Santarelli et al., 2003). Reduced levels of the $5\text{-}HT_{1A}$ receptor have been reported in the DS brain at birth (Bar-Peled et al., 1991), in hippocampal neurospheres and in the hippocampus of newborn Ts65Dn mice (Bianchi et al., 2010b). Thus, reduced $5\text{-}HT_{1A}$ receptor expression may also partially underlie the defective neurogenesis found in Ts65Dn mice (Bianchi et al., 2010b).

The selective serotonin reuptake inhibitor fluoxetine is an antidepressant that has been shown to increase neurogenesis in the mouse DG and SVZ (Malberg et al., 2000; Shankaran et al., 2006). Chronic treatment with fluoxetine restored proliferation in the DG and SVZ, differentiation and survival. Furthermore, this treatment restored brain derived neurotrophic factor (BDNF) expression, total granule cell number and had a pro-cognitive effect (Bianchi et al., 2010b). Moreover, a recent report (Begenisic et al., 2014) demonstrated that fluoxetine administration normalizes GABA release and rescues hippocampal synaptic plasticity in Ts65Dn mice. Several reports have demonstrated in other animal models that the enhancement of 5-HT release induced by this antidepressant is accompanied by reduced levels of GABAergic inhibition (Hajszan et al., 2005; Li et al., 2010; Malberg et al., 2000; Maya Vetencourt et al., 2008). 5-HT inhibits GABA release in interneurons via a presynaptic mechanism mediated by $5\text{-}HT_{1/2}$ receptor families (Koyama et al., 1999; Xiang and Prince, 2003), most likely regulating the availability of transmitter vesicles (Wang and Zucker, 1998).

Fluoxetine modulates GABA release in the hippocampus independently of evoked IPSCs (Méndez et al., 2012). Thus, it is possible that the two mechanisms, i.e., a modulation of GABA release promoted by increased levels of 5-HT and a direct action of fluoxetine at GABAergic synapses, may converge together to promote a normalization of the excessive inhibition state in the hippocampal circuitries of Ts65Dn mice. Although it cannot be excluded that fluoxetine might improve memory and synaptic plasticity through other mechanisms such as enhancement of neurogenesis and/or increased BDNF expression.

### 3.3.3. Noradrenaline

Noradrenaline (NA) has also been shown to play a role in neurogenesis, as neuron proliferation is enhanced or impaired following increases or reductions in NA transmission, respectively (Duman et al., 2001). Therefore, altered NA transmission in the trisomic condition (Bartesaghi et al., 2011; Rueda et al., 2012b) may also play a role in the impairment of adult hippocampal neurogenesis.

There is evidence linking $GABA_B$ receptors to the activity of the noradrenergic system. Administration of a $GABA_B$ receptor antagonist induces downregulation of β-adrenoceptors (Bowery, 1993; Pratt and Bowery, 1993). In addition, $GABA_A$ and $GABA_B$ receptors are involved in the control of NA release in the median preoptic nucleus (Sakamaki et al., 2003).

Noradrenergic afferents from the locus coeruleus to hippocampal neurons have a role in contextual learning (Murchison et al., 2004), a cognitive process impaired in individuals with DS (Nadel, 2003) and in Ts65Dn mice (Salehi et al., 2009). Salehi et al. (2009) demonstrated that enhancing NA transmission through the administration of L-threo-3,4-dihydroxyphenylserine (L-DOPS), a synthetic amino acid that is metabolized by NA-containing neurons to produce NA, or xamoterol, a ß1-adrenergic receptor partial agonist, rescued contextual learning in Ts65Dn mice. These authors hypothesized that, given that NA can activate or inhibit GABAergic neurons and that GABA can increase the release of NA, there could be an overlap in the mechanisms by which $GABA_A$ antagonists and NA-enhancing drugs improve learning in Ts65Dn mice.

### 3.3.4. Neurotrophins

Neurotrophic factors promote neuronal survival, neurite outgrowth and synaptic plasticity (Campenot and MacInnis, 2004; Chao et al., 2006; Sofroniew et al., 2001). Consequently, alterations in their expression may alter many aspects of neurodevelopment.

Reduced expression of Brain Derived Neurotrophic factor (BDNF) has been reported in the hippocampus and cortices of DS fetuses (Guedj et al., 2009; Toiber et al., 2010) and in young and adult Ts65Dn mice (Bianchi et al., 2010b; Bimonte-Nelson et al., 2003; Fukuda et al., 2010).

Fukuda et al. (2010) demonstrated that the chronic administration of the analgesic neurotropin to Ts65Dn mice prevents the age-dependent decline in hippocampal BDNF expression. This treatment also enhanced the cognitive abilities of trisomic mice. Because the analgesic action of neurotropin is mediated by the noradrenergic and GABAergic systems (Hata et al., 1988), its cognitive-enhancing effects in Ts65Dn mice could also be determined by improvements in the function of these transmitter systems.

### 3.3.5. Environmental Enrichment

Active care programs are one of the most successful therapeutic interventions used in DS individuals. In rodents, environmental enrichment has been associated with morphological, physiological and cognitive improvements. These changes include increases in cortical weight and thickness, hippocampal neurogenesis, dendritic branching, length, number and size of dendritic spines (Greenough et al., 1973; Nilsson et al., 1999; van Praag et al., 1999a), facilitation of LTP (Hargreaves et al., 1992; Paylor et al., 1992) and more efficient learning (Boehm et al., 1996; Kolb et al., 1983; Schwartz, 1964).

In the Ts65Dn mouse, environmental enrichment has been shown to improve cognitive abilities, enhance adult hippocampal neurogenesis and LTP (Chakrabarti et al., 2011; Martínez-Cué et al., 2002). Interestingly, environmental enrichment also reduces the release of GABA in the hippocampus and visual cortex of Ts65Dn mice (Begenisic et al., 2011). Therefore, these studies provide support for the hypothesis of the interplay between GABAergic over-inhibition, neurogenesis alterations and cognitive deficits in Ts65Dn mice.

## Conclusion

Most of the knowledge we have gained in the last few years about the neurobiological correlations of the altered cognitive abilities found in DS comes from studies performed in mouse models, especially in the Ts65Dn mouse. Based on these studies, two main mechanisms have been proposed to underlie DS impaired cognition: i) the hypocellularity found in different brain areas due to altered neurogenesis and ii) enhanced inhibition.

Enhanced inhibition might be directly compromising Ts65Dn cognitive abilities by altering synaptic efficacy. In addition, the altered GABAergic activity might play a role in the reduced neurogenesis found in DS and in the Ts65Dn mouse. Alterations in GABAergic activity during pre- and early post-natal stages might be responsible for the impairments in neural development and, during later life stages; they might be altering synaptic plasticity and adult hippocampal neurogenesis that would also lead to altered learning and memory. In addition, GABA-mediated over-inhibition might be directly responsible for the functional alterations found during adulthood and indirectly, it could be affecting the function of different transmitter systems that also play a role in the neuromorphological and behavioral DS phenotypes.

However, although there is a wide body of evidence demonstrating the neuromorphological alterations in both DS individuals and in mouse models of DS, so far GABA-mediated over-inhibition during adulthood has only been demonstrated in mouse models. Therefore, there is a need to confirm that this phenotype, which is consistently found in the Ts65Dn mouse, is also a hallmark in DS brains.

Finally, in the last few years, much attention has been provided to different therapeutic strategies targeting over-inhibition, neuromorphological alterations or changes in the function of different transmitter systems or molecular pathways. Many of them have proven to enhance learning and memory in the Ts65Dn mouse. Because in many cases, their targets are apparently unrelated, and most of them improve cognitive abilities in these mice, an effort should be made to elucidate whether there is a common mechanism inducing their pro-cognitive effect or whether the observed improvements are unrelated.

## References

Atack JR, Bayley PJ, Seabrook GR, Wafford KA, McKernan RM, Dawson GR (2006) L-655,708 enhances cognition in rats but is not proconvulsant at a dose selective for alpha5-containing GABAA receptors. *Neuropharmacology,* 51: 1023-1029.

Ballard TM, Knoflach F, Prinssen E, Borroni E, Vivian JA, Basile J, Gasser R, Moreau JL, Wettstein JG, Buettelmann B, et al. (2009) RO4938581, a novel cognitive enhancer acting at GABAA alpha5 subunit-containing receptors. *Psychopharmacology (Berl)* 202: 207-223.

Bar-Peled O, Gross-Isseroff R, Ben-Hur H, Hoskins I, Groner Y, Biegon A (1991) Fetal human brain exhibits a prenatal peak in the density of serotonin 5-HT1A receptors. *Neurosci. Lett.,* 127: 173-176.

Bartesaghi R, Guidi S, Ciani E (2011) Is it possible to improve neurodevelopmental abnormalities in Down syndrome? *Rev. Neurosci.,* 22: 419-455.

Begenisic T, Baroncelli L, Sansevero G, Milanese M, Bonifacino T, Bonanno G, Cioni G, Maffei L, Sale A (2014) Fluoxetine in adulthood normalizes GABA release and rescues hippocampal synaptic plasticity and spatial memory in a mouse model of Down syndrome. *Neurobiol. Dis.,* 63: 12-19.

Begenisic T, Spolidoro M, Braschi C, Baroncelli L, Milanese M, Pietra G, Fabbri ME, Bonanno G, Cioni G, Maffei L, et al. (2011) Environmental enrichment decreases GABAergic inhibition and improves cognitive abilities, synaptic plasticity, and visual functions in a mouse model of Down syndrome. *Front Cell Neurosci.,* 5: 29.

Belichenko NP, Belichenko PV, Kleschevnikov AM, Salehi A, Reeves RH, Mobley WC (2009a) The "Down syndrome critical region" is sufficient in the mouse model to confer behavioral, neurophysiological, and synaptic phenotypes characteristic of Down syndrome. *J. Neurosci.,* 29: 5938-5948.

Belichenko PV, Kleschevnikov AM, Masliah E, Wu C, Takimoto-Kimura R, Salehi A, Mobley WC (2009b) Excitatory-inhibitory relationship in the fascia dentata in the Ts65Dn mouse model of Down syndrome. *J. Comp. Neurol.,* 512: 453-466.

Belichenko PV, Kleschevnikov AM, Salehi A, Epstein CJ, Mobley WC (2007) Synaptic and cognitive abnormalities in mouse models of Down syndrome: exploring genotype-phenotype relationships. *J. Comp. Neurol.,* 504: 329-345.

Belichenko PV, Masliah E, Kleschevnikov AM, Villar AJ, Epstein CJ, Salehi A, Mobley WC (2004) Synaptic structural abnormalities in the Ts65Dn mouse model of Down Syndrome. *J. Comp. Neurol.,* 480: 281-298.

Ben-Ari Y (2002) Excitatory actions of gaba during development: the nature of the nurture. *Nat. Rev. Neurosci.,* 3: 728-739.

Best TK, Cramer NP, Chakrabarti L, Haydar TF, Galdzicki Z (2012) Dysfunctional hippocampal inhibition in the Ts65Dn mouse model of Down syndrome. *Exp. Neurol.,* 233: 749-757.

Best TK, Siarey RJ, Galdzicki Z (2007) Ts65Dn, a mouse model of Down syndrome, exhibits increased GABAB-induced potassium current. *J. Neurophysiol.,* 97: 892-900.

Bhattacharyya A, McMillan E, Chen SI, Wallace K, Svendsen CN (2009) A critical period in cortical interneuron neurogenesis in down syndrome revealed by human neural progenitor cells. *Dev. Neurosci.,* 31: 497-510.

Bianchi P, Ciani E, Contestabile A, Guidi S, Bartesaghi R (2010a) Lithium restores neurogenesis in the subventricular zone of the Ts65Dn mouse, a model for Down syndrome. *Brain Pathol.,* 20: 106-118.

Bianchi P, Ciani E, Guidi S, Trazzi S, Felice D, Grossi G, Fernandez M, Giuliani A, Calzà L, Bartesaghi R (2010b) Early pharmacotherapy restores neurogenesis and cognitive performance in the Ts65Dn mouse model for Down syndrome. *J. Neurosci.,* 30: 8769-8779.

Bimonte-Nelson HA, Hunter CL, Nelson ME, Granholm AC (2003) Frontal cortex BDNF levels correlate with working memory in an animal model of Down syndrome. *Behav. Brain Res.,* 139: 47-57.

Boehm GW, Sherman GF, Hoplight BJ, Hyde LA, Waters NS, Bradway DM, Galaburda AM, Denenberg VH (1996) Learning and memory in the autoimmune BXSB mouse: effects of neocortical ectopias and environmental enrichment. *Brain Res.,* 726: 11-22.

Bonin RP, Martin LJ, MacDonald JF, Orser BA (2007) Alpha5GABAA receptors regulate the intrinsic excitability of mouse hippocampal pyramidal neurons. *J. Neurophysiol.,* 98: 2244-2254.

Bonnert TP, McKernan RM, Farrar S, le Bourdelles B, Heavens RP, Smith DW, Hewson L, Rigby MR, Sirinathsinghji DJ, Brown N, et al. (1999) theta, a novel gamma-aminobutyric acid type A receptor subunit. *Proc. Natl. Acad. Sci. USA,.* 96: 9891-9896.

Bowery NG (1993) GABAB receptor pharmacology. *Annu. Rev. Pharmacol. Toxicol.,* 33: 109-147.

Braudeau J, Delatour B, Duchon A, Pereira PL, Dauphinot L, de Chaumont F, Olivo-Marin JC, Dodd RH, Herault Y, Potier MC (2011) Specific targeting of the GABA-A receptor alpha5 subtype by a selective inverse agonist restores cognitive deficits in Down syndrome mice. *J. Psychopharmacol.,* 25: 1030-1042.

Brun VH, Otnass MK, Molden S, Steffenach HA, Witter MP, Moser MB, Moser EI (2002) Place cells and place recognition maintained by direct entorhinal-hippocampal circuitry. *Science,* 296: 2243-2246.

Campenot RB, MacInnis BL (2004) Retrograde transport of neurotrophins: fact and function. *J. Neurobiol.,* 58: 217-229.

Cancedda L, Fiumelli H, Chen K, Poo MM (2007) Excitatory GABA action is essential for morphological maturation of cortical neurons in vivo. *J. Neurosci.,* 27: 5224-5235.

Caraiscos VB, Elliott EM, You-Ten KE, Cheng VY, Belelli D, Newell JG, Jackson MF, Lambert JJ. Rosahl TW, Wafford KA, et al. (2004) Tonic inhibition in mouse hippocampal CA1 pyramidal neurons is mediated by alpha5 subunit-containing gamma-aminobutyric acid type A receptors. *Proc. Natl. Acad. Sci. USA,* 101: 3662-3667.

Carlesimo GA, Marotta L, Vicari S (1997) Long-term memory in mental retardation: evidence for a specific impairment in subjects with Down's syndrome. *Neuropsychologia,* 35: 71-79.

Chakrabarti L, Best TK, Cramer NP, Carney RS, Isaac JT, Galdzicki Z, Haydar TF (2010) Olig1 and Olig2 triplication causes developmental brain defects in Down syndrome. *Nat. Neurosci.,* 13: 927-934.

Chakrabarti L, Galdzicki Z, Haydar TF (2007) Defects in embryonic neurogenesis and initial synapse formation in the forebrain of the Ts65Dn mouse model of Down syndrome. *J. Neurosci.,* 27: 11483-11495.

Chakrabarti L, Scafidi J, Gallo V, Haydar TF (2011) Environmental enrichment rescues postnatal neurogenesis defect in the male and female Ts65Dn mouse model of Down syndrome. *Dev. Neurosci.,* 33: 428-441.

Chambers MS, Atack JR, Carling RW, Collinson N, Cook SM, Dawson GR, Ferris P, Hobbs SC, O'Connor D, Marshall G, et al. (2004) An orally bioavailable, functionally selective inverse agonist at the benzodiazepine site of GABAA alpha5 receptors with cognition enhancing properties. *J. Med. Chem.,* 47: 5829-5832.

Chao MV, Rajagopal R, Lee FS (2006) Neurotrophin signalling in health and disease. *Clin. Sci. (Lond).* 110: 167-173.

Chapman RS, Hesketh LJ (2000) Behavioral phenotype of individuals with Down syndrome. *Ment. Retard. Dev. Disabil. Res. Rev.,* 6: 84-95.

Cole, S.O. (1986) Effects of benzodiazepines on acquisition and performance: a critical assessment. *Neurosci. Biobehav. Rev.,* 10: 265-272.

Collinson N, Atack JR, Laughton P, Dawson GR, Stephens DN (2006) An inverse agonist selective for alpha5 subunit-containing GABAA receptors improves encoding and recall but not consolidation in the Morris water maze. *Psychopharmacology (Berl).* 188: 619-628.

Collinson N, Kuenzi FM, Jarolimek W, Maubach KA, Cothliff R, Sur C, Smith A, Otu FM, Howell O, Atack JR, et al. (2002) Enhanced learning and memory and altered GABAergic synaptic transmission in mice lacking the alpha 5 subunit of the GABAA receptor. *J. Neurosci.,* 22: 5572-5580.

Contestabile A, Fila T, Ceccarelli C, Bonasoni P, Bonapace L, Santini D, Bartesaghi R, Ciani E (2007) Cell cycle alteration and decreased cell proliferation in the hippocampal dentate gyrus and in the neocortical germinal matrix of fetuses with Down syndrome and in Ts65Dn mice. *Hippocampus,* 17: 665-678.

Cramer NP, Best TK, Stoffel M. Siarey RJ, Galdzicki Z (2010) GABAB-GIRK2-mediated signaling in Down syndrome. *Adv. Pharmacol.,* 58: 397-426.

Crestani F, Keist R, Fritschy JM, Benke D, Vogt K, Prut L, Blüthmann H, Möhler H, Rudolph U (2002) Trace fear conditioning involves hippocampal alpha5 GABA(A) receptors. *Proc. Natl. Acad. Sci. USA,* 99: 8980-8985.

Dawson GR, Maubach KA, Collinson N, Cobain M, Everitt BJ, MacLeod AM, Choudhury HI, McDonald LM, Pillai G, Rycroft W, et al. (2006) An inverse agonist selective for alpha5 subunit-containing GABAA receptors enhances cognition. *J. Pharmacol. Exp. Ther.,* 316: 1335-1345.

del Cerro S, Jung M, Lynch G (1992) Benzodiazepines block long-term potentiation in slices of hippocampus and piriform cortex. *Neuroscience,* 49: 1-6.

Doischer D, Hosp JA, Yanagawa Y, Obata K, Jonas P, Vida I, Bartos M (2008) Postnatal differentiation of basket cells from slow to fast signaling devices. *J. Neurosci.,* 28: 12956-12968.

Dorow R, Horowski R, Paschelke G, Amin M (1983) Severe anxiety induced by FG 7142, a beta-carboline ligand for benzodiazepine receptors. *Lancet,* 2: 98-99.

Driscoll LL, Carroll JC, Moon J, Crnic LS, Levitsky DA, Strupp BJ (2004) Impaired sustained attention and error-induced stereotypy in the aged Ts65Dn mouse: a mouse model of Down syndrome and Alzheimer's disease. *Behav. Neurosci.,* 118: 1196-1205.

Duman RS, Nakagawa S, Malberg J (2001) Regulation of adult neurogenesis by antidepressant treatment. *Neuropsychopharmacology,* 25: 836-844.

Earnheart JC, Schweizer C, Crestani F, Iwasato T, Itohara S, Mohler H, Luscher B. (2007) GABAergic control of adult hippocampal neurogenesis in relation to behavior indicative of trait anxiety and depression states. *J. Neurosci.,* 27: 3845-3854.

Encinas JM, Vaahtokari A, Enikolopov G (2006) Fluoxetine targets early progenitor cells in the adult brain. Pr*oc. Natl. Acad. Sci. USA,* 103: 8233-8238.

Escorihuela RM, Vallina IF, Martinez-Cue C, Baamonde C, Dierssen M, Tobena A, Florez J, Fernandez-Teruel A (1998) Impaired short- and long-term memory in Ts65Dn mice, a model for Down syndrome. *Neurosci. Lett.,* 247: 171-174.

Fernandez F, Morishita W, Zuniga E, Nguyen J, Blank M, Malenka RC, Garner CC (2007) Pharmacotherapy for cognitive impairment in a mouse model of Down syndrome. *Nat. Neurosci.,* 10: 411-413.

Fernandez F, Trinidad JC, Blank M, Feng DD, Burlingame AL, Garner CC (2009) Normal protein composition of synapses in Ts65Dn mice: a mouse model of Down syndrome. *J. Neurochem.,* 110: 157-169.

Fritschy JM, Mohler H (1995) GABAA-receptor heterogeneity in the adult rat brain: differential regional and cellular distribution of seven major subunits. *J. Comp. Neurol.,* 359: 154-194.

Fukuda Y, Berry TL, Nelson M, Hunter CL, Fukuhara K, Imai H, Ito S, Granholm-Bentley AC, Kaplan AP, Mutoh T (2010) Stimulated neuronal expression of brain-derived neurotrophic factor by Neurotropin. *Mol. Cell Neurosci.,* 45: 226-233.

Gaiarsa JL, Porcher C (2013) Emerging neurotrophic role of GABAB receptors in neuronal circuit development. *Front Cell Neurosci.,* 7: 206.

Ge S, Goh EL, Sailor KA, Kitabatake Y, Ming GL, Song H (2006) GABA regulates synaptic integration of newly generated neurons in the adult brain. *Nature,* 439: 589-593.

Ghoneim MM, Mewaldt SP (1990) Benzodiazepines and human memory: a review. *Anesthesiology,* 72: 926-938.

Glykys J, Mody I (2006) Hippocampal network hyperactivity after selective reduction of tonic inhibition in GABAA receptor alpha5 subunit-deficient mice. *J. Neurophysiol.,* 95: 2796-2807.

Godridge H, Reynolds GP, Czudek C, Calcutt NA, Benton M (1987) Alzheimer-like neurotransmitter deficits in adult Down's syndrome brain tissue. *J. Neurol. Neurosurg. Psychiatry,* 50: 775-778.

Greenough WT, Volkmar FR, Juraska JM (1973) Effects of rearing complexity on dendritic branching in frontolateral and temporal cortex of the rat. *Exp. Neurol.,* 41: 371-378.

Guedj F, Sébrié C, Rivals I, Ledru A, Paly E, Bizot JC, Smith D, Rubin E, Gillet B, Arbones M, et al. (2009) Green tea polyphenols rescue of brain defects induced by overexpression of DYRK1A. *PLoS One.* 4: e4606.

Guidi S, Bonasoni P, Ceccarelli C, Santini D, Gualtieri F, Ciani E, Bartesaghi R (2008) Neurogenesis impairment and increased cell death reduce total neuron number in the hippocampal region of fetuses with Down syndrome. *Brain Pathol.,* 18: 180-197.

Hajszan T, MacLusky NJ, Leranth C (2005) Short-term treatment with the antidepressant fluoxetine triggers pyramidal dendritic spine synapse formation in rat hippocampus. *Eur. J. Neurosci.,* 21: 1299-1303.

Hanson JE, Blank M, Valenzuela RA, Garner CC, Madison DV (2007) The functional nature of synaptic circuitry is altered in area CA3 of the hippocampus in a mouse model of Down's syndrome. *J. Physiol.,* 579: 53-67.

Hargreaves EL, Boon F, Cain DP (1992) Rats housed in a complex environment exhibit greater hilar LTP tan individually housed littermates. In Society for Neuroscience - Abstracts. p. abstract: 344.

Hata T, Kita T, Itoh E, Oyama R, Kawabata A (1988) Mechanism of the analgesic effect of neurotropin. *Jpn. J. Pharmacol.,* 48: 165-173.

Haydar TF, Reeves RH (2012) Trisomy 21 and early brain development. *Trends Neurosci.,* 35: 81-91.

Huang W, Galdzicki Z, van Gelderen P, Balbo A, Chikhale EG, Schapiro MB, Rapoport, SI (2000) Brain myo-inositol level is elevated in Ts65Dn mouse and reduced after lithium treatment. *Neuroreport,* 11: 445-448.

Jensen S, Kirkegaard L, Anderson BN (1987) Randomized clinical investigation of Ro 15-1788, a benzodiazepine antagonist, in reversing the central effects of flunitrazepam. *Eur. J. Anaesthesiol.,* 4: 113-118.

Kempermann G, Gast D, Gage FH (2002) Neuroplasticity in old age: sustained fivefold induction of hippocampal neurogenesis by long-term environmental enrichment. *Ann. Neurol.,* 52: 135-143.

Kempermann G, Kuhn HG, Gage FH (1997) More hippocampal neurons in adult mice living in an enriched environment. *Nature,* 386: 493-495.

Kilb W (2012) Development of the GABAergic system from birth to adolescence. *Neuroscientist,* 18: 613-630.

Klausberger T (2009) GABAergic interneurons targeting dendrites of pyramidal cells in the CA1 area of the hippocampus. *Eur. J. Neurosci.,* 30: 947-957.

Kleschevnikov AM, Belichenko PV, Faizi M, Jacobs LF, Htun K, Shamloo M, Mobley WC (2012a) Deficits in cognition and synaptic plasticity in a mouse model of Down syndrome ameliorated by GABAB receptor antagonists. *J. Neurosci.,* 32: 9217-9227.

Kleschevnikov AM, Belichenko PV, Gall J, George L, Nosheny R, Maloney MT, Salehi A, Mobley WC (2012b) Increased efficiency of the GABAA and GABAB receptor-mediated neurotransmission in the Ts65Dn mouse model of Down syndrome. *Neurobiol. Dis.,* 45: 683-691.

Kleschevnikov AM, Belichenko PV, Villar AJ, Epstein CJ, Malenka RC, Mobley WC (2004) Hippocampal long-term potentiation suppressed by increased inhibition in the Ts65Dn mouse, a genetic model of Down syndrome. *J. Neurosci.,* 24: 8153-8160.

Kobayashi T, Washiyama K, Ikeda K (2003) Inhibition of G protein-activated inwardly rectifying K+ channels by fluoxetine (Prozac). *Br. J. Pharmacol.,* 138: 1119-1128.

Kolb B, Sutherland RJ, Whishaw IQ (1983) A comparison of the contributions of the frontal and parietal association cortex to spatial localization in rats. Behav Neurosci. 97: 13-27.

Koyama S, Kubo C, Rhee JS, Akaike N (1999) Presynaptic serotonergic inhibition of GABAergic synaptic transmission in mechanically dissociated rat basolateral amygdala neurons. *J. Physiol.,* 518 ( Pt 2): 525-538.

Kurt MA, Kafa MI, Dierssen M, Davies DC (2004) Deficits of neuronal density in CA1 and synaptic density in the dentate gyrus, CA3 and CA1, in a mouse model of Down syndrome. *Brain Res.,* 1022: 101-109.

Laurie DJ, Wisden W, Seeburg PH (1992) The distribution of thirteen GABAA receptor subunit mRNAs in the rat brain. III. Embryonic and postnatal development. *J. Neurosci.,* 12: 4151-4172.

Li IH, Huang WS, Shiue CY, Huang YY, Liu RS, Chyueh SC, Hu SH, Liao MH, Shen LH, Liu JC, et al. (2010) Study on the neuroprotective effect of fluoxetine against MDMA-induced neurotoxicity on the serotonin transporter in rat brain using micro-PET. *Neuroimage,* 49: 1259-1270.

Lingford-Hughes A, Hume SP, Feeney A, Hirani E, Osman S, Cunningham VJ, Pike VW, Brooks DJ, Nutt DJ (2002) Imaging the GABA-benzodiazepine receptor subtype containing the alpha5-subunit in vivo with [11C]Ro15 4513 positron emission tomography. *J. Cereb. Blood Flow Metab.,* 22: 878-889.

Lister RG (1985) The amnesic action of benzodiazepines in man. *Neurosci. Biobehav. Rev.,* 9: 87-94.

Lockstone HE, Harris LW, Swatton JE, Wayland MT, Holland AJ, Bahn S (2007) Gene expression profiling in the adult Down syndrome brain. *Genomics,* 90: 647-660.

Lu QR, Sun T, Zhu Z, Ma N, Garcia M, Stiles CD, Rowitch DH (2002) Common developmental requirement for Olig function indicates a motor neuron/oligodendrocyte connection. *Cell,* 109: 75-86.

Lüscher C, Jan LY, Stoffel M, Malenka RC, Nicoll RA (1997) G protein-coupled inwardly rectifying K+ channels (GIRKs) mediate postsynaptic but not presynaptic transmitter actions in hippocampal neurons. *Neuron,* 19: 687-695.

Macdonald RL, Olsen RW (1994) GABAA receptor channels. *Annu. Rev. Neurosci.,* 17: 569-602.

Malberg JE, Eisch AJ, Nestler EJ, Duman RS (2000) Chronic antidepressant treatment increases neurogenesis in adult rat hippocampus. *J. Neurosci.,* 20: 9104-9110.

Manent JB, Demarque M, Jorquera I, Pellegrino C, Ben-Ari Y, Aniksztejn L, Represa A (2005) A noncanonical release of GABA and glutamate modulates neuronal migration. *J. Neurosci.,* 25: 4755-4765.

Markwardt S, Overstreet-Wadiche L (2008) GABAergic signalling to adult-generated neurons. *J. Physiol.,* 586: 3745-3749.

Martinez-Cue C, Martinez P, Rueda N, Vidal R, Garcia S, Vidal V, Corrales A, Montero JA, Pazos A, Florez J, et al. (2013) Reducing GABAA alpha5 receptor-mediated inhibition rescues functional and neuromorphological deficits in a mouse model of down syndrome. *J. Neurosci.,* 33: 3953-3966.

Martinez-Cue C, Rueda N, Garcia E, Florez J (2006) Anxiety and panic responses to a predator in male and female Ts65Dn mice, a model for Down syndrome. *Genes Brain Behav., 5*: 413-422.

Martínez-Cué C, Baamonde C, Lumbreras M, Paz J, Davisson MT, Schmidt C, Dierssen M, Flórez J (2002) Differential effects of environmental enrichment on behavior and learning of male and female Ts65Dn mice, a model for Down syndrome. *Behav. Brain Res.,* 134: 185-200.

Martínez-Cué C, Delatour B, Potier MC (2014) Treating enhanced GABAergic inhibition in Down syndrome: Use of GABA α5-selective inverse agonists. *Neurosci. Biobehav. Rev.,* In press.

Marty A, Llano I (2005) Excitatory effects of GABA in established brain networks. Trends *Neurosci.,* 28: 284-289.

Maya Vetencourt JF, Sale A, Viegi A, Baroncelli L, De Pasquale R, O'Leary OF, Castrén E, Maffei L (2008) The antidepressant fluoxetine restores plasticity in the adult visual cortex. *Science,* 320: 385-388.

Mitra A, Blank M, Madison DV (2012) Developmentally altered inhibition in Ts65Dn, a mouse model of Down syndrome. *Brain Res.,* 1440: 1-8.

Mohler H, Fritschy JM, Luscher B, Rudolph U, Benson J, Benke D (1996) The GABAA receptors. From subunits to diverse functions. Ion Channels. 4: 89-113.

Murchison CF, Zhang XY, Zhang WP, Ouyang M, Lee A, Thomas SA (2004) A distinct role for norepinephrine in memory retrieval. *Cell,* 117: 131-143.

Méndez P, Pazienti A, Szabó G, Bacci A (2012) Direct alteration of a specific inhibitory circuit of the hippocampus by antidepressants. *J. Neurosci.,* 32: 16616-16628.

Nadel L (2003) Down's syndrome: a genetic disorder in biobehavioral perspective. *Genes Brain Behav,* 2: 156-166.

Nilsson M, Perfilieva E, Johansson U, Orwar O, Eriksson PS (1999) Enriched environment increases neurogenesis in the adult rat dentate gyrus and improves spatial memory. *J. Neurobiol.,* 39: 569-578.

Nutt DJ, Besson M, Wilson SJ, Dawson GR, Lingford-Hughes AR (2007) Blockade of alcohol's amnestic activity in humans by an alpha5 subtype benzodiazepine receptor inverse agonist. *Neuropharmacology,* 53: 810-820.

O'Doherty A, Ruf S, Mulligan C, Hildreth V, Errington ML, Cooke S, Sesay A, Modino S, Vanes L, Hernandez D, et al. (2005) An aneuploid mouse strain carrying human chromosome 21 with Down syndrome phenotypes. *Science,* 309: 2033-2037.

Okaty BW, Miller MN, Sugino K, Hempel CM, Nelson SB (2009) Transcriptional and electrophysiological maturation of neocortical fast-spiking GABAergic interneurons. *J. Neurosci.,* 29: 7040-7052.

Olsen RW, Bureau M, Khrestchatisky M, MacLennan AJ, Chiang MY, Tobin AJ, Xu W, Jackson M, Sternini C, Brecha N (1990) Isolation of pharmacologically distinct GABA-benzodiazepine receptors by protein chemistry and molecular cloning. *Adv. Biochem. Psychopharmacol.,* 46: 35-49.

Olsen RW, Sieghart W (2009) GABA A receptors: subtypes provide diversity of function and pharmacology. *Neuropharmacology,* 56: 141-148.

Owens,DF, Kriegstein AR (2002) Is there more to GABA than synaptic inhibition? *Nat. Rev. Neurosci., 3*: 715-727.

Pathania M, Yan LD, Bordey A (2010) A symphony of signals conducts early and late stages of adult neurogenesis. *Neuropharmacology,* 58: 865-876.

Paylor R, Morrison SK, Rudy JW, Waltrip LT, Wehner JM (1992) Brief exposure to an enriched environment improves performance on the Morris water task and increases hippocampal cytosolic protein kinase C activity in young rats. *Behav. Brain Res.,* 52: 49-59.

Perez-Cremades D, Hernandez S, Blasco-Ibanez JM, Crespo C, Nacher J, Varea E (2010) Alteration of inhibitory circuits in the somatosensory cortex of Ts65Dn mice, a model for Down's syndrome. *J. Neural. Transm.,* 117: 445-455.

Pham TM, Nurse S, Lacaille JC (1998) Distinct GABAB actions via synaptic and extrasynaptic receptors in rat hippocampus in vitro. *J. Neurophysiol.,* 80: 297-308.

Pollonini G, Gao V, Rabe A, Palminiello S, Albertini G, Alberini CM (2008) Abnormal expression of synaptic proteins and neurotrophin-3 in the Down syndrome mouse model Ts65Dn. *Neuroscience,* 156: 99-106.

Popov VI, Kleschevnikov AM, Klimenko OA, Stewart MG, Belichenko PV (2011) Three-dimensional synaptic ultrastructure in the dentate gyrus and hippocampal area CA3 in the Ts65Dn mouse model of Down syndrome. *J. Comp. Neurol.,* 519, 1338-1354.

Pratt GD, Bowery NG. (1993). Repeated administration of desipramine and a GABAB receptor antagonist, CGP 36742, discretely up-regulates GABAB receptor binding sites in rat frontal cortex. *Br. J. Pharmacol.,* 110: 724-735.

Rabow LE, Russek SJ, Farb DH (1995) From ion currents to genomic analysis: recent advances in GABAA receptor research. *Synapse,* 21: 189-274.

Represa A, Ben-Ari Y (2005) Trophic actions of GABA on neuronal development. *Trends Neurosci.,* 28: 278-283.

Reynolds GP, Warner CE (1988) Amino acid neurotransmitter deficits in adult Down's syndrome brain tissue. *Neurosci. Lett.,* 94: 224-227.

Risser D, Lubec G, Cairns N, Herrera-Marschitz M (1997) Excitatory amino acids and monoamines in parahippocampal gyrus and frontal cortical pole of adults with Down syndrome. *Life Sci.,* 60: 1231-1237.

Ross MH, Galaburda AM, Kemper TL (1984) Down's syndrome: is there a decreased population of neurons? *Neurology,* 34: 909-916.

Rudolph U, Mohler H (2006) GABA-based therapeutic approaches: GABAA receptor subtype functions. *Curr. Opin. Pharmacol.,* 6: 18-23.

Rueda N, Flórez J, Martínez-Cué C (2012) Mouse models of Down syndrome as a tool to unravel the causes of mental disabilities. *Neural Plast.,* 2012: 584071.

Rueda N, Llorens-Martín M, Flórez J, Valdizán E, Banerjee P, Trejo JL, Martínez-Cué C (2010) Memantine normalizes several phenotypic features in the Ts65Dn mouse model of Down syndrome. *J. Alzheimers Dis.,* 21: 277-290.

Sairanen M, Lucas G, Ernfors P, Castrén M, Castrén E (2005) Brain-derived neurotrophic factor and antidepressant drugs have different but coordinated effects on neuronal turnover, proliferation, and survival in the adult dentate gyrus. *J. Neurosci.,* 25: 1089-1094.

Sakamaki K, Nomura M, Hatakenaka S, Miyakubo H, Tanaka J (2003) GABAergic modulation of noradrenaline release in the median preoptic nucleus area in the rat. *Neurosci. Lett.,* 342: 77-80.

Salehi A, Faizi M, Colas D, Valletta J, Laguna J, Takimoto-Kimura R, Kleschevnikov A, Wagner SL, Aisen P, Shamloo M, et al. (2009) Restoration of norepinephrine-modulated contextual memory in a mouse model of Down syndrome. *Sci. Transl Med.,* 1: 7ra17.

Santarelli L, Saxe M, Gross C, Surget A, Battaglia F, Dulawa S, Weisstaub N, Lee J, Duman R, Arancio O, et al. (2003) Requirement of hippocampal neurogenesis for the behavioral effects of antidepressants. *Science,* 301: 805-809.

Sarter M, Bruno JP, Berntson GG (2001) Psychotogenic properties of benzodiazepine receptor inverse agonists. *Psychopharmacology (Berl).* 156: 1-13.

Schwartz S (1964) Effect of neonatal cortical lesions and early environmental factors on adult rat behavior. *J. Comp. Physiol. Psychol.,* 57: 72-77.

Scott-McKean JJ, Costa AC (2011) Exaggerated NMDA mediated LTD in a mouse model of Down syndrome and pharmacological rescuing by memantine. *Learn Mem.,* 18: 774-778.

Seabrook GR, Easter A, Dawson GR, Bowery BJ (1997) Modulation of long-term potentiation in CA1 region of mouse hippocampal brain slices by GABAA receptor benzodiazepine site ligands. *Neuropharmacology,* 36: 823-830.

Serwanski DR, Miralles CP, Christie SB, Mehta AK, Li X, De Blas AL (2006) Synaptic and nonsynaptic localization of GABAA receptors containing the alpha5 subunit in the rat brain. *J. Comp. Neurol.,* 499: 458-470.

Shankaran M, King C, Lee J, Busch R, Wolff M, Hellerstein MK (2006) Discovery of novel hippocampal neurogenic agents by using an in vivo stable isotope labeling technique. *J. Pharmacol. Exp. Ther.,* 319: 1172-1181.

Shin M, Besser LM, Kucik JE, Lu C, Siffel C, Correa A, Collaborative CAMPaS. (2009) Prevalence of Down syndrome among children and adolescents in 10 regions of the United States. *Pediatrics,* 124: 1565-1571.

Shors TJ, Townsend DA, Zhao M, Kozorovitskiy Y, Gould E (2002) Neurogenesis may relate to some but not all types of hippocampal-dependent learning. *Hippocampus,* 12: 578-584.

Siarey RJ, Carlson EJ, Epstein CJ, Balbo A, Rapoport SI, Galdzicki Z (1999) Increased synaptic depression in the Ts65Dn mouse, a model for mental retardation in Down syndrome. *Neuropharmacology,* 38: 1917-1920.

Siddiqui A, Lacroix T, Stasko MR, Scott-McKean JJ, Costa AC, Gardiner KJ (2008) Molecular responses of the Ts65Dn and Ts1Cje mouse models of Down syndrome to MK-801. *Genes Brain Behav.,* 7: 810-820.

Smigielska-Kuzia J, Bockowski L, Sobaniec W, Kulak W, Sendrowski K (2010) Amino acid metabolic processes in the temporal lobes assessed by proton magnetic resonance spectroscopy (1H MRS) in children with Down syndrome. *Pharmacol. Rep.,* 62: 1070-1077.

Smigielska-Kuzia J, Sobaniec W (2007) Brain metabolic profile obtained by proton magnetic resonance spectroscopy HMRS in children with Down syndrome. *Adv. Med. Sci.,* 52 Suppl 1: 183-187.

Sofroniew MV, Howe CL, Mobley WC (2001) Nerve growth factor signaling, neuroprotection, and neural repair. *Annu. Rev. Neurosci.,* 24: 1217-1281.

Sternfeld F, Carling RW, Jelley RA, Ladduwahetty T, Merchant KJ, Moore KW, Reeve AJ, Street LJ, O'Connor D, Sohal B, et al. (2004) Selective, orally active gamma-aminobutyric acidA alpha5 receptor inverse agonists as cognition enhancers. *J. Med. Chem.,* 47: 2176-2179.

Sturgeon X, Gardiner KJ (2011) Transcript catalogs of human chromosome 21 and orthologous chimpanzee and mouse regions. *Mamm Genome.,* 22: 261-271.

Sybirska E, Davachi L, Goldman-Rakic PS (2000) Prominence of direct entorhinal-CA1 pathway activation in sensorimotor and cognitive tasks revealed by 2-DG functional mapping in nonhuman primate. *J. Neurosci.,* 20: 5827-5834.

Szemes M, Davies RL, Garden CL, Usowicz MM (2013) Weaker control of the electrical properties of cerebellar granule cells by tonically active GABAA receptors in the Ts65Dn mouse model of Down's syndrome. *Mol. Brain,* 6: 33.

Takebayashi H, Yoshida S, Sugimori M, Kosako H, Kominami R, Nakafuku M, Nabeshima Y (2000) Dynamic expression of basic helix-loop-helix Olig family members: implication of Olig2 in neuron and oligodendrocyte differentiation and identification of a new member, Olig3. *Mech. Dev.,* 99: 143-148.

Toiber D, Azkona G, Ben-Ari S, Torán N, Soreq H, Dierssen M (2010) Engineering DYRK1A overdosage yields Down syndrome-characteristic cortical splicing aberrations. *Neurobiol. Dis.,* 40: 348-359.

Tozuka Y, Fukuda S, Namba T, Seki T, Hisatsune T (2005) GABAergic excitation promotes neuronal differentiation in adult hippocampal progenitor cells. *Neuron,* 47: 803-815.

van Praag H, Christie BR, Sejnowski TJ, Gage FH (1999a) Running enhances neurogenesis, learning, and long-term potentiation in mice. *Proc. Natl. Acad. Sci. USA,* 96: 13427-13431.

van Praag H, Kempermann G, Gage FH (1999b) Running increases cell proliferation and neurogenesis in the adult mouse dentate gyrus. *Nat. Neurosci.,* 2: 266-270.

van Praag H, Schinder AF, Christie BR, Toni N, Palmer TD, Gage FH (2002) Functional neurogenesis in the adult hippocampus. *Nature,* 415: 1030-1034.

Venault P, Chapouthier G (2007) From the behavioral pharmacology of beta-carbolines to seizures, anxiety, and memory. *ScientificWorldJournal.,* 7: 204-223.

Venault P, Chapouthier G, Simiand J, Dodd RH, Rossier J (1987) Enhancement of performance by methyl beta-carboline-3-carboxylate, in learning and memory tasks. *Brain Res. Bull.,* 19: 365-370.

Vicari S (2006) Motor development and neuropsychological patterns in persons with Down syndrome. *Behav. Genet.,* 36: 355-364.

Vidal V, García S, Martínez P, Corrales A, Flórez J, Rueda N, Sharma A, Martínez-Cué C (2012) Lack of behavioral and cognitive effects of chronic ethosuximide and gabapentin treatment in the Ts65Dn mouse model of Down syndrome. Neuroscience. 220: 158-168.

Wang C, Zucker RS (1998) Regulation of synaptic vesicle recycling by calcium and serotonin. *Neuron,* 21: 155-167.

Wang DD, Kriegstein AR (2008) GABA regulates excitatory synapse formation in the neocortex via NMDA receptor activation. *J. Neurosci.,* 28: 5547-5558.

Wang DD, Kriegstein AR (2009) Defining the role of GABA in cortical development. *J. Physiol.,* 587: 1873-1879.

Whiting PJ, Bonnert TP, McKernan RM, Farrar S, Le Bourdelles B, Heavens RP, Smith DW, Hewson L, Rigby MR, Sirinathsinghji DJ, et al. (1999) Molecular and functional diversity of the expanding GABA-A receptor gene family. *Ann. NY Acad. Sci. USA,* 868: 645-653.

Whittle N, Sartori SB, Dierssen M, Lubec G, Singewald N (2007) Fetal Down syndrome brains exhibit aberrant levels of neurotransmitters critical for normal brain development. *Pediatrics,* 120: 1465-1471.

Xiang Z, Prince DA (2003) Heterogeneous actions of serotonin on interneurons in rat visual cortex. *J. Neurophysiol.,* 89: 1278-1287.

Yates CM, Simpson J, Gordon A (1986) Regional brain 5-hydroxytryptamine levels are reduced in senile Down's syndrome as in Alzheimer's disease. *Neurosci. Lett.,* 65: 189-192.

Zhou Q, Anderson DJ (2002) The bHLH transcription factors OLIG2 and OLIG1 couple neuronal and glial subtype specification. *Cell,* 109: 61-73.

In: Gamma-Aminobutyric Acid (GABA) ISBN: 978-1-63321-838-3
Editors: Josipa Vlainić and Maja Jazvinšćak Jembrek 

*Chapter 8*

# BEHAVIORAL AND PSYCHOLOGICAL SYMPTOMS OF DEMENTIA AND GABAERGIC SYSTEM: IMPLICATIONS FOR TREATMENT

***Maite Solas and Maria J. Ramirez*** [*]
Dpt of Pharmacology and Toxicology, University of Navarra, Pamplona, Spain

## ABSTRACT

Alzheimer's disease (AD) is the most common form of dementia in the elderly, currently affecting more than 35 million people worldwide. Research into AD therapy has been only successful in terms of developing symptomatic treatments. Neurone and synapse loss together with neurotransmitter dysfunction have, along with Aβ deposition and neurofibrillary tangles, been recognized as hallmarks of AD. Furthermore, clinical and preclinical studies point to this neurotransmitter dysfunction as a main factor underlying both cognitive and neuropsychiatric symptoms of the illness. In fact, cholinergic dysfunction, together with glutamatergic deficits, is considered to underlie cognitive disturbance of AD. GABA is the primary inhibitory neurotransmitter in the central nervous system and GABAergic neurons provide extensive innervation to cholinergic and glutamatergic neurons. It has been shown that dysfunction of the GABAergic system may contribute to cognitive impairment in humans and significant reductions in GABA levels have been described in severe cases of AD. Furthermore, in humans, GABA levels decrease with aging -the strongest risk factor for AD- and alterations in this neurotransmission can be underlying the behavioral and psychological symptoms of AD. This chapter examines the involvement of the GABAergic system in both cognitive and non-cognitive behavioural symptoms in AD and provides some pointers for rational drug development

**Keywords:** Cognition; memory deficits; behavioral symptoms of dementia; glutamate

[*] Dpt of Pharmacology and Toxicology, University of Navarra, Pamplona, Spain. Email: mariaja@unav.es.

## THE GABAERGIC SYSTEM

The amino acid GABA (γ-Aminobutyric acid) was first identified and described in the vertebrate brain in 1950. Due to lack of investigative reagents and its omnipresence throughout the brain, GABA was not classified as an amino acid neurotransmitter until 1970. GABA is now considered the primary inhibitory neurotransmitter in the mammalian brain occurring in 30-40% of all synapses and it plays a role in regulating neuronal excitability throughout the nervous system.

In the GABAergic neuron, as well as in the glutamatergic neuron, glutamine is retrieved and transformed into glutamate by the phosphate-activated glutaminase. Then, in the GABAergic neuronal population, glutamate is further converted into GABA by decarboxylation catalyzed with glutamic acid decarboxylase (GAD) (Liang et al., 2006) for which there are two gene products of different molecular weight, GAD65 and GAD67. GAD-mediated GABA synthesis occurs in the cytosol, and GABA is transported into synaptic vesicles by the vesicular GABA transporter (VGAT). When GABA is released from the neuron, is taken up into astrocytes and transaminated to succinic acid semialdehyde or oxidized to succinate and then either exits the tricarboxylic acid (TCA) cycle as malate or is converted via α-ketoglutarate into glutamate (Hertz et al., 1978). Regarding GABA uptake, four transporters have been described (Guastella et al., 1990). The four cloned transporters are products of the slc6al (mouse, GAT1; rat and human, GAT-1), slc6a12 (mouse, GAT2; rat and human, BGT-1), slc6a13 (mouse, GAT3; rat, GAT-2; human not cloned) and slc6a11 genes (mouse, GAT4; rat and human, GAT-3). GAT-1 seems to be the predominant neuronal GABA transporter whereas the others show a more ubiquitous distribution.

Although the inhibitory actions of GABA can be conferred mainly through two distinct receptor classes ($GABA_A$ and $GABA_B$), the ligand-gated $GABA_A$ receptor mediates the majority of fast inhibitory neurotransmission in the vertebrate brain.

## GABA RECEPTORS

The neurotransmitter receptors of amino acids are split into several types, most broadly demarcated as ionotropic and metabotropic.

Ionotropic receptors are constituted as transmembrane ion channels that open or close in response to the binding of a ligand. These receptors convert the chemical signal of a presynaptically released Neurotransmitter directly and very quickly into a postsynaptic electrical signal (Olsen and Sieghart, 2008), inducing the inhibitory or excitatory postsynaptic potentials, thus inhibiting or activating the neuron. Until now, two ionotropic receptors for GABA ($GABA_A$ and $GABA_A$-ρ) have been described. The $GABA_A$-ρ receptor, was originally designated a distinct subtype, $GABA_C$. Because $GABA_A$-ρ receptors are exclusively composed of the ρ subunit of the $GABA_A$ receptor, the International Union of Basic and Clinical Pharmacology now recommend that '$GABA_C$' no longer be used (Olsen and Sieghart, 2008).

Metabotropic receptors are connected with second messenger systems and exert a rather modulatory role in the CNS (Parmentier et al., 2002). GABA metabotropic receptors are linked to the G-proteins system and, opposite to the ionotropic ligand-gated channels, their action is slow and long-lasting (Bockaert et al., 2010). There is one metabotropic receptor for GABA ($GABA_B$ receptor).

Both $GABA_A$ and $GABA_B$ receptors are localized in the central nervous system (CNS). $GABA_A$-ρ is specific for the retina (Bormann et al., 2000) and will not be discussed further in this chapter.

# $GABA_A$ RECEPTORS

$GABA_A$ receptors contain an intrinsic ligand-gated $Cl^-$ channel, formed by the pentameric assembly of many types of subunits. GABA binds extracellularly to increase the probability of the channel opening. The receptor also contains a number of different allosteric binding sites which modulate the activity of the receptor indirectly. These allosteric sites are the targets of various other drugs, including the benzodiazepines, barbiturates, ethanol, neuroactive steroids, inhaled anaesthetics, and picrotoxin, among others. The flow of chloride ions hyperpolarizes the cell, decreasing the likelihood of the neuron firing an action potential. Based on the presence of seven subunit families comprising at least 18 subunits in the central nervous system ($\alpha_{1-6}$, $\beta_{1-3}$, $\gamma_{1-3}$, δ, ε, θ, $\rho_{1-3}$,), the $GABA_A$-receptors display extraordinary structural heterogeneity (Figure 1) (for review see Barnard et al., 1998; Fritschy et al., 2004; Möhler ,2001, 2002, 2006; Möhler et al., 2002, 2005; Rudolph and Möhler, 2006; Sieghart and Sperk, 2002; Sieghart, 2006; Whiting et al., 2000). Although the precise composition of subunits intrinsic to a particular $GABA_A$ receptor may be quite heterogeneous, most $GABA_A$ receptors subtypes **in vivo** are generally comprised of two α and β subunits (Farrar et al., 1999; Jechlinger et al., 1998; Li and De Blas, 1997), and one γ subunit. Receptors containing $\alpha_1$, $\alpha_2$, $\alpha_3$ or $\alpha_5$ subunits in combination with $\gamma_2$ and $\beta_2$ or $\beta_3$ are benzodiazepine-sensitive, whereas those containing $\alpha_4$ or $\alpha_6$ or δ instead of $\gamma_2$, fail to be responsive to these drugs (Barnard et al., 1998) (Table 1). Besides their structural diversity, $GABA_A$ receptor subtypes display strikingly different expression patterns, which points to specific functional roles for receptor subtypes in distinct neuronal networks.

## Benzodiazepine-Sensitive $GABA_A$ Receptors

Receptors containing the $\alpha_1$, $\alpha_2$, $\alpha_3$ or $\alpha_5$ subunits in combination with any of the β subunits and the $\gamma_2$ subunit are most prevalent in the brain (Table 1). These receptors are sensitive to benzodiazepine modulation with the drug-binding site located at the interface between the α and the $\gamma_2$ subunit. The major receptor subtype is assembled from the subunits $\alpha_1\beta_2\gamma_2$, with only a few brain regions lacking this receptor (Fritschy and Brünig, 2003; Fritschy and Möhler, 1995; Pirker et al., 2000).

Receptors containing the $\alpha_5$ subunit are of minor abundance in the brain but are expressed to a significant extent in the hippocampus, where they comprise 15–20% of the benzodiazepine-sensitive $GABA_A$ receptor population, predominately co-assembled with the $\beta_3$ and $\gamma_2$ subunits (Möhler et al., 1996). Pharmacological studies indicate that α5 subunit is a key subunit involved in learning and memory (Collinson et al., 2002; Dawson et al., 2006; Ballard et al., 2009).

**Table 1. GABA$_A$ receptor subtypes**

| Subunits | Localization | Pharmacology |
|---|---|---|
| $\alpha_1\beta_2\gamma_2$ | Major subtype (60%). Synaptic and extrasynaptic | Benzodiazepine-sensitive. Mediates sedative and anti-convulsant activity |
| $\alpha_2\beta_3\gamma_2$ | Minor subtype (15–20%). Synaptic | Benzodiazepine-sensitive. Mediates anxiolytic activity |
| $\alpha_3\beta_n\gamma_2$ | Minor subtype (10-15%) | Benzodiazepine-sensitive. Pharmacology yet unclear |
| $\alpha_5\beta_{1,3}\gamma_2$ | <5% of receptors. Extrasynaptic (cerebral cortex, hippocampus, olf. bulb) | Benzodiazepine-sensitive. Mediates modulation of temporal and spatial memory |
| $\alpha_4\beta_n\delta$ | <5% of receptors. Extrasynaptic | Insensitive to benzodiazepines. Sensitive to low concentration of ethanol |
| $\alpha_4\beta_n\gamma$ | <5% of receptors. Extrasynaptic | Insensitive to benzodiazepines |
| $\alpha_6\beta_n\delta$ | Small population. Extrasynaptic (only in cerebellum) | Insensitive to benzodiazepines. Sensitive to low concentration of ethanol |
| $\alpha_6\beta_{2,3}\gamma_2$ | <5% of receptors. Synaptic (only in cerebellum) | Insensitive to benzodiazepines |

The % values are estimates taking all brain GABA$_A$ receptors as 100%. Adapted from Möhler, 2007.

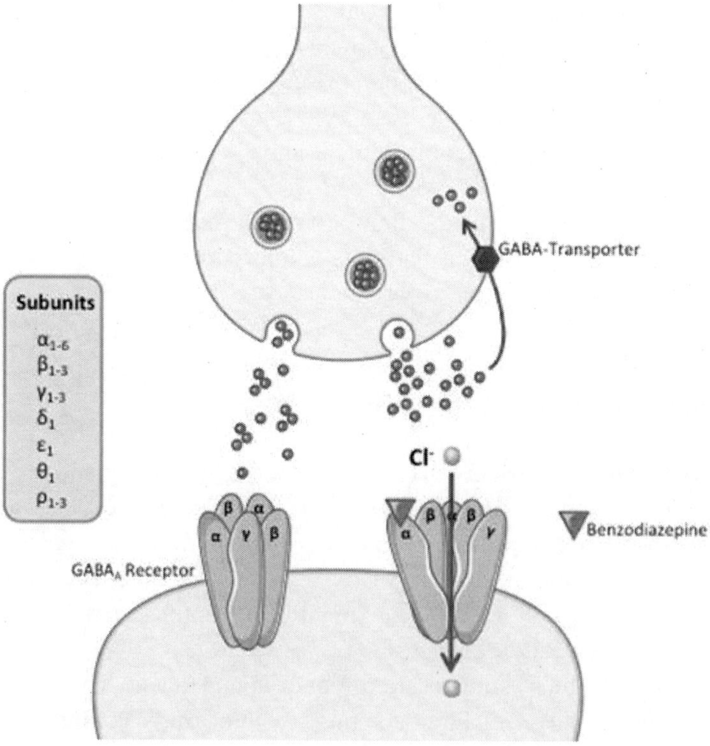


Figure 1. Scheme of GABAergic synapse depicting major elements of signal transduction. GABA$_A$ receptors are GABA-gated pentameric $Cl^-$ channels and they display an extraordinary structural heterogenicity. However, most GABA$_A$ receptor subtypes in vivo are considered to be heteropentamers composed of isoforms of α, β and γ subunits (Adapted from Möhler, 2007).

### Benzodiazepine-Insensitive $GABA_A$ Receptors

$GABA_A$ receptors that do not respond to benzodiazepines such as diazepam, flunitrazepam, clonazepam and zolpidem are of low abundance in the brain and are largely characterized by the $\alpha_4$ and $\alpha_6$ subunits (Table 1). Receptors containing the $\alpha_4$ subunit are generally expressed at very low abundance but more prominently in thalamus and dentate gyrus (Pirker et al., 2000); those containing the $\alpha_6$ subunit are restricted to the granule cell layer of the cerebellum (Nusser et al., 1996; Pöltl et al., 2003).

## $GABA_B$ Receptors

The $GABA_B$ receptor is not widely distributed in the brain, compared with $GABA_A$ (Zorumski et al., 1991). $GABA_B$ is linked to G proteins and a second-messenger system that mediates calcium or potassium channels, producing slow inhibitory postsynaptic potentials in several brain regions (Chebib et al., 1999). $GABA_B$ receptors are heterooligomeric and are made up of a $GABA_B$ R1a or $GABA_B$ R1b subunit and a $GABA_B$ R2 subunit (Chebib et al., 1999). Although both receptors bind GABA, $GABA_B$ is not modulated by benzodiazepines, barbiturates, or steroids, unlike $GABA_A$ (Chebib et al., 1999). Instead, it is distinguished from $GABA_A$ through selective affinity for baclofen (Lloyd et al., 1987).

## GABA and Cognition

Spatial and temporal learning and memory are linked to oscillatory neuronal activity in the hippocampus, where the NMDA (N-methyl-D-aspartate)-type glutamate receptors on principal neurons have attracted most attention in modulating memory performance. However, there is a balancing control by GABAergic inhibition. Learning triggers a rapid increase in inhibitory synaptogenesis and the GABA content of inhibitory synapses (Jasinska et al., 2010), accompanied by long-lasting enhancement of synaptic inhibition onto excitatory neurons in mice (Brosh and Barkai, 2009). Therefore, the GABAergic system appears to be important in the neuronal control of learning and memory.

Activity-induced modulation of inhibitory synaptic transmission has been shown in several brain regions of the mammalian brain (Grunze et al., 1996; Holmgren and Zilberter, 2001; Komatsu and Yoshimura, 2000). Such long-lasting plasticity of GABAergic synaptic transmission is crucially dependent on calcium entry into the postsynaptic neuron (for review, see Gaiarsa et al., 2002). For example, activity-induced enhancement in the number of $GABA_A$ receptors was shown in the hippocampus after kindling (Nusser et al., 1998), and enhanced GABA release was shown after brain-derived neurotrophic factor (BDNF) application (Ohba et al., 2005). In addition, a novel environment and spatial learning also trigger a lasting increase in GABA release from hippocampal GABAergic neurons in mice (Cui et al., 2008; Nitz and McNaughton, 2004). Conversely, decreasing GABA levels in the hippocampus by overexpressing GABA transporter 1 (GAT1), which is responsible for GABA reuptake after its synaptic release, impairs learning and memory in mice (Hu et al., 2004). Thus, changes in GABAergic function may have a role in orchestrating the circuit changes involved in synaptic plasticity, learning and memory (Crestani et al., 2002; Introini-Collison et al., 1994; McElroy and Korol, 2005; Wiltgen et al., 2005).

The functions of $GABA_A$ receptors containing α5 subunit are less well defined. Nevertheless, α5-containing $GABA_A$ receptors are preferentially expressed in the hippocampus (Quirk et al., 1996), suggesting that they play a key role in hippocampal functions such as learning and memory (Maubach, 2003). While other types of $GABA_A$ receptors are largely synaptic, $\alpha_5GABA_A$ receptors are located extrasynaptically at the base of the dendritic spines, which receive the excitatory input. The $\alpha_5GABA_A$ receptors are therefore in a privileged position to modulate the excitatory input arising at the spines via NMDA receptors. Mice with a partial deficit of $\alpha_5GABA_A$ receptors in hippocampus showed an improved performance in fear conditioning, a hippocampus-dependent memory task (Crestani et al., 2002). Similarly, in a mouse line in which $\alpha_5GABA_A$ receptors were deleted in the entire brain (Collinson et al., 2002; Whiting, 2003), an improved performance in the water maze model of spatial learning was observed. Furthermore, a partial inverse agonist acting at $\alpha_5GABA_A$ receptors enhanced the performance of wild-type rats in the water maze test (Chambers et al., 2004). Thus, neuronal inhibition in the hippocampus mediated via $\alpha_5$ $GABA_A$ receptors is a critical element in the regulation of the acquisition and memory (Fritschy et al., 1997). Based upon this evidences and its preferential hippocampal location, it was hypothesized that a compound with antagonism or inverse agonism selective for α5-containing $GABA_A$ receptors might enhance hippocampally mediated cognitive function (Maubach, 2003).

## The GABAergic System in Alzheimer's Disease

Alzheimer's disease (AD) is a progressive neurodegenerative disorder that leads to the loss of mental functions such as learning and memory. Neurochemically, the classical hallmark of AD is the disruption of basal forebrain cholinergic pathways and consequent cortical cholinergic denervation of the neocortex and hippocampus. This cholinergic dysfunction, together with glutamatergic deficits, is considered to underlie cognitive disturbance of AD (Francis et al., 1999; Francis, 2003; Perry et al., 1999; Terry Jr. et al., 2003). Deficiencies in central noradrenergic (Matthews et al., 2002), serotonergic (Chen et al., 1996, 2000; Garcia-Alloza et al., 2004), and perhaps dopaminergic (Minger et al., 2000; Storga et al., 1996) neural transmission may also play a critical role in some of the clinical manifestations of AD. Interestingly, in contrast to the marked deficits seen in cholinergic and glutamatergic systems, the current literature supports the claim that GABAergic neurons and receptors appear more resistant to neurodegeneration and is generally thought that this neurotransmission is well preserved (reviewed in refs. Armstrong et al., 2003; Bahn et al., 2001).

The precise mechanisms underlying selective neuronal vulnerability are currently unknown but using several methods, investigations demonstrate that despite resistance of the GABAergic system to neurodegeneration, particular subunits of the $GABA_A$ receptor are altered with age and AD, which can induce compensatory increases in $GABA_A$ receptor subunits within surrounding cells. Thus, pharmacological modulation of the $GABA_A$ receptor has gained increasing attention as a potential treatment for central processes affected in AD, including neuronal survival and cognition.

## ALTERATIONS IN THE GABAERGIC SYSTEM IN ALZHEIMER´S DISEASE

Although riddled with limitations, postmortem studies in AD comprise the bulk of evidence attempting to establish altered GABA in patients with AD. These postmortem investigations include, first, studies measuring GABA (Nägga et al., 1999; Seidl et al., 2001; Tarbit et al., 1980; Yew et al., 1999), GAD and GABA-T (Aoyagi et al., 1990; Boissiere et al., 1998; Davies et al., 1979; Nakamura et al., 1990; Perry et al., 1978; Sherif et al., 1992, 1995; Yates et al., 1990) concentrations; and second, GABA receptor ligand-binding studies that use GABA-specific ligands (Chu et al., 1987a, 1987b; Hardy et al., 1987; Reisine et al., 1978) or benzodiazepines (Carlson et al., 1993; Cross et al., 1986; Greenamyre et al., 1987; Griffiths et al., 1994; Jansen et al., 1990; Owen et al., 1983; Sedvall et al., 1987; Shimohama et al., 1988). Moreover, as putative markers of CNS GABA, cerebrospinal fluid (CSF) and plasma GABA levels have been measured.

Postmortem studies on cortical areas have, for the most part, shown that the frontal, temporal, and parietal regions have reduced GABA concentration in AD. GAD and GABA-T have also been measured centrally postmortem. GAD is located only within neurons and can therefore be used as a marker for GABA localization in the brain. Potential alterations in GABA-T in AD patients may reflect differences in the rate at which GABA undergoes catabolism. Several studies have examined GAD activity in AD patients postmortem (Boissiere, 1998; Davies, 1979; Nakamura et al., 1990; Perry et al., 1978; Yates et al., 1990). Despite differing methodologies and design issues, studies suggest decreased GAD activity with compensatory increases in mRNA expression. Studies that have examined whether GABA-T activity is altered in AD patients show a possible disease-dependent effect of AD on GABA-T activity (Aoyagi et al., 1990; Sherif et al., 1992, 1995).

Binding studies using GABA or benzodiazepines suggest that the temporal region is affected in AD patients. The limbic regions that appear to have reduced GABA in patients with AD include the cingulate, amygdala and thalamus. GABA in the hippocampus, caudate, putamen, and nucleus accumbens does not appear to be affected by AD, though there have been some positive results found within the hippocampus and caudate. Despite the relative sparing of $GABA_A$ receptors in AD, it is possible that the specific subunit composition of these receptors may undergo alterations with disease progression. Radioligand binding studies demonstrate mild reductions in $GABA_A$/or benzodiazepine binding sites in the AD brain (Chu et al., 1987a, 1987b; Vogt et al., 1991). $GABA_A$ subunit expression in hippocampus and prefrontal cortex has been analyzed during the course of AD in humans in several studies. In the hippocampus, protein or mRNA for $GABA_A$ subunits $\alpha1$, $\alpha5$ and $\beta3$ decrease in AD patients with severe neuropathology (Rissman et al., 2007). In prefrontal cortex reduced amount of $\alpha1$ and $\alpha2$ $GABA_A$ subunit expression in early and late AD stages while a downregulation of $GABA_A$ receptor subunits $\alpha4$, $\beta2$ and $\delta$ has been observed during the late stages of AD (Luchetti et al., 2011).

CSF is in direct contact with the brain and, therefore, may contain endogenous chemical constituents found in cortical and subcortical areas. Of published studies (Bareggi et al., 1982; Enna et al., 1977; Jimenez-Jimenez et al., 1998; Kuroda et al., 1983; Manyam et al., 1980; Mohr et al., 1986; Oishi et al., 1996; Pomara et al., 1989; Tohgi et al., 1992; Tosca et al., 1992; Weiner et al., 1996; Zimmer et al., 1984), only 4 found significant reductions in CSF GABA among AD patients, compared with control subjects (Enna et al., 1977; Manyam et al., 1980; Mohr et al., 1986; Zimmer et al., 1984).

Although GABA cannot cross the blood–brain barrier, some investigators have considered whether GABA concentrations are altered in the plasma of patients with AD. Among the studies in the medical literature, only 1 found AD patients to have a significant reduction in GABA (Jimenez-Jimenez et al., 1998) while others (Oishi et al., 1996; Weiner et al., 1996) were unable to detect a significant difference. The validity of these measurements as biological markers of AD remains uncertain.

In summary, with regard to AD-related changes, while there are inconsistencies, the literature generally supports the view that GABA levels as well as $GABA_A$ receptor subunits in the brain of AD patients are relatively altered, leading to a GABAergic dysfunction in AD.

## Glutamate-GABA Imbalance in Alzheimer´s Disease

The proper functioning of the CNS depends on the physiological homeostasis, which is itself maintained and regulated by glutamatergic (excitatory) and GABAergic (inhibitory) forces acting dependently to each other, flowing into a natural cycle and always seeking the balance. However, neurons are metabolically handicapped in the sense that they are not able to perform de novo synthesis of these two neurotransmitters. Therefore, a metabolite shuttle known as the glutamate/GABA-glutamine cycle is necessary for the release of neurotransmitter glutamate or GABA from neurons and subsequent uptake into astrocytes. In return, astrocytes release glutamine to be taken up into neurons for use as neurotransmitter precursor. Among others, discoveries of intercellular glutamine and glutamate pools, related to astrocytes and neurons, respectively, led to the suggestion of a glutamate/GABA glutamine cycle working between neurons and astrocytes (Benjamin et al., 1972; Ottersen et al., 1992; Van den Berg and Garfinkel, 1971). Thus, the circle of glutamate/GABA transformations is closed in the tripartite synapse (composed by the glutamatergic neuron, the GABAergic neuron and the astrocyte), with no beginning and no end, as schematically shown in Figure 2. In a glutamatergic synapse glutamate is released and taken up into surrounding astrocytes, through the excitatory amino acid transporters (EAAT 1/2). In the astrocyte, glutamate is transformed into glutamine by the astrocyte-specific enzyme glutamine synthetase (GS) (Arriza et al., 1994; Norenberg et al., 1979; Pines et al., 1992) and released into the extracellular space. From there, glutamine is taken up into glutamatergic neurons (Chaudhry et al., 2002) and transformed back to glutamate by phosphate-activated glutaminase (Kvamme et al., 1982). In the GABAergic neuron, as well as in the glutamatergic neuron, glutamine is transformed into glutamate and further converted into GABA. When GABA is released from the neuron, is taken up into astrocytes and metabolized into glutamate (Hertz et al., 1978). This glutamate is then converted to glutamine and returned to neurons, closing the glutamate/GABA- glutamine cycle.

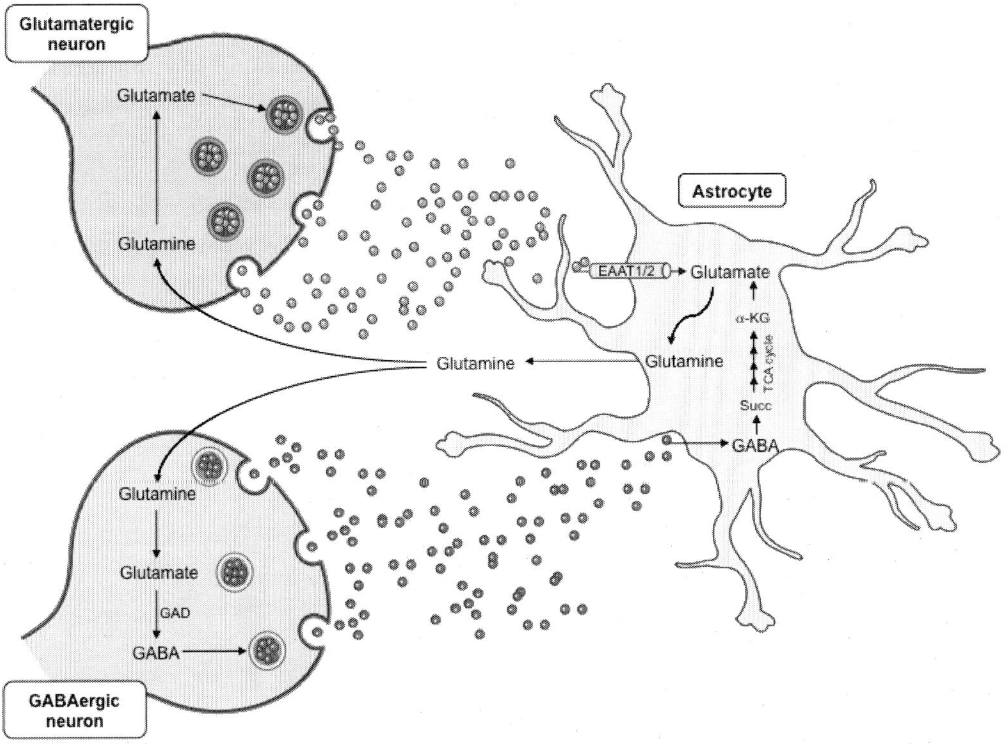


Figure 2. Schematic representation of the glutamate/GABA-glutamine cycle. GS: glutamine synthetase; EAAT1/2: excitatory amino acid transporter; Succ: succinate; α-KG: α-ketoglutarate; TCA cycle: tricarboxylic acid cycle; GAD: glutamate descarboxylase (Adapted from Puerta et al., 2014).

The AD brain is characterized by extensive neuronal and synaptic loss in areas of the brain essential for cognitive and memory functions, such as the cerebral cortex and hippocampus. Approximately 90% of hippocampal neurons confer excitatory glutamatergic neurotransmission; the remaining 10% of hippocampal neurons are inhibitory in nature, of which the majority is GABAergic. It has been suggested that the dysfunction in GABA signaling in AD is accompanied by an aberrant glutamatergic signaling (Lanctôt et al., 2004; Rissman and Mobley, 2011). Therefore, this could lead to an excitatory/inhibitory imbalance in the AD brain (Figure 3). Moreover, a long-standing hypothesis in the AD field suggests that increasing oxidative or metabolic stress can lead to excessive glutamatergic tone, which is thought to lead neuronal loss in AD. Considerable research has focused on the role of calcium-permeable glutamate receptors in promoting glutamate-mediated excitotoxicity in AD. An over-stimulation of NMDA and α-amino-3-hydroxy-5-methyl-4-isoxazolepropionic acid (AMPA) receptors by glutamate has been demonstrated to induce cell death by calcium-dependent pathways (Arundine and Tymianski, 2004; Pellegrini-Giampietro et al., 1997). In line with this hypothesis, many studies of the AD brain have found reductions both in glutamate-releasing cells (Hyman et al., 1984) and in glutamate receptor subunits (Carter et al., 2004; Ikonomovic et al., 1999, 2000; Mishizen-Eberz et al., 2004), reviewed in (Armstrong et al., 2003; Mishizen et al., 2000). Accepting that stimulation of ionotropic glutamate receptors contribute to the pathogenesis of AD, and the view that this could serve to disrupt excitatory/inhibitory balance, it is important to also consider that disruptions or alterations in GABA neurotransmission or inhibitory $GABA_A$ receptors may significantly worsen this situation and impact hippocampal structure and function. Interestingly, GABA is physiologically released by neurons in response to glutamate excitotoxicty (Saransaari and Oja, 2006; Vignes, 2001), suggesting that it may take part in neuronal defense mechanisms to compensate for glutamatergic overactivation. Different classes of GABA receptor agonists have been shown to decrease neuronal vulnerability to excitotoxic damage in several models (Lapchak et al. 2000; Pisani et al. 2006; Schwartz-Bloom et al. 2000; Velasco and Tapia 2002; Zhang et al., 2007). Moreover, AD is characterized by increased seizure activity (Abou-Khalil, 2010; De Simone et al., 2010; Menendez, 2005; Palop and Mucke, 2009a, 2009b), which not only suggests a disruption of excitatory/inhibitory balance, but begs the question of which neurotransmitter systems are responsible.

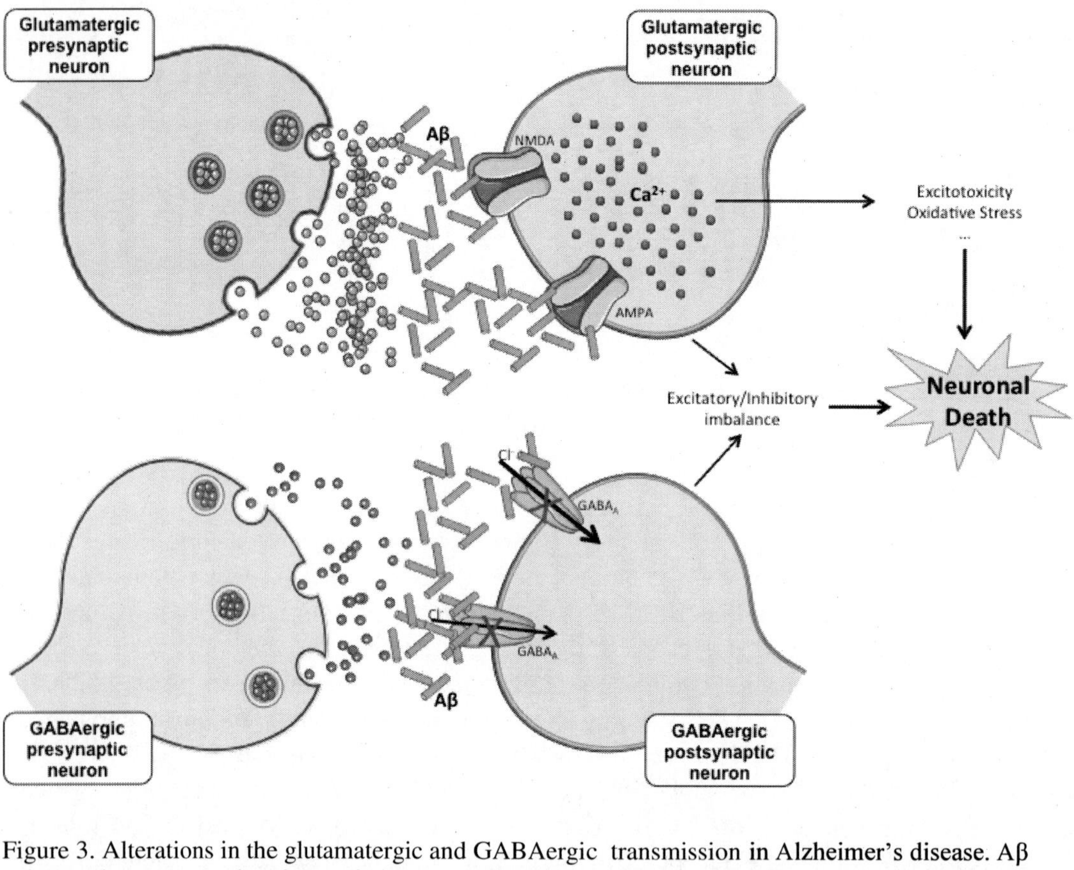


Figure 3. Alterations in the glutamatergic and GABAergic transmission in Alzheimer's disease. Aβ enhance the pre-synaptic release of glutamate, due to this, glutamate concentration in synaptic cleft increases. Activation of NMDA and AMPA receptors increases the influx of calcium and activates several signaling pathways responsible for processes such as neuronal excitotoxicity or oxidative stress, leading to neuronal death. Moreover, Aβ may increase neuronal excitability by inhibiting GABA-induced Cl- current in the neurons, decreasing the inhibitory neurotransmission, and producing aberrant excitatory/inhibitory network synchronization. This glutamatergic/GABAergic imbalance also leads to a neuronal death.

## GABA AND AMYLOID PATHOLOGY

AD is characterized neuropathologically by the extracellular deposition of the 4 kDa β-amyloid peptide (Aβ), a 39–43 amino acid peptide that is neurotoxic (Borchelt et al., 1996) and accumulates in neuritic plaques (Wahrle et al., 2002). Amyloid precursor protein (APP) is the precursor of Aβ and can be processed via alternative pathways. A non-amyloidogenic secretory pathway includes cleavage of APP to soluble APP (sAPPα) by α-secretases within the Aβ peptide sequence, thus precluding the formation of Aβ. In contrast, the formation of the amyloidogenic Aβ peptides is regulated by the sequential action of β- and γ- secretases (Checler, 1995; Nunan and Small, 2000). Both in vitro (Iversen et al., 1995) and in vivo (Chen et al., 1994) studies have reported the toxic effects of Aβ or Aβ peptide fragments suggesting an important role of Aβ in the pathogenesis of AD and it has been proposed that Aβ causes neuronal dysfunction and cognitive impairments characteristic of both familiar and sporadic forms of AD (Selkoe and Wolfe, 2007). Indeed, a leading hypothesis in the AD field is the Aβ cascade hypothesis, which suggests that overproduction of Aβ is an initiator of multiple neurotoxic pathways, including excitotoxicity, oxidative stress, and cell death (Robinson and Bishop, 2002).

Work on the GABA system in AD has uncovered crucial links between Aβ and alterations in GABA signaling. These data not only serve to link GABA to the Aβ cascade hypothesis, but may shed light on the mechanisms behind increased seizure activity in AD. As a potential mechanism underlying this epileptic activity, studies demonstrate that Aβ can induce synaptic depression and aberrant excitatory/inhibitory network synchronization (Palop and Mucke, 2010) (Figure 3). Although the relationship between these mechanisms and AD-related events are unclear, it seems likely that resultant synaptic depression and/or aberrations in excitatory/inhibitory balance can lead to deficits in learning and memory and synaptic vulnerability in AD mouse models (Palop and Mucke, 2010). Moreover, it has been suggested that Aβ may increase neuronal excitability by inhibiting GABA-induced $Cl^-$ current in the neurons of mammalian central nervous system (Masashi and Mituyuki, 1996) (Figure 3) and vulnerability of GABAergic neurons to human Aβ has been demonstrated (Pakaski et al., 1998). Interestingly, several studies demonstrated that selective $GABA_A$ receptor agonists protective against Aβ-induced toxicity in rodents (Gu et al., 2003; Lee et al., 2005; Lin and Jun-Tian, 2004; Louzada et al., 2004; Marcade et al., 2008). These neuroprotective effects could be blocked in culture by $GABA_A$ receptor antagonists (Marcade et al., 2008). In contrast, it has been (Lee et al., 2005) shown that baclofen, a $GABA_B$ receptor agonist, does not exhibit any protective effect against Aβ, indicating a $GABA_A$ receptor specific subtype requirement for neuroprotection.

Accepting that GABAergic tone is relatively preserved in AD, future therapeutics aimed at increasing GABAergic activity may reduce production of Aβ, which can have two important disease-modifying effects; reducing or alleviating Aβ plaque development and Aβ-induced excitotoxity, both of which increase cognition.

## GABAergic System and Behavioural and Psychological Symptoms of Alzheimer´s Disease

AD is a chronic progressive disorder characterised by dementia but often featuring behavioral and psychological syndromes referred to as behavioural and psychological symptoms of dementia (BPSD) (IPA, 1996). The extent and nature of BPSD in AD is varied and includes aggressive behavior, overactivity, depression or psychosis (Hope et al., 1997) all of which are major contributory factors to early institutionalisation of the patient (Levy et al., 1999).

Although deficits in the cholinergic system have been associated with both cognitive changes (Whitehouse et al., 1981) and BPSD (Cummings et al., 1996, 1998), manipulation of the cholinergic system has limited effectiveness. Hence, given the complexities of the BPSD of AD, symptomatic relief may require multiple transmitter replacement (Mohr et al., 1994). Glutamate and GABA systems are emerging as targets for development of medications for mood disorders.

Several lines of emerging evidence suggest that dysfunction of GABA systems is associated with major depression. In animal studies it has been shown that increasing GABAergic tone exerts an antidepressant effect (Lloyd et al., 1989). Furthermore, several studies employing magnetic resonance spectroscopy suggest that in humans unipolar depression is associated with reductions in cortical GABA levels (Sanacora et al., 1999). In addition, antidepressant and mood-stabilizing treatments appear to raise cortical GABA levels and to ameliorate GABA deficits in patients with mood disorders (Krystal et al., 2002).

Besides a role in anxiolysis, there is evidence that $GABA_A$/benzodiazepine recognition (BZ) sites mediate the antidepressant effects of certain benzodiazepines and are altered in the cortex of patients with clinical depression (Cheetham et al., 1898; Pandey et al., 1997; Taylor et al., 2003). In contrast, receptor and functional studies of $GABA_B$ receptors have yielded conflicting results, with some studies showing an upregulation of $GABA_B$ receptor binding with antidepressant treatment, while others do not (see Shiah and Yatham, 1998 for a review).

It has been also shown that drugs that increase plasma GABA levels can decrease aggression and GABA levels may correlate with some aspects of aggressive behaviour (Bjork et al., 2001). However, cholinergic deficiency in cortical regions may be linked not only to cognitive deficits, but also to BPSD observed in AD patients (Minger et al., 2000) and treatment with cholinergic compounds often improves behavior (Cummings, 2000; Levy et al., 1999). It has been previously described (Garcia-Alloza et al., 2005) that there was a strong correlation between aggressive behavior and MMSE. Therefore, the correlation found between the ChAT to GABA ratio with aggressive behavior may be linked to an imperfect integration of cognitive processes that may contribute to BPSD in AD (Parnetti et al., 2001).

Clinical experience supports GABA as a therapeutic target for symptomatic treatment of BPSD. Aggression and agitation are drug-responsive symptoms. Benzodiazepines, for example, are commonly used in clinical practice to reduce agitation and aggression exhibited by patients with dementia (Conn et al., 1999). Although benzodiazepines such as lorazepam have been reported to work in some cases (Fritz et al., 1990), the potential therapeutic effect may be outweighed by adverse events, such as sedation (Ancill et al., 1991; Sunderland et al., 1989). Other GABAergic therapies, including anti-convulsants, show greater promise in managing behaviours such as aggression but are limited by toxicity.

In conclusion, GABA's association with such neuropsychiatric symptoms as depression (Keverne 1999), aggression (Adams et al., 1993; Delgado, 1973; Eichelman et al., 1987; Funderburk et al., 1970; Keverne, 1999; Malick and Goldberg, 1970; Panksepp, 1971; Roeling et al., 1993), and psychosis (Keverne, 1999), as well as its ability to regulate acetylcholine, dopamine, and serotonin (Decker and McGaugh, 1991; Zorumski and Isenberg, 1991), make it a therapeutic target for controlling BPSD.

## IMPLICATIONS IN THE TREATMENT OF ALZHEIMER'S DISEASE

There are currently no effective clinical treatments to cure or to arrest the progression of AD (De Felice and Ferreira, 2002; Schneider et al., 2014). Therefore, studies aimed at finding novel therapeutic targets or approaches capable of interrupting neuronal dysfunction and brain degeneration in AD are of great current interest.

Drugs that interact at the $GABA_A$ receptor can possess a spectrum of pharmacological activities, depending on their ability to modify the actions of GABA. For example, $GABA_A$ receptor agonists such as diazepam enhance the inhibitory effects of GABA at the $GABA_A$ receptor and show effects that translate into, for example, the anxiolytic, sedative, and amnesia promoting properties observed clinically. By contrast, non-selective inverse agonists show opposing effects and could be beneficial clinically in terms of enhancing cognition. Moreover, $GABA_A$ receptor agonists protect neurons in culture against the neurotoxicity of Aβ and of various glutamate receptor agonists (Paula-Lima et al., 2003, 2005; Louzada et al., 2004). It is, thus, tempting to propose that stimulation of GABAergic signaling could represent an effective alternative therapeutic approach in AD. Stimulating GABAergic transmission has indeed been attempted to treat AD (Lanctôt et al., 2004; Möhler, 2011). Most of the interventions using GABAergic agents aimed to manage behavioral and psychological dysfunctions associated with dementia, including aggression and agitation. In this regard, benzodiazepines have demonstrated efficacy, but they are limited by tolerance after long-term use and other side effects such as sedation, dizziness, and ataxia (Wallace, 2001; Lanctôt et al., 2004). Antiepileptic drugs such as vigabatrin, topiramate, and THIP (4,5,6,7-tetrahydroisoxazolo[5,4-c]pyridin-3-ol) offer novel possibilities to interrupt or retard AD progression in light of their neuroprotective actions against excitotoxicity (Kristensen et al., 2003; Eleuteri et al., 2009). Interestingly, a recent study demonstrated that Aβ–induced aberrant network activity contributes to synaptic and cognitive deficits, and showed that treatment of AD mouse models with levetiracetam, an antiepileptic drug, reduced abnormal spike activity detected by electroencephalography, reversed hippocampal remodeling, behavioral abnormalities, synaptic dysfunction, and deficits in learning and memory (Sanchez et al., 2012).

Consistent with the idea that abnormal network activity is crucial to synaptic and cognitive deficits in AD, endogenous molecules such as melatonin and taurine were found to attenuate or block Aβ-induced excitotoxicity **in vitro** by mechanisms related to $GABA_A$ receptor activation (Louzada et al., 2004; Paula-Lima et al., 2005). Indeed, Brito-Moreira et al. (2011) have recently demonstrated that pre-treatment of neurons with taurine, as well as with the NMDAR blocker MK-801, prevents the release of glutamate induced by non-lethal concentrations of Aβ in primary hippocampal neurons. Collectively, results suggest that the beneficial effects of $GABA_A$ receptor activation may occur at a stage previous to neuronal death.

## Conclusion

The role of GABA in dementia has yet to be fully elucidated. Given its function as the major inhibitory neurotransmitter in the CNS, it is highly probable that behavioural and cognitive symptoms associated with neurodegenerative diseases such as AD may be a direct or indirect result of GABAergic dysfunction.

The general literature indicates that $GABA_A$ receptors are potential targets for treatment of both cognitive deficits and BPSD in AD. In the future, ligands are needed which differentiate $GABA_A$ receptors by selective affinity and display full agonistic activity at a preferred receptor subtype. Such agents are expected to show stronger clinical efficacy than partial agonists in the treatment of CNS diseases, ranging from anxiety disorders, insomnias and memory dysfunctions to cognitive deficits and pain, based on the modulation of inhibitory control.

## References

Abou-Khalil BW *(*2010*)* How important is Alzheimer's disease as a risk factor for unprovoked seizures and epilepsy in the elderly? *Epilepsy Curr.* 10*,* 36–37.

Adams DB, Boudreau W, Cowan CW, Kokonowski C, Oberteuffer K, Yohay K (1993) Offense produced by chemical stimulation of the anterior hypothalamus of the rat. *Physiol Behav.* 53:1127–32.

Ancill RJ, Carlyle WW, Liang RA, Holliday SG (1991) Agitation in the demented elderly: a role for benzodiazepines? *Int Clin Psychopharmacol.* 6:141–6.

Aoyagi T, Wada T, Nagai M, Kojima F, Harada S, Takeuchi T, Takahashi H, Hirokawa K, Tsumita T (1990) Increased gamma-aminobutyrate aminotransferase activity in brain of patients with Alzheimer's disease. *Chem Pharm Bull (Tokyo).* 38:1748–9.

Armstrong DM, Sheffield R, Mishizen-Eberz AJ, Carter TL, Rissman RA, Mizukami K, Ikonomovic M D. *(*2003*)* Plasticity of glutamate and GABAA receptors in the hippocampus of patients with Alzheimer's disease. Cell. Mol. Neurobiol. 23*,* 491–505.

Arriza JL, Fairman WA, Wadiche JI, Murdoch GH, Kavanaugh MP, Amara SG (1994) Functional comparisons of three glutamate transporter subtypes cloned from human motor cortex. *J Neurosci.* 14:5559-5569.

Arundine M, Tymianski M *(*2004*)* Molecular mechanisms of glutamate-dependent neurodegeneration in ischemia and traumatic brain injury. *Cell Mol Life Sci.* 61*:* 657–668.

Bahn SJ, Augood M, Ryan DG, Standaert M, Starkey PC, Emson PC (2001) Gene expression profiling in the post-mortem human brain--no cause for dismay. *J Chem Neuroanat.* 22: 79–94

Ballard TM, Knoflach F, Prinssen E, Borroni E, Vivian JA, Basile J, Gasser R, Moreau JL, Wettstein JG, Buettelmann B, Knust H, Thomas AW, Trube G, Hernandez MC (2009)

RO4938581, a novel cognitive enhancer acting at GABAA alpha5 subunit-containing receptors. *Psychopharmacology (Berl).* 202(1-3):207-23.

Bareggi SR, Franceschi M, Bonini L, Zecca L, Smirne S (1982) Decreased CSF concentrations of homovanillic acid and gamma- aminobutyric acid in Alzheimer's disease. Age or disease-related modifications? *Arch Neurol. 39*:709–12.

Barnard EA, Skolnick P, Olsen RW, Möhler H, Sieghart W, Biggio G, Braestrup C, Bateson AN, Langer SZ *(*1998*)* Subtypes of $\gamma$-aminobutyric acid$_A$ receptors: classification on the bases of subunit structure and receptor function. *Pharmacol Reviews.* 50: 291–313.

Benjamin AM, Quastel JH (1972) Locations of amino acids in brain slices from the rat. Tetrodotoxin-sensitive release of amino acids. *Biochem J.* 128:631-646.

Bjork JM, Moeller FG, Kramer GL, Kram M, Suris A, Rush AJ, Petty F (2001) Plasma GABA levels correlate with aggressiveness in relatives of patients with unipolar depressive disorder. *Psychiatry Res.* 101:131–136.

Bockaert J, Perroy J, Becamel C, Marin P, Fagni L (2010) GPCR interacting proteins (GIPs) in the nervous system: Roles in physiology and pathologies. *Ann Rev Pharmacol Toxicol.* 50:89-109.

Boissiere F, Faucheux B, Duyckaerts C, Hauw JJ, Agid Y, Hirsch EC (1998) Striatal expression of glutamic acid decarboxylase gene in Alzheimer's disease. *J Neurochem.* 71:767–74.

Borchelt DR, Thinakaran G, Eckman CB, Lee MK, Davenport F, Ratovitsky T, Prada CM, Kim G, Seekins S, Yager D, Slunt HH, Wang R, Seeger M, Levey AI, Gandy SE, Copeland NG, Jenkins NA, Price DL, Younkin SG, Sisodia SS (1996) Familial Alzheimer's disease-linked presenilin 1 variants elevate Abeta1-42/1-40 ratio in vitro and in vivo. *Neuron.* 17(5):1005-13.

Bormann J (2000) The 'ABC' of GABA receptors. *Trends Pharmacol Sci.* 21:16–9.

Brito-Moreira J, Paula-Lima AC, Bomfim T R, Oliveira FB, Sepúlveda FJ, De Mello FG, Aguayo LG, Panizzutti R, Ferreira ST *(*2011*)* A$\beta$ oligomers induce glutamate release from hippocampal neurons. *Curr Alzheimer Res.* 8: 552–562.

Brosh I, Barkai E (2009) Learning-induced enhancement of feedback inhibitory synaptic transmission. *Learn Mem.* 16:413–416.

Carlson MD, Penney JB, Jr, Young AB (1993) NMDA, AMPA, and benzodiazepine binding site changes in Alzheimer's disease visual cortex. *Neurobiol Aging.* 14:343–52.

Carter TL, Rissman RA, Mishizen-Eberz AJ, Wolfe BB, Hamilton RL, Gandy S, Armstrong DM *(*2004*)* Differential preservation of AMPA receptor subunits in the hippocampi of Alzheimer's disease patients according to Braak stage. *Exp Neurol.* 187, 299–309.

Chambers MS, Atack JR, Carling RW, Collinson N, Cook SM, Dawson GR, Ferris P, Hobbs SC, O'connor D, Marshall G, Rycroft W, Macleod AM (2004) An orally bioavailable, functionally selective inverse agonist at the benzodiazepine site of GABAA alpha5 receptors with cognition enhancing properties. *J Med Chem.* 47(24):5829-32.

Chaudhry FA, Reimer RJ, Edwards RH (2002) The glutamine commute: take the N line and transfer to the A. *J Cell Biol.* 157:349-355.

Chebib M, Johnston GA (1999) The 'ABC' of GABA receptors: a brief review. *Clin Exp Pharmacol Physiol.* 26:937–40.

Checler F (1995) Processing of the beta-amyloid precursor protein and its regulation in Alzheimer's disease. *J Neurochem.* 65(4):1431-44.

Cheetham SC, Crompton MR, Katona CL, Parker SJ, Horton RW (1998) Brain GABAA/benzodiazepine binding sites and glutamic acid decarboxylase activity in depressed suicide victims. *Brain Res.* 460: 114–123

Chen CP, Alder JT, Bowen DM, Esiri MM, McDonald B, Hope T, Jobst KA, Francis PT (1996) Presynaptic serotonergic markers in community-acquired cases of Alzheimer's disease: correlations with depression and neuroleptic medication. *J Neurochem.* 66: 1592–1598

Chen CP, Eastwood SL, Hope T, McDonald B, Francis PT, Esiri MM (2000) Immnunocytochemical study of the dorsal and median raphe nuclei in patients with Alzheimer's disease prospectively assessed for behavioural changes. *Neuropathol Appl Neurobiol.* 26: 1–10

Chen SY, Harding JW, Barnes CD (1994) Neuropathology of synthetic β-amyloid peptide analogs in vivo. *Brain Res.* 715: 44–50

Chu DC, Penney JB Jr, Young AB *(*1987a*)* Cortical $GABA_B$ and $GABA_A$ receptors in Alzheimer's disease: a quantitative autoradiographic study. Neurology. 37:1454–1459.

Chu DC, Penney JB Jr, Young AB *(*1987b*)* Quantitative autoradiography of hippocampal GABAB and GABAA receptor changes in Alzheimer's disease. *Neurosci Lett.* 82: 246–252.

Collinson N, Kuenzi FM, Jarolimek W, Maubach KA, Cothliff R, Sur C, Smith A, Otu FM, Howell O, Atack JR, McKernan RM, Seabrook GR, Dawson GR, Whiting PJ, Rosahl TW (2002) Enhanced learning and memory and altered GABAergic synaptic transmission in mice lacking the alpha 5 subunit of the GABAA receptor. *J Neurosci.* 22(13):5572-80.

Conn DK, Ferguson I, Mandelman K, Ward C (1999) Psychotropic drug utilization in long-term care facilities for the elderly in Ontario, Canada. *Int Psychogeriatr.* 11:223–33.

Crestani F, Keist R, Fritschy JM, Benke D, Vogt K, Prut L, Blüthmann H, Möhler H, Rudolph U (2002) Trace fear conditioning involves hippocampal alpha5 GABA(A) receptors. *Proc Natl Acad Sci U S A.* 99(13):8980-5.

Cross AJ, Crow TJ, Ferrier IN, Johnson JA (1986) The selectivity of the reduction of serotonin S2 receptors in Alzheimer-type dementia. *Neurobiol Aging.* 7:3–7.

Cui Y, Costa RM, Murphy GG, Elgersma Y, Zhu Y, Gutmann DH, Parada LF, Mody I, Silva AJ (2008) Neurofibromin regulation of ERK signaling modulates GABA release and learning. *Cell.* 135:549 –560.

Cummings JL (2000) The role of cholinergic agents in the management of behavioural disturbances in Alzheimer's disease. *Int J Neuropsychopharmacol.* 3: 21–29

Cummings JL, Back C (1998) The cholinergic hypothesis of neuropsychiatric symptoms in Alzheimer's disease. *Am J Geriatr Psychiatry.* 6:S64 –S78.

Cummings JL, Kaufer D (1996) Neuropsychiatric aspects of Alzheimer's disease: the cholinergic hypothesis revisited. *Neurology.* 47:876 –83.

Davies P (1979) Neurotransmitter-related enzymes in senile dementia of the Alzheimer type. *Brain Res.* 171:319–27.

Dawson GR, Maubach KA, Collinson N, Cobain M, Everitt BJ, MacLeod AM, Choudhury HI, McDonald LM, Pillai G, Rycroft W, Smith AJ, Sternfeld F, Tattersall FD, Wafford KA, Reynolds DS, Seabrook GR, Atack JR (2006) An inverse agonist selective for alpha5 subunit-containing GABAA receptors enhances cognition. *J Pharmacol Exp Ther.* 316(3):1335-45.

De Felice FG, Ferreira ST (2002) Beta-amyloid production, aggregation, and clearance as targets for therapy in Alzheimer's disease. *Cell Mol Neurobiol.* 22(5-6):545-63.

De Simone R, Puig XS, Gelisse P, Crespel A, Genton P (2010) Senile myoclonic epilepsy: delineation of a common condition associated with Alzheimer's disease in Down syndrome. *Seizure.* 19:383–389.

Decker MW, McGaugh JL (1991) The role of interactions between the cholinergic system and other neuromodulatory systems in learning and memory. *Synapse.* 7:151–68.

Delgado JMR (1973) Antiaggressive effects of chlordiazepoxide. New York: Raven Press.

Eichelman B (1987) Neurochemical basis of aggressive behavior. *Psychiatri Ann.* 17:371–4.

Eleuteri S, Monti B, Brignani S, Contestabile A (2009) Chronic dietary administration of valproic acid protects neurons of the rat nucleus basalis magnocellularis from ibotenic acid neurotoxicity. *Neurotox Res.* 15:127–132.

Enna SJ, Stern LZ, Wastek GJ, Yamamura HI (1977) Cerebrospinal fluid gamma-aminobutyric acid variations in neurological disorders. *Arch Neurol.* 34:683–5.

Farrar SJ, Whiting PJ, Bonnert TP, McKernan RM (1999) Stoichiometry of a ligand-gated ion channel determined by fluorescence energy transfer. *J Biol Chem.* 274: 10100–10104.

Francis PT (2003) Glutamatergic systems in Alzheimer's disease. *Int J Geriatr Psychiatry.* 18: 15–21

Francis PT, Palmer AM, Snape M, Wilcock GK (1999) The cholinergic hypothesis of Alzheimer's disease: a review of progress. *J Neurol Neurosurg Psychiatry.* 66:137–147

Fritschy JM, Benke D, Johnson DK, Mohler H, Rudolph U (1997) GABAA-receptor alpha-subunit is an essential prerequisite for receptor formation in vivo. *Neuroscience.* 81(4):1043-53.

Fritschy JM, Brünig I (2003) Formation and plasticity of GABAergic synapses: physiological mechanisms and pathophysiological implications. *Pharmacol Ther.* 98:299-323.

Fritschy JM, Crestani F, Rudolph U, Möhler H (2004) $GABA_A$ receptor subtypes with special reference to memory function and neurological disorders, *in* Excitatory Inhibitory Balance: Synapses, Circuits and Systems Plasticity (Hensch TK *and* Fagiolini M, *eds.*), 215–228. *Kluwer Academic/Plenum Publishers, New York.*

Fritschy JM, Mohler H (1995) GABAA-receptor heterogeneity in the adult rat brain: differential regional and cellular distribution of seven major subunits. *J Comp Neurol.* 359:154-94.

Fritz J, Stewart JT (1990) Lorazepam treatment of resistive aggression in dementia [letter]. *Am J Psychiatry.* 147:1250.

Funderburk WH, Foxwell MH, Hakala MW (1970) Effects of psychotherapeutic drugs on hypothalamic-induced hissing in cats. *Neuropharmacology.* 9:1–7.

Gaiarsa JL, Caillard O, Ben-Ari Y (2002) Long-term plasticity at GABAergic and glycinergic synapses: mechanisms and functional significance. *Trends Neurosci.* 25(11):564-70.

Garcia-Alloza M, Gil-Bea FJ, Diez-Ariza M, Chen CPLH, Francis PT, Lasheras B, Ramirez MJ (2005) Cholinergic-serotonergic imbalance contributes to cognitive and behavioral symptoms in Alzheimer's disease. *Neuropsychologia.* 43:442–449

Garcia-Alloza M, Hirst WD, Chen CP, Lasheras B, Francis PT, Ramirez MJ (2004) Differential involvement of 5-HT(1B/1D) and 5-HT6 receptors in cognitive and noncognitive symptoms in Alzheimer's disease. *Neuropsychopharmacology.* 29:410–416

Greenamyre JT, Penney JB, D'Amato CJ, Young AB (1987) Dementia of the Alzheimer's type: changes in hippocampal L-[3H]glutamate binding. *J Neurochem.* 48:543–51.

Griffiths PD, Perry RH, Crossman AR (1994) A detailed anatomical analysis of neurotransmitter receptors in the putamen and caudate in Parkinson's disease and Alzheimer's disease. *Neurosci Lett.* 169:68–72.

Grunze HC, Rainnie DG, Hasselmo ME, Barkai E, Hearn EF, McCarley RW, Greene RW (1996) NMDA-dependent modulation of CA1 local circuit inhibition. *J Neurosci.* 16(6):2034-43.

Gu Z, Zhong P, Yan Z (2003) Activation of muscarinic receptors inhibits beta-amyloid peptide-induced signaling in cortical slices. *J Biol Chem.* 278: 17546–17556.

Guastella J, Nelson N, Nelson H, Czyzyk L, Keynan S, Miedel MC, Davidson N, Lester HA, Kanner BI (1990) Cloning and expression of a rat brain GABA transporter. *Science.* 249:1303-1306.

Hardy J, Cowburn R, Barton A, Reynolds G, Dodd P, Wester P, O'Carroll AM, Lofdahl E, Winblad B (1987) A disorder of cortical GABAergic innervation in Alzheimer's disease. *Neurosci Lett.* 73:192–6.

Hertz L, Wu PH, Schousboe A (1978) Evidence for net uptake of GABA into mouse astrocytes in primary cultures--its sodium dependence and potassium independence. *Neurochem Res.* 3:313-323.

Holmgren CD, Zilberter Y (2001) Coincident spiking activity induces long-term changes in inhibition of neocortical pyramidal cells. *J Neurosci.* 21(20):8270-7.

Hope T, Keene J, Gedling K, Cooper S, Fairburn C, Jacoby R (1997) Behaviour changes in dementia. *Int J Geriatr Psychiatry.* 12:1062–1078

Hu JH, Ma YH, Jiang J, Yang N, Duan SH, Jiang ZH, Mei ZT, Fei J, Guo LH (2004) Cognitive impairment in mice over-expressing gammaaminobutyric acid transporter 1 (GAT1). *Neuroreport.* 15:9 –12.

Hyman BT, Van Hoesen GW, Damasio AR, Barnes CL (1984) Alzheimer's disease: cell-specific pathology isolates the hippocampal formation. Science. 225: 1168–1170.

Ikonomovic MD, Mizukami K, Warde D, Sheffield R, Hamilton R, Wenthold RJ, Armstrong DM (1999) Distribution of glutamate receptor subunit NMDAR1 in the hippocampus of normal elderly and patients with Alzheimer's disease. *Exp Neurol.* 160:194–204.

Ikonomovic MD, Nocera R, Mizukami K, Armstrong DM (2000) Age-related loss of the AMPA receptor subunits GluR2/3 in the human nucleus basalis of Meynert. *Exp Neurol.* 166: 363–375.

Introini-Collison IB, Castellano C, McGaugh JL (1994) Interaction of GABAergic and beta-noradrenergic drugs in the regulation of memory storage. *Behav Neural Biol.* 61(2):150-5.

IPA (1996) Behavioral and Psychological signs and symptoms in demenia (BPSSD): implications for research and treatment. *Int Psychogeriatr.* 8:215–552

Iversen LL, Mortishire-Smith RJ, Pollack SJ, Shearman MS (1995) The toxicity in vitro of beta-amyloid protein. *Biochem J.* 311:1-16.

Jansen KL, Faull RL, Dragunow M, Synek BL (1990) Alzheimer's disease: changes in hippocampal N-methyl-D-aspartate, quisqualate, neurotensin, adenosine, benzodiazepine, serotonin and opioid receptors an autoradiographic study. *Neuroscience.* 39:613–27.

Jasinska M, Siucinska E, Cybulska-Klosowicz A, Pyza E, Furness DN, Kossut M, Glazewski S (2010) Rapid, learning-induced inhibitory synaptogenesis in murin barrel field. *J Neurosci.* 30:1176–1184.

Jechlinger M, Pelz R, Tretter V, Klausberger T, Sieghart W (1998) Subunit composition and quantitative importance of hetero-oligomeric receptors: $GABA_A$ receptors containing alpha6 subunits. *J. Neurosci.* 18:2449–2457.

Jiménez-Jiménez FJ, Molina JA, Gómez P, Vargas C, de Bustos F, Benito-León J, Tallón-Barranco A, Ortí-Pareja M, Gasalla T, Arenas J (1998) Neurotransmitter amino acids in cerebrospinal fluid of patients with Alzheimer's disease. *J Neural Transm.* 105:269–77.

Keverne EB (1999) GABA-ergic neurons and the neurobiology of schizophrenia and other psychoses. *Brain Res Bull.* 48:467–73.

Komatsu Y, Yoshimura Y (2000) Activity-dependent maintenance of long-term potentiation at visual cortical inhibitory synapses. *J Neurosci.* 20:7539-46.

Kristensen BW, Noraberg J, Zimmer J (2003) The GABAA receptor agonist THIP is neuroprotective in organotypic hippocampal slice cultures. *Brain Res.* 973:303–306.

Krystal JH, Sanacora G, Blumberg H, Anand A, Charney DS, Marek G, Epperson CN, Goddard A, Mason GF (2002) Glutamate and GABA systems as targets for novel antidepressant and mood-stabilizing treatments. *Mol Psychiatry.* 7:71–80

Kuroda H (1983) Gamma-aminobutyric acid (GABA) in cerebrospinal fluid. *Acta Med Okayama.* 37:167–77.

Kvamme E, Svenneby G, Hertz L, Schousboe A (1982) Properties of phosphate activated glutaminase in astrocytes cultured from mouse brain. *Neurochem Res.* 7:761-770.

Lanctôt KL, Herrmann N, Mazzotta P, Khan LR, Ingber N (2004) GABAergic function in Alzheimer's disease: evidence for dysfunction and potential as a therapeutic target for the treatment of behavioural and psychological symptoms of dementia. *Can J Psychiatry.* 49(7):439-53.

Lapchak PA, Chapman DF, Nunez SY, Zivin JA (2000) Dehydroepiandrosterone sulfate is neuroprotective in a reversible spinal cord ischemia model: possible involvement of GABA(A) receptors. *Stroke.* 31:1953–1956.

Lee BY, Ban JY, Seong YH (2005) Chronic stimulation of GABAA receptor with muscimol reduces amyloid beta protein (25–35)-induced neurotoxicity in cultured rat cortical cells. *Neurosci Res.* 52:347–356.

Levy ML, Cummings JL, Kahn-Rose R (1999) Neuropsychiatric symptoms and cholinergic therapy for Alzheimer's disease. *Gerontology.* 45: 15–22.

Li M, De Blas AL (1997) Coexistence of two beta subunit isoforms in the same gamma-aminobutyric acid type A receptor. J Biol Chem. 272:1654–1659.

Liang SL, Carlson GC, Coulter DA (2006) Dynamic regulation of synaptic GABA release by the glutamate-glutamine cycle in hippocampal area CA1. *J Neurosci.* 26:8537-8548.

Lin X, Jun-Tian Z (2004) Neuroprotection by d-securinine against neurotoxicity induced by beta-amyloid (25–35). *Neurol Res.* 26:792–796.

Lloyd K, Morselli P. (1987) Psychopharmacology of GABAergic drugs, *in. Psychopharmacology: the third generation of progress* (Meltzer H and Meltzer HS, eds), 183-195. Raven Press, New York.

Lloyd KG, Zivkovic B, Scatton B, Morselli PL, Bartholini G (1989) The gabaergic hypothesis of depression. *Prog Neuropsychopharmacol Biol Psychiatry.* 13: 341–351

Louzada PR, Paula Lima AC, Mendonca-Silva DL, Noel F, De Mello FG, Ferreira ST (2004) Taurine prevents the neurotoxicity of beta-amyloid and glutamate receptor agonists: activation of GABA receptors and possible implications for Alzheimer's disease and other neurological disorders. *FASEB J.* 18:511–518.

Luchetti S, Bossers K, Van de Bilt S, Agrapart V, Morales RR, Frajese GV, Swaab DF (2011) Neurosteroid biosynthetic pathways changes in prefrontal cortex in Alzheimer's disease. *Neurobiol Aging.* 32(11):1964-76.

Malick JB, Goldberg ME (1970) Effects of a choline acetyltransferase inhibitor on self-stimulatory behavior in the rat. *Arch Int Pharmacodyn Ther.* 184:252–6.

Manyam NV, Katz L, Hare TA, Gerber JC, Grossman MH (1980) Levels of gamma-aminobutyric acid in cerebrospinal fluid in various neurologic disorders. *Arch Neurol.* 37:352–5.

Marcade M, Bourdin J, Loiseau N, Peillon H, Rayer A, Drouin D, Schweighoffer F, Desire L *(*2008*)* Etazolate, a neuroprotective drug linking GABA(A) receptor pharmacology to amyloid precursor protein processing. *J Neurochem.* 106:392–404.

Masashi S, Mituyuki I (1996) Amyloid β proteins reduce the GABA-induced $Cl^-$ current in identified Aplasia neurons. *Neurosci Lett.* 213:213–215

Matthews KL, Chen CP, Esiri MM, Keene J, Minger SL, Francis PT (2002) Noradrenergic changes, aggressive behavior, and cognition in patients with dementia. *Biol Psychiatry.* 51:407–416

Maubach KP (2003) sychiatric drug discovery and development. *Expert Opin Investig Drugs.* 12(9):1571-1575.

McElroy MW, Korol DL (2005) Intrahippocampal muscimol shifts learning strategy in gonadally intact young adult female rats. *Learn Mem.* 12(2):150-8.

Menendez M *(*2005*)* Down syndrome, Alzheimer's disease and seizures. *Brain Dev.* 27:246–252.

Minger SL, Esiri MM, McDonald B, Keene J, Carter J, Hope T, Francis PT (2000) Cholinergic deficits contribute to behavioral disturbance in patients with dementia. *Neurology.* 55:1460–1467

Mishizen AJ, Ikonomovic I, Armstrong DM (2000) *Glutamate receptors in aging and Alzheimer's disease, in Functional Neurobiology of Aging* (Hof P and Mobbs C eds), 283–314. Academic Press, San Diego, CA.

Mishizen-Eberz AJ, Rissman RA, Carter TL, Ikonomovic MD, Wolfe BB, Armstrong DM *(*2004*)* Biochemical and molecular studies of NMDA receptor subunits NR1/2A/2B in hippocampal subregions throughout progression of Alzheimer's disease pathology. Neurobiol Dis. 15:80–92.

Möhler H (2001*) Functions of GABA receptors: pharmacology and pathophysiology, in Pharmacology of GABA and Glycine Neurotransmission* (MöhlerH, ed.), pp. 101–116. Springer Publishers, New York.

Möhler H (2002) Pathophysiological aspects of diversity in neuronal inhibition: a new benzodiazepine pharmacology. *Dialogues Clin Neurosci.* 4:261–269.

Möhler H (2006) GABAA receptor diversity and pharmacology. *Cell Tissue Res.* 326:505–516.

Möhler H (2011) The rise of a new GABA pharmacology. *Neuropharmacology.* 60:1042–1049.

Mohler H, Fritschy JM, Luscher B, Rudolph U, Benson J, Benke D (1996) The $GABA_A$ receptors. From subunits to diverse functions. *Ion Channels.* 4:89–113.

Möhler H, Fritschy JM, Rudolph U *(*2002*)* A new benzodiazepine pharmacology. *J Pharm Exptl Ther.* 30:2–8.

Möhler H, Fritschy JM, Vogt K, Crestani F, Rudolph U (2005) Pathophysiology and pharmacology of GABAA receptors, in Anxiety and Anxiolytic Drugs, *Handbook of Experimental Pharmacology,* Vol. 169 (Holsboer F. and Ströhle A, eds.), 225–247. Springer Publishers, New York.

Mohr E, Bruno G, Foster N, Gillespie M, Cox C, Hare TA, Tamminga C, Fedio P, Chase TN (1986) GABA-agonist therapy for Alzheimer's disease. *Clin Neuropharmacol.* 9:257–63.

Mohr E, Mendis T, Rusk IN, Grimes JD (1994) Neurotransmitter replacement therapy in Alzheimer's disease. *J Psychiatry Neurosci.* 19:17–23.

Nägga K, Bogdanovic N, Marcusson J (1999) GABA transporters (GAT-1) in Alzheimer's disease. *J Neural Transm.* 106:1141–9.

Nakamura S (1990) Senile dementia and presenile dementia. *Tohoku J Exp Med.* 161(Suppl):49–60.

Nitz D, McNaughton B (2004) Differential modulation of CA1 and dentate gyrus interneurons during exploration of novel environments. *J Neurophysiol.* 91:863– 872.

Norenberg MD, Martinez-Hernandez A (1979) Fine structural localization of glutamine synthetase in astrocytes of rat brain. *Brain Res.* 161:303-310.

Nunan J, Small DH (2000) Regulation of APP cleavage by alpha-, beta- and gamma-secretases. *FEBS Lett.* 13:483(1):6-10.

Nusser Z, Hájos N, Somogyi P, Mody I (1998) Increased number of synaptic GABA(A) receptors underlies potentiation at hippocampal inhibitory synapses. *Nature.* 395(6698):172-7.

Nusser Z, Sieghart W, Benke D, Fritschy JM, Somogyi P (1996) Differential synaptic localization of two major gamma-aminobutyric acid type A receptor alpha subunits on hippocampal pyramidal cells. *Proc Natl Acad Sci U S A.* 93(21):11939-44.

Ohba S, Ikeda T, Ikegaya Y, Nishiyama N, Matsuki N, Yamada MK (2005) BDNF locally potentiates GABAergic presynaptic machineries: target-selective circuit inhibition. *Cereb Cortex.* 15(3):291-8.

Oishi M, Mochizuki Y, Yoshihashi H, Takasu T, Nakano E (1996) Laboratory examinations correlated with severity of dementia. *Ann Clin Lab Sci.* 26:340–5.

Olsen RW, Sieghart W (2008) International Union of Pharmacology. LXX. Subtypes of gamma-aminobutyric acid(A) receptors: classification on the basis of subunit composition, pharmacology, and function. Update. *Pharmacological Rev.* 60:243-260.

Ottersen OP, Zhang N, Walberg F (1992) Metabolic compartmentation of glutamate and glutamine: morphological evidence obtained by quantitative immunocytochemistry in rat cerebellum. *Neuroscience.* 46:519-534.

Owen F, Poulter M, Waddington JL, Mashal RD, Crow TJ (1983) [3H]R05-4864 and [3H]flunitrazepam binding in kainate-lesioned rat striatum and in temporal cortex of brains from patients with senile dementia of the Alzheimer type. *Brain Res.* 278:373–5.

Pakaski M, Farkas Z, Kasa P Jr, Forgon M, Papp H, Zarandi M, Penke B, Kasa P Sr (1998) Vulnerability of small GABAergic neurons to human beta-amyloid pentapeptide. *Brain Res.* 796(1-2):239-46.

Palop JJ, Mucke L (2009a) Epilepsy and cognitive impairments in Alzheimer disease. *Arch Neurol.* 66:435–440.

Palop JJ, Mucke L (2009b) Synaptic depression and aberrant excitatory network activity in Alzheimer's disease: two faces of the same coin? *Neuromol Med.* 12:48–55.

Palop JJ, Mucke L (2010) Amyloid-beta-induced neuronal dysfunction in Alzheimer's disease: from synapses toward neural networks. *Nat Neurosci.* 13:812–818.

Pandey GN, Conley RR, Pandey SC, Goel S, Roberts RC, Tamminga CA, Chute D, Smialek J (1997) Benzodiazepine receptors in the post-mortem brain of suicide victims and schizophrenic subjects. *Psychiatry Res.* 71:137–149

Panksepp J (1971) Drugs and stimulus-bound attack. Physiol Behav. 6:317–20.

Parmentier ML, Prezeau L, Bockaert J, Pin JP (2002) A model for the functioning of family 3 GPCRs. *Trends in pharmacological sciences.* 23:268-274.

Parnetti L, Amici S, Lanari A,Gallai V (2001) Pharmacological treatment of non-cognitive disturbances in dementia disorders. *Mech Ageing Dev.* 122:2063–2069

Paula-Lima AC, De Felice FG, Brito-Moreira J, Ferreira ST (2005) Activation of GABA(A) receptors by taurine and muscimol blocks the neurotoxicity of beta-amyloid in rat hippocampal and cortical neurons. *Neuropharmacol.* 49:1140–1148.

Paula-Lima AC, Louzada PR, De Mello FG, Ferreira ST (2003) Neuroprotection against Abeta and glutamate toxicity by melatonin: are GABA receptors involved? *Neurotox Res.* 5:323–327.

Pellegrini-Giampietro DE, Gorter JA, Bennett MV, Zukin RS (1997) The GluR2 (GluR-B) hypothesis: Ca(2+)-permeable AMPA receptors in neurological disorders. *Trends Neurosci.* 20:464–470.

Perry EK, Tomlinson BE, Blessed G, Bergmann K, Gibson PH, Perry RH (1978) Correlation of cholinergic abnormalities with senile plaques and mental test scores in senile dementia. *BMJ* 2:1457–9.

Perry E, Walker M, Grace J, Perry R (1999) Acetylcholine in mind: a neurotransmitter correlate of consciousness? *Trends Neurosci.* 22:273–280

Pines G, Danbolt NC, Bjørås M, Zhang Y, Bendahan A, Eide L, Koepsell H, Storm-Mathisen J, Seeberg E, Kanner BI (1992) Cloning and expression of a rat brain L-glutamate transporter. *Nature.* 360:464-467.

Pirker S, Schwarzer C, Wieselthaler A, Sieghart W, Sperk G (2000) GABA(A) receptors: immunocytochemical distribution of 13 subunits in the adult rat brain. *Neuroscience.* 101(4):815-50.

Pisani F, Costa C, Caccamo D, Mazzon E, Gorgone G, Oteri G, Calabresi P, Ientile R (2006) Tiagabine and vigabatrin reduce the severity of NMDA-induced excitotoxicity in chick retina. *Exp Brain Res.* 171:511–515.

Pöltl A, Hauer B, Fuchs K, Tretter V, Sieghart W (2003) Subunit composition and quantitative importance of GABA(A) receptor subtypes in the cerebellum of mouse and rat. *J Neurochem.* 87(6):1444-55.

Pomara N, Deptula D, Galloway MP, LeWitt PA, Stanley M (1989) CSF GABA in caregiver spouses of Alzheimer patients. *Am J Psychiatry.* 146:787–8.

Puerta E, Tordera RM, Ramirez MJ, Solas M (2014) *Glutamate and GABA: Partners in Crime in Stress Induced Cognitive Dysfunction, in Cognitive Dysfunctions: Biological Basis, Management of Symptoms and Long-Term Neurological Implications* (Burgess EN and Thornton LA, eds), 63-86. Nova publisher, New York.

Quirk K, Blurton P, Fletcher S, Leeson P, Tang F, Mellilo D, Ragan CI, McKernan RM (1996) [3H]L-655,708, a novel ligand selective for the benzodiazepine site of $GABA_A$ receptors which contain the alpha 5 subunit. *Neuropharmacol.* 35(9-10):1331-5.

Reisine TD, Yamamura HI, Bird ED, Spokes E, Enna SJ (1978) Pre- and postsynaptic neurochemical alterations in Alzheimer's disease. *Brain Res.* 159:477–81.

Rissman RA, De Blas AL, Armstrong DM (2007) GABA(A) receptors in aging and Alzheimer's disease. *J Neurochem.* 103(4):1285-92.

Rissman RA, Mobley WC (2011) Implications for treatment: GABAA receptors in aging, Down syndrome and Alzheimer's disease. *J Neurochem.* 117:613-622.

Robinson SR, Bishop GM (2002) The search for an amyloid solution. *Science.* 298(5595):962-4

Roeling TA, Kruk MR, Schuurmans R, Veening JG (1993) Behavioural responses of bicucculline methiodide injections into the ventral hypothalamus of freely moving, socially interacting rats. *Brain Res.* 615:121–7.

Rudolph U, Möhler H (2006) GABA-based therapeutic approaches: $GABA_A$ receptor subtype functions. *Curr Opin Pharmacol.* 6:18–23.

Sanacora G, Mason GF, Rothman DL, Behar KL, Hyder F, Petroff OA, Berman RM, Charney DS, Krystal JH (1999) Reduced cortical gamma-aminobutyric acid levels in depressed patients determined by proton magnetic resonance spectroscopy. *Arch Gen Psychiatry.* 56:1043–1047

Sanchez PE, Zhu L, Verret L, Vossel KA, Orr AG, Cirrito JR, Devidze N, Ho K, Yu GQ, Palop JJ, Mucke L. (2012) Levetiracetam suppresses neuronal network dysfunction and reverses synaptic and cognitive deficits in an Alzheimer's disease model. *Proc Natl Acad Sci USA.* 109:2895–2903.

Saransaari P, Oja SS (2006) Taurine release in mouse brain stem slices under cell-damaging conditions. *Amino Acids.* 32:439–446.

Schneider LS, Mangialasche F, Andreasen N, Feldman H, Giacobini E, Jones R, Mantua V, Mecocci P, Pani L, Winblad B, Kivipelto M (2014) Clinical trials and late-stage drug development for Alzheimer's disease: an appraisal from 1984 to 2014. *J Intern. Med.* 275(3):251-83

Schwartz-Bloom RD, Miller KA, Evenson DA, Crain BJ, Nadler JV (2000) Benzodiazepines protect hippocampal neurons from degeneration after transient cerebral ischemia: an ultrastructural study. *Neuroscience.* 98:471–484.

Schousboe A, Sarup A, Bak LK, Waagepetersen HS, Larsson OM (2004) Role of astrocytic transport processes in glutamatergic and GABAergic neurotransmission. *Neurochem Int.* 45:521-527.

Sedvall G, Nyback H, Farde L, Persson A (1987) Neurotransmitter receptor imaging in Alzheimer's disease. *J Neural Transm Suppl.* 24:43–8.

Seidl R, Cairns N, Singewald N, Kaehler ST, Lubec G (2001) Differences between GABA levels in Alzheiemer's disease and Down syndrome with Alzheimer-like neuropathology. *Naunyn-Schmiedeberg's Arch Pharmacol.* 363:139–45.

Selkoe DJ, Wolfe MS (2007) Presenilin: running with scissors in the membrane. *Cell.* 131(2):215-21.

Sherif F, Ahmed SS, Eriksson L (1995) Brain aminobutyrate aminotransferase activity in Alzheimer's disease [letter]. *Neurodegeneration.* 4:114–5.

Sherif F, Gottfries CG, Alafuzoff I, Oreland L (1992) Brain gamma-aminobutyrate aminotransferase (GABA-T) and monoamine oxidase (MAO) in patients with Alzheimer's disease. *J Neural Transm Park Dis Dement Sect.* 4:227–40.

Shiah IS, Yatham LN (1998) GABA function in mood disorders: an update and critical review. *Life Sci,* 63: 1289–1303

Shimohama S, Taniguchi T, Fujiwara M, Kameyama M (1998) Changes in benzodiazepine receptors in Alzheimer-type dementia. *Ann Neurol.* 23:404–6.

Sieghart W (2006) *Subunit composition and structure of GABAA receptor subtypes, in GABA Receptor* (Enna SJ and Möhler H, eds). Humana Press, Totowa, NJ.

Sieghart W, Sperk G (2002) Subunit composition, distribution and function of GABAA receptor subtypes. *Curr Topics Med Chem.* 2:795–816.

Storga D, Vrecko K, Birkmayer JG, Reibnegger G (1996) Monoaminergic neurotransmitters, their precursors and metabolites in brains of Alzheimer patients. *Neurosci Lett,* 203:29–32

Sunderland T, Weingartner H, Cohen RM, Tariot PN, Newhouse PA, Thompson KE, Lawlor BA, Mueller EA (1989) Low-dose oral lorazepam administration in Alzheimer subjects and age- matched controls. *Psychopharmacology.* 99:129–133.

Tarbit I, Perry EK, Perry RH, Blessed G, Tomlinson BE (1980) Hippocampal free amino acids in Alzheimer's disease. *J Neurochem.* 35:1246–9.

Taylor M, Bhagwagar Z, Cowen PJ, Sharp T (2003) GABA and mood disorders. *Psychol Med.* 33:387–393

Terry AV Jr, Buccafusco JJ (2003) The cholinergic hypothesis of age and Alzheimer's disease-related cognitive deficits: recent challenges and their implications for novel drug development. *J Pharmacol Exp Ther*. 306:821–827

Tohgi H, Abe T, Takahashi S, Kimura M (1992) A selective reduction of excitatory amino acids in cerebrospinal fluid of patients with Alzheimer type dementia compared with vascular dementia of the Binswanger type. *Neurosci Lett.* 141:5–8.

Tosca P, Canevari L, Di Paolo E, Ferrari R, Verze S, Zerbi F, Dagani F (1992) Glutamate and GABA levels in CSF from patients affected by dementia and olivo-ponto-cerebellar atrophy. *Acta Neurol Scand.* 85:430–435.

Van den Berg CJ, Garfinkel D (1971) A stimulation study of brain compartments. Metabolism of glutamate and related substances in mouse brain. *Biochem J.* 123:211-218.

Velasco I, Tapia R *(*2002*)* High extracellular gamma-aminobutyric acid protects cultured neurons against damage induced by the accumulation of endogenous extracellular glutamate. *J Neurosci Res.* 67:406–410.

Vignes M *(*2001*)* Regulation of spontaneous inhibitory synaptic transmission by endogenous glutamate via non-NMDA receptors in cultured rat hippocampal neurons. *Neuropharmacol.* 40:737–748.

Vogt BA, Crino PB, Volicer L (1991) Laminar alterations in gamma-aminobutyric acidA, muscarinic, and beta adrenoceptors and neuron degeneration in cingulate cortex in Alzheimer's disease. *J Neurochem.* 57:282–290.

Wahrle S, Das P, Nyborg AC, McLendon C, Shoji M, Kawarabayashi T, Younkin LH, Younkin SG, Golde TE (2002) Cholesterol-dependent gamma-secretase activity in buoyant cholesterol-rich membrane microdomains. *Neurobiol Dis.* 9(1):11-23.

Wallace SJ *(*2001*)* Newer antiepileptic drugs: advantages and disadvantages. *Brain Dev.* 23:277–283.

Weiner MF, Speciale SG, Risser RC, Kramer GL, Petty F (1996) Cerebrospinal fluid and plasma gamma-aminobutyric acid in Alzheimer's disease. *Biol Psychiatry.* 40:933–4.

Whitehouse PJ, Price DL, Clark AW, Coyle JT, DeLong MR (1981) Alzheimer disease: evidence for selective loss of cholinergic neurons in the nucleus basalis. *Ann Neurol.* 10:122–6.

Whiting PJ (2003) The $GABA_A$ receptor gene family: new opportunities for drug development. *Curr Opin Drug Discov Devel.* 6(5):648-57.

Whiting P, Wafford KA, McKernan RM (2000) *Pharmacologic subtypes of GABAA receptors based on subunit composition, in GABA in the Nervous System: The View At Fifty Years* (Martin DL and Olsen RW, eds.), 113–126. Lippincott, Philadelphia.

Wiltgen BJ, Sanders MJ, Ferguson C, Homanics GE, Fanselow MS (2005) Trace fear conditioning is enhanced in mice lacking the delta subunit of the GABAA receptor. *Learn Mem.* 12(3):327-33.

Yates CM, Butterworth J, Tennant MC, Gordon A (1990) Enzyme activities in relation to pH and lactate in postmortem brain in Alzheimer-type and other dementias. *J Neurochem.* 55:1624–30.

Yew DT, Li WP, Webb SE, Lai HW, Zhang L (1999) Neurotransmitters, peptides, and neural cell adhesion molecules in the cortices of normal elderly humans and Alzheimer patients: a comparison. *Exp Gerontol.* 34:117–33.

Zhang F, Li C, Wang R, Han D, Zhang QG, Zhou C, Yu HM, Zhang GY (2007) Activation of GABA receptors attenuates neuronal apoptosis through inhibiting the tyrosine phosphorylation of NR2A by Src after cerebral ischemia and reperfusion. Neuroscience. 150:938–949.

Zimmer R, Teelken AW, Trieling WB, Weber W, Weihmayr T, Lauter H (1984) Gamma-aminobutyric acid and homovanillic acid concentration in the CSF of patients with senile dementia of Alzheimer's type. *Arch Neurol.* 41:602–4.

Zorumski CF, Isenberg KE (1991) Insights into the structure and function of GABA-benzodiazepine receptors: ion channels and psychiatry. *Am J Psychiatry.* 148:162–73.

In: Gamma-Aminobutyric Acid (GABA)
Editors: Josipa Vlainić and Maja Jazvinšćak Jembrek
ISBN: 978-1-63321-838-3


*Chapter 9*

# GABAERGIC SYSTEM AND ALZHEIMER'S DISEASE

***Claudio De Piazza****
Neurology Unit, Valduce Hospital, Como, Italy

## ABSTRACT

Neuropsychiatric symptoms in dementia, commonly addressed as behavioural and psychological symptoms in dementia (BPSD), are a matter of major clinical relevance. The use of antipsychotics, though evidence for their efficacy is better than for any other drug class, is heavily counterbalanced by safety concerns and therefore alternative effective treatments are needed. Amongst others, drugs targeting the GABAergic system are gaining attention as attractive candidates for treating behavioural disorders in dementia patients. Notably, the emerging literature highlights GABAergic system involvement in neurodegenerative diseases, such as Alzheimer's disease (AD), which may ultimately lead to excessive glutamatergic tone. This is known to mediate neuronal death. Furthermore, altered GABA neurotransmission is thought to account for behavioural and cognitive disruption. The aim of this article is to review the available evidence on the therapeutic potential and rationale for the use of drugs with GABAergic activity, namely benzodiazepines, gabapentin, carbamazepine and valproate.

**Keywords**: GABA, dementia, behavioural and psychological symptoms of dementia (BPSD), gabapentin, benzodiazepines, carbamazepine, valproate

## OVERVIEW OF THE $GABA_A$ RECEPTOR CLASS

Gamma-aminobutyric acid (GABA) is the primary inhibitory neurotransmitter in the mammalian central nervous system (CNS). Originally three distinct receptor classes were identified ($GABA_A$, $GABA_B$ and $GABA_C$ receptors), hence, the $GABA_A$ receptor was subsequently recognized as of prominent importance in the vertebrate brain, mediating the

* Corresponding Author address: Neurology Unit, Valduce Hospital, via Dante Alighieri 11, 22100 Como, Italy. Email: claudio.depiazza@gmail.com.

majority of fast inhibitory neurotransmissions (Rissman et al., 2007). The $GABA_A$ receptor is a ligand-gated chloride channel, formed as a pentameric assembly of multiple subunits. In the mature brain, the opening of this channel induces a chloride influx (ions entering the cell), resulting in the hyperpolarization/inhibition of the neuron. On the other hand, in the developing brain, the different gradient in chloride concentrations across the cell membrane leads to the efflux of $Cl^-$ ions when the channel is opened, conferring excitatory properties on the GABA acting at the $GABA_A$ receptor (Li and Xu, 2008).

The subunits of the $GABA_A$ receptor are classified according to their degree of sequence identity, and include: α1-6, β1-4, γ1-3, ρ1-3, δ, ε, π, and θ subunits (Barnard et al., 1998; Bonnert et al., 1999; Whiting et al., 1999). Subunit composition may differ among $GABA_A$ receptors, although the most common type is the pentamer comprised of two α, two β and one γ subunit. The different subunit composition, as shown by genetic, molecular and pharmacological tools, may explain the behavioural and cognitive contribution of individual $GABA_A$ receptors. As an example, the α5 subunit is abundant in the hippocampus, and is thought to be critically involved in learning and memory (Ballard et al., 2009; Collinson et al., 2002; Dawson et al., 2006). Even some of the pharmacological properties of the $GABA_A$ receptors rely upon their specific subunit composition. Regarding benzodiazepine activity, it has been reported that whereas receptors containing α1, β2-3 and γ2 subunits mediate sedative, anterograde amnestic and anticonvulsant actions, receptors containing α1, β2-3 and γ2 subunits mediate an anxiolytic effect and muscle relaxation (Olsen and Sieghart, 2009). Furthermore, the specific subunit composition accounts for the enhanced responsiveness to benzodiazepines frequently seen in the elderly. It has been reported that the presence of the α1 subunit within the receptor complex confers increased affinity to benzodiazepines, whereas the α2, α3 and α5 subunits are lower affinity receptors (Ruano et al., 1991; Ruano et al., 1995). Thus, considering that an increase in α1-containing $GABA_A$ receptors has been found in the elderly (Gutierrez et al., 1996), it is likely that alterations in the composition of $GABA_A$ receptor subunits may account for altered age-related sensitiveness to benzodiazepines.

## GABAergic Involvement in Alzheimer's Disease

Due to the increasingly ageing population, dementia and related complications are becoming an unavoidable issue of both medical and social relevance. Projections estimate that there will be approximately 135 million people with dementia worldwide by 2050 (Alzheimer's Disease International, 2014). Among the various aetiologies, Alzheimer's disease (AD) represents the most common type of dementia, accounting for approximately 60-80% of all cases (Reitz et al., 2011). Cognitive and/or behavioural decline, which involves a minimum of two domains (including impaired ability to acquire and remember new information, impaired reasoning and handling of complex tasks/poor judgement, impaired visual and spatial abilities, impaired language functions and changes in personality or behaviour), is the clinical feature common to all-cause dementias. Interference with the ability to function during daily activities, especially a decline from previous levels of functioning, which cannot be explained by delirium or a major psychiatric disorder, is a further feature required for diagnosis of AD.

In 1983, the National Institute of Neurological and Communicative Disorders and Stroke (NINCDS) and the Alzheimer's Disease and Related Disorders Association (ADRDA) established a set of criteria for the diagnosis of AD (McKhann et al., 1984). These criteria, commonly referred to as the NINCDS-ADRDA criteria, have been quite successful in the past three decades, and have been widely used both in clinical practice and research. More recently, the National Institute on Aging and the Alzheimer's Association updated the 1984 criteria (McKhann et al., 2011). According to these newly published recommendations, once it has been determined that the criteria for all-cause dementia have been met, further evaluation of the patient's history, observation, neuropsychological testing, imaging and laboratory findings (including biomarkers of AD pathology) will enable the distinction into "probable AD dementia", "possible AD dementia" or "probable or possible AD dementia with evidence of the AD pathophysiological process". In more detail, so called "probable AD dementia" requires insidious onset, a clear cut history of worsening of cognition and initial deficits most prominent in memory or, depending on the particular presentation, in linguistic, visual and spatial or executive function; "possible AD dementia" is characterized by an atypical course or an aetiologically mixed presentation; the "probable or possible AD dementia with evidence of the AD pathophysiological process" identifies the subset of patients with biomarker evidence of an underlying AD pathophysiological process. Nevertheless, to date, neither satisfying therapy nor preventative cures have been available.

The pathological hallmarks of the disease in the brain, required for a definite post-mortem diagnosis, are amyloid plaques, consisting predominantly of the amyloid-β peptide, and neurofibrillary tangles, formed by hyperphosphorylated tau protein. A leading theory in AD research is the so-called "amyloid hypothesis", which suggests that aggregation of the amyloid-β peptide could act as an initiator of multiple neurotoxic pathways, including the glutamate excitotoxicity, oxidative stress, tau hyperphosphorylation, disturbances in ion homeostasis and mitochondrial function, synaptotoxicity and cell death (Finder, 2010; Robinson and Bishop, 2002). As a result of all these pathophysiological processes, the brain regions critically involved in learning and memory, such as the hippocampus and the association cortices of the frontal, temporal and parietal lobes, show extensive atrophy and reactive gliosis.

Another long-standing hypothesis in the field of AD supports the idea of the selective vulnerability of certain neuronal populations within the specific brain regions. Particularly, massive cell loss affects the basal forebrain cholinergic neurons, the noradrenergic and serotonergic brainstem neurons and the hippocampal glutamatergic neurons. On the other hand, several initial studies have sustained the idea that the GABAergic system is relatively spared by these involutive brain changes (Lowe et al., 1988; Mountjoy et al., 1984; Reinikainen et al., 1988; Rossor, 1982).

More recently, this idea has been partly revised by the emerging literature highlighting evidence of GABAergic system involvement in neurodegenerative diseases, such as AD, as well as in the healthy-aging brain (Rissman et al., 2007; Rissman and Mobley, 2011). Despite decrease in the total number and the affinity of the $GABA_A$ receptors in aged brain, disease-related changes in the receptor subunit composition have been also recognized. Subsequent alteration of the excitatory/inhibitory (E/I) balance may result in excessive glutamatergic tone, which is known to mediate neuronal death. Indeed, Palop and Mucke (2010) reported the alterations in E/I balance related to learning and memory deficits and synaptic vulnerability in AD mouse models. Whether and to what extent these changes assume a causative role in humans is yet to be fully elucidated. Furthermore, altered GABA neurotransmission is thought to account for the non-cognitive behavioural disturbances in dementia (Garcia-Alloza et al., 2006; Lanctôt et al., 2004; Lanctôt et al., 2007). It has been shown that a decrease in the GABA content and the upregulation of $GABA_A$ receptors into the frontal and temporal cortex, correlates significantly with depression in AD patients (Garcia-Alloza et al., 2006). These findings are consistent with previous observations with respect to clinically depressed non-demented patients (Cheetham et al., 1988; Pandey et al., 1997; Taylor et al., 2003). It has also been shown that pharmacological agents that increase GABA levels are able to reduce aggression and that GABA levels correlate to some aspects of aggressive behaviour (Bjork et al., 2001).

Given these hypotheses, the GABAergic system is increasingly gaining attention as a potential target for therapeutic interventions aimed at reverting the pathological E/I imbalance (Louzada et al., 2004) as well as treating behavioural disorders in dementia patients. The latter, which has recently gained attention in clinical practice, will be discussed in this chapter.

## Behavioural and Psychological Symptoms of Dementia

Neuropsychiatric symptoms, commonly addressed as behavioural and psychological symptoms in dementia (BPSD), are a matter of a major clinical relevance. The term BPSD is used to indicate an extremely wide spectrum of clinical features, consisting of: mood disturbances, agitation, irritability, restlessness with semi-purposeful motor activity, wandering, heightened responsiveness to internal and external stimuli, resistance in cooperating in daily activities and sleep disorders.

It has been reported that an outburst of these problems, more than cognitive dysfunction and physical dependence, may account for the greatest burden for family caregivers (Machnicki et al., 2009; Pinquart and Sörensen, 2003) and may predict the likelihood of institutionalization of the patient (Chan et al., 2003; De Vugt et al., 2005). Furthermore, it is worth considering that BPSD are extremely common, with approximately two thirds of these patients experiencing them during the course of their illness (Lyketsos et al., 2000), and are relatively persistent, particularly in the later stages of the disease (Eustace et al., 2002).

Management of BPSD is challenging and, provided that no underlying cause is responsible for their appearance, generally requires a non-pharmacological approach as the first choice. Positive and robust data exist supporting the effectiveness of non-pharmacological or psychosocial treatment in residential care (Livingston et al., 2005; O'Connor et al., 2009). Furthermore, a recent meta-analysis (Brodaty and Arasaratnam, 2012) also validated the efficacy of non-pharmacological intervention when delivered in a community setting. Specifically, Brodaty and Arasaratnam (2012) reported that psychosocial interventions delivered to patients by family caregivers were able to reduce the frequency and severity of BPSD to an extent at least equal to that provided by pharmacotherapy.

Nonetheless, pharmacotherapy is frequently an unavoidable option to keep the behavioural bursts under control. Overall, the largest number of randomized controlled trials (RCTs) has focused on antipsychotics and several systematic reviews have concluded that the evidence for their efficacy is better than for any other drug class (Alexopoulos et al., 1998;

Alexopoulos et al., 2004; Herrmann, 2001; Sink et al., 2005). Unfortunately safety concerns counterbalance their efficacy, thus limiting their use. Indeed, both typical and atypical antipsychotic medications have been associated with an increased risk of cerebrovascular accidents and mortality when used in demented patients (Herrmann et al., 2004; Herrmann and Lanctôt, 2005; Layton et al., 2005; Liperoti et al., 2005; Nasrallah et al., 2004; Schneeweiss et al., 2007; Schneider et al., 2005; Suh and Shah, 2005). These data, as well as recommendations from some health regulatory agencies to curtail the use of the antipsychotic medications in patients with BPSD (American Geriatrics Society and American Association for Geriatric Psychiatry, 2003; Banerjee, 2009), have shown the urgent need for safer and effective alternative treatments. Among the various therapeutic options, cognitive enhancers appear to have beneficial effects on behaviour solely in patients with mild to moderate BPSD (Cummings et al., 2006; Gauthier et al., 2005; Trinh et al., 2003). Therefore, initial treatment with cholinesterase inhibitors or memantine would seem a reasonable option (even a preferable option considering their efficacy on cognition). On the other hand, their use in more seriously disturbed patients requires further evaluation (Herrmann and Lanctôt, 2007). Regarding antidepressants, positive data are available indicating they are safe and effective in treating depression in dementia (Thompson et al., 2007). On the other hand, additional studies are required to support their use in the treatment of agitation and other BPSD (Herrmann and Lanctôt, 2007). Other drug classes considered for the treatment of BPSD are benzodiazepines, anticonvulsants, lithium and beta-blockers. Even if some evidence exists that these drugs may play a role in certain situations, data are lacking to recommend their routine use in demented patients (APA Work Group on Alzheimer's Disease and other Dementias, 2007).

In this chapter we will focus on drugs with GABAergic activity. Namely, the aim of the present chapter is to review the available evidence on their therapeutic potential and rationale for their use.

## GABAPENTIN

Gabapentin is an antiepileptic agent structurally analogue of the neurotransmitter GABA. Initially approved for use as an add-on therapy for patients with partial seizures, it is currently used for a wider range of indications, including neuropathic pain, anxiety and sleep disorders. Various theories have been proposed to explain its cellular and molecular action, which is still not fully understood. Initial studies have supported the idea that gabapentin does not bind to either the $GABA_A$ or the $GABA_B$ receptor (Sauman-Chauhan et al., 1993), nor is it converted metabolically into GABA (Taylor et al., 1998). One theory has postulated that the drug may act by modulating the GABA transporter function. Redistribution of specific GABA transporter proteins from intracellular locations to the plasma membrane could explain the increased GABA uptake and the subsequent increase in GABA synaptic levels, as observed in vitro in hippocampal cultures exposed to gabapentin (Whitworth and Quick, 2001). Other proposed biochemical events that may explain its pharmacological action are the enhanced activity of the enzyme glutamic acid decarboxylase involved in GABA production, and/or the decreased breakdown of GABA by GABA decarboxylase, which ultimately leads to increased extracellular GABA concentrations within the CNS (Löscher et al., 1991). Indeed, nuclear magnetic resonance spectroscopy studies have shown that GABA concentrations are elevated in patients taking gabapentin, and that this elevation of GABA is related to seizure control (Mattson et al., 1997; Petroff et al., 1996). However, the potentiation of inhibitory GABAergic pathways is insufficient to explain fully the therapeutic effect of gabapentin. Other complex intracellular signalling pathways and various neurotransmitter release systems (dopamine, noradrenaline and serotonin) have also been implicated as possible sites of action of gabapentin (Maneuf et al., 2003). Among the various binding sites of the drug, the α2δ voltage-dependent calcium channel subunit is worth mentioning, as it appears to have particular therapeutic relevance in explaining the action of gabapentin. Remarkably, differences in the α2δ binding affinities of stereoselective analogues of gabapentin have been reported to correlate well with their structure-activity relationships in animal models of epilepsy (Taylor et al., 1993) and pain (Field et al., 2000).

To date there is still limited evidence to support the use of gabapentin in BPSD, since no randomized controlled trials (RCTs) have ever been conducted. Nonetheless, over the last two decades, emerging literature, consisting of several case reports and case series, has been compiled and testifies to the strong interest this drug arouses, as a potential alternative to antipsychotics. In particular, its relatively benign adverse-effect profile and its limited potential for drug-drug interactions are major advantages, which make gabapentin particularly suitable for use in the geriatric population.

The first case report regarding the use of gabapentin for treatment of BPSD was by Regan and Gordon, published in 1997 (Regan and Gordon, 1997). They reported the case of a 68 year-old woman with AD, showing troublesome agitation, unresponsive to treatment with buspirone, fluoxetine, trazodone and haloperidol. Three weeks after commencing treatment with gabapentin, 300 mg twice daily, the patient was much less agitated according to a clinician, nursing home staff and family assessment. Sustained improvement was still apparent nine weeks later, and therefore the therapy was continued.

A twelve-patient, prospective, open-label case series was published by Herrmann et al., 2000. The patients were reported to have moderate to severe dementia with severe behavioural disorders, and not to have responded to previous treatment with neuroleptics. Gabapentin was commenced at an initial dose of 100 mg twice a day, and the dose was later increased to a maximum of 1200 mg a day. Analyses of the ten patients who completed at least four weeks of the treatment revealed no significant changes on the Neuropsychiatric Inventory (NPI) and the Cohen-Mansfield Agitation Inventory (CMAI) scales. However, on the Clinical Global Impression (CGI) scale, two patients had improved, three had minimally improved, six were unchanged, and one was minimally worse. In 2000, Hawkins et al., examined the use of gabapentin for the treatment of aggressive behaviour in nursing home patients with a DSM-IV diagnosis of dementia. Of the twenty-four patients included in this retrospective, open-label case series, twenty-two were much or greatly improved, on the basis of the CGI scale, four were minimally improved, one remained unchanged, and in two patients treatment was discontinued due to excessive sedation. Gabapentin was administered at an initial dose of 100-300 mg daily, and it was subsequently titrated up to a maximum of 3600 mg daily, for better control of the patients' agitated or aggressive behaviour. A twenty-patient open-label case series was reported by Moretti et al. in 2003. The patients were all diagnosed with probable AD with behavioural alterations and serious comorbidities (paralytic ileus, open-angle glaucoma, ischaemic cardiopathy, hepatic failure or severe prostatic hyperplasia). Gabapentin was initiated at a dose of 300 mg, three times per day. The highest dose administered was 1800 mg a day, and patients were permitted to continue any previous therapy for concurrent diseases, other than antipsychotics and benzodiazepines, which were discontinued. Assessment of their behavioural symptoms using the NPI and CMAI scales, as well as the assessment of the caregiver's stress level, using the Caregiver Burden Inventory scale, demonstrated a significant and sustained benefit. In 2004, Raudino and colleagues reported a series of nine patients with AD and major behavioural symptoms. All of them were treated with gabapentin, starting at a dose of 300 mg at bedtime, and this was subsequently increased every two to three days, up to a maximum of 1200 mg a day. After one month, psychiatric symptoms, assessed by the NPI scale, were improved in seven out of nine patients. At six months, improvement was maintained in only two patients, whereas the remainder showed worsening of behavioural symptoms, despite an increase in the drug dose.

A comprehensive review of the available literature on the use of gabapentin in BPSD was published by Kim and colleagues in 2008 (Kim et al., 2008). Search of PubMed, PsycINFO, Ovid MEDLINE, Cochrane Library and ClinicalTrials.gov yielded eleven case reports and four case series (mentioned above) but no RCTs. As stated by Kim and colleagues, several limitations undermine the quality of the available data, such as the inherent risk of a bias favouring gabapentin. Namely, cases in which the behavioural disturbances were unaffected or aggravated by medication are less likely to be reported. Moreover, there is a lack of congruency in the type of scales used to assess the clinical response, which makes comparison of different studies difficult. Finally, the overestimation of the drug's efficacy is possible given the fact that some cases of agitation may have resolved either spontaneously or secondary to drug-induced sedation. In addition, Kim et al. (2008) reported that neither a specific dosage recommendation, nor a specific target plasma concentration may be suggested, because of the lack of consensus. The adverse effects reported were: excessive sedation, gait instability, mild drowsiness, headache, dizziness, reduced ambulation, disorientation, confusion, hallucinations, fatigue, apathy and decreased appetite. In some cases of Lewy body dementia treated with gabapentin, increased agitation was reported, suggesting that the drug might not be appropriate for all types of dementia-related behavioural symptoms. The authors concluded that, although gabapentin may be considered for the treatment of BPSD, the lack of RCTs limits support for the off-label use of this drug in dementia.

Following the review by Kim et al. two other original articles relevant to the topic were published. In 2011, Buskova and colleagues reported the case of a 77 year-old woman with incipient vascular dementia, with recurrent episodes of nocturnal agitation and wandering. After an initial non pharmacological approach had proven ineffective, 400 mg gabapentin was initiated at bedtime. In the subsequent nine month follow-up of the patient, no recurrence of the previous episodes occurred. Cooney et al. (2013) reported a retrospective case series on seven patients with vascular or mixed vascular/Alzheimer dementia, treated with gabapentin over a six-month period. All patients were referred due to agitation/aggressive behaviour, which was creating serious concerns for their caregivers, who reported that they were likely to transfer their relatives to inpatient care if these neuropsychiatric symptoms were not brought under control. Gabapentin was started at a dose of 100 mg twice a day and increased to a maximum of 600 mg daily. Even though no standardized behavioural rating scale was used to assess the effectiveness of the treatment, the authors reported a clinically significant improvement in the aggressive behaviour of all patients. Notably, antipsychotic drugs were uneventfully discontinued in three patients after the initiation of gabapentin treatment (in the other four patients they were stopped before the initiation of gabapentin because they were clearly ineffective). As underscored in this paper, in these cases gabapentin proved effective in a much lower dosage than reported in other studies.

In the last few years, several review articles have been published addressing the use of anticonvulsants for the treatment of BPSD (Amann et al., 2009; Guay, 2007; Konovalov et al., 2008; Pinheiro, 2008; Yeh and Ouyang, 2012). Thus far, carbamazepine has the most promising evidence of efficacy among the mood stabilizers. Its benefit, anyway, is heavily counterbalanced by the high risk of drug-drug interaction and tolerability concerns. However, Guay (2007) was more supportive regarding the use of gabapentin, indicating it as qualitatively similar in efficacy to carbamazepine, in the management of agitation in demented patients. In addition, several authors have agreed that the studies published to date have numerous design flaws. In conclusion, there is not enough evidence to support the routine use of gabapentin in BPSD, and RCTs are mandatory to find stronger evidence of its efficacy. Moreover, there is also a general consensus that it is worthwhile to investigate it further, given its good tolerability profile and its limited potential for drug-drug interaction.

## BENZODIAZEPINES

Benzodiazepines are positive allosteric modulators of the $GABA_A$ receptor. Each receptor bears one binding site for benzodiazepines and two for the neurotransmitter GABA. Binding of the drug induces a conformational change in the receptor complex, resulting in the increased conduction of chloride ions across the neuronal cell membrane. The consequent hyperpolarization of the cells accounts for GABA's inhibitory effect throughout the CNS (Griffin et al., 2013). As already mentioned in this chapter, the differing subunit compositions of the $GABA_A$ receptor, encompassing high or low-affinity subtypes, account for the individual responsiveness to benzodiazepines (and therefore for the enhanced responsiveness commonly seen in the elderly).

In 2012, the American Geriatrics Society (AGS) updated Beers Criteria for Potentially Inappropriate Medication Use in Older Adults (American Geriatrics Society Beers Criteria Update Expert Panel, 2012), which now encompasses fifty-three medications or medication classes, divided into three categories: "potentially inappropriate medications and classes to avoid in older adults", "potentially inappropriate medications and classes to avoid in older adults with certain diseases and syndromes that the drugs listed can exacerbate", and finally "medications to be used with caution in older adults". According to this classification, benzodiazepines are included in the "potentially inappropriate medications and classes to avoid in older adults". AGS Updated Beers Criteria recommend avoiding benzodiazepines (any type), especially for treatment of insomnia, agitation, or delirium. The quality of the evidence is rated as "high" and, consequently, the strength of the recommendation is rated as "strong". The rationale for this indication is increased drug sensitivity, the slower metabolism of long-acting agents and an increased risk of cognitive impairment, delirium, falls, fractures, and motor vehicle accidents in older adults. The Panel reported that the use of benzodiazepines may be appropriate in selected circumstances, such as seizure disorders, rapid eye movement sleep disorders, benzodiazepine withdrawal, ethanol withdrawal, severe generalized anxiety disorder, periprocedural anaesthesia, and end-of-life care use. The AGS Updated Beers Criteria also include benzodiazepines in the category "potentially inappropriate medications to avoid in older adults with certain diseases and syndromes that the drugs listed can exacerbate", considering cognitive impairment and dementia as threatening diseases. Again, avoiding them in such situations is a recommendation that reaches the level of "strong" on the basis of the "high" quality of evidence.

The American Psychiatric Association practice guidelines for treatment of patients with Alzheimer's disease and other dementias (APA Work Group on Alzheimer's Disease and other Dementias, 2007) reports for benzodiazepines a higher likelihood of side effects and a lower likelihood of benefit than for antipsychotics. It is advised that long term use should be avoided, whereas on an occasional as-needed basis they may be useful (particularly in treating episodes of agitation in patients with prominent anxiety features). Regarding dosage, it is recommended to start low and titrate slowly upward to the minimum effective dose, while monitoring for adverse effects (e.g., oral lorazepam may be given in doses from 0.5 to 1.0 mg every 4-6 hours). Regarding the variety of benzodiazepines, the APA practice guidelines indicate that agents that do not require oxidative metabolism in the liver and have no active metabolites, such as lorazepam and oxazepam, are preferable. The guidelines also cautions about the use of benzodiazepines with long half-lives (e.g. clonazepam) or with long-lived metabolites (e.g. diazepam, chlordiazepoxide, lorazepate, flurazepam) since it can take weeks until they reach steady-state levels in the plasma, especially in elderly patients. Moreover, the use of these drugs is associated with a higher risk of falls and hip fractures than short-acting agents (Grad, 1995).

A recently published systematic review (Tampi and Tampi, 2014) of the available RCTs evaluating the use of benzodiazepines in patients with dementia identified five studies relevant to the topic. In the study by Covington (1975), it was shown that thioridazine is superior to diazepam for the treatment of BPSD. In the study by Coccaro et al., (1990), comparing haloperidol, oxazepam and diphenhydramine, no significant difference was noted in terms of efficacy in the management of agitated behaviours in severely demented patients. Ancill et al. (1991) compared alprazolam to lorazepam and no significant difference was demonstrated between the efficacy of the two drugs. Moreover, the authors concluded that even recognizing that benzodiazepines are effective in the treatment of agitation in dementia, a risk benefit assessment is essential in deciding whether or not to use them. Christensen and Benfield (1998) demonstrated the equal efficacy of alprazolam to low dose haloperidol, offering a practical alternative to antipsychotic medication in treating behavioural symptoms in older adults with dementia. Finally, in the study by Meehan et al., 2002, no differences were noted between intramuscular (IM) lorazepam, IM olanzapine and an IM placebo. Compared to the placebo, the active drugs proved to be superior in terms of efficacy, without significant treatment-emergent adverse effects. Overall, four of the five studies indicated that there was no significant difference in efficacy between the active drugs for treatment of BPSD (one study indicated that thioridazine may be better than diazepam) and all five studies reported no significant difference between the active agents in terms of tolerability. In conclusion, recognizing that there is a dearth of controlled data, the authors stated that their review does not provide additional information which may contradict the recommendations of the AGS Updated Beers Criteria or the APA practice guidelines. Given the data available, they agreed that the routine use of benzodiazepines for treatment of BPSD cannot be recommended, and their use may only be justified in selected circumstances, e.g. when other psychotropic agents are unsafe or overtly contraindicated.

## Carbamazepine and Valproate

It is widely accepted that the majority of antiepileptic drugs (AEDs) act through multiple mechanisms involving different targets at various levels (channels, receptors and signalling pathways). It is also true that even for those AEDs for which a main molecular or cellular activity has been documented, it remains difficult to clearly attribute a given therapeutic effect to a particular mechanism of action. This heterogeneous biological activity of AEDs may account for their widespread use in several disorders (i.e. epilepsy, mood disorders, migraine headaches and neuropathic pain) but also for their tolerability concerns. In the following paragraphs, the use of carbamazepine and valproate in BPSD is discussed briefly, given the fact that they share indirect GABAergic properties and have been considered for treating behavioural disturbances in elderly demented patients.

Carbamazepine acts primarily as a blocker of voltage-dependent sodium channels, stabilizing their inactivated state. Additionally, it shows the blockade of calcium L-type channels and potentiates GABAergic pathways. Finally, adenosine receptor antagonism, an increase in extracellular serotonin concentration, an increase in dopaminergic transmission, and the inhibition of glutamate release have also been reported as the mechanisms of carbamazepine action (Ambrósio et al., 2002).

The first reports of carbamazepine use for the treatment of behavioural disturbances date back to the 1970s (Dalby, 1971; Monroe, 1975). After these single case reports provided initial evidence of efficacy, a negative, placebo-controlled, double-blind study was published in 1982 (Chambers et al., 1982). Nineteen elderly demented patients treated with 100-300 mg carbamazepine daily failed to show a response in their behavioural disturbances, and, instead the worsening of their cognitive functioning was observed, as assessed by means of the Behavioural Rating Scale and the Clifton Assessment Schedule. The low plasma levels of the drug (medium serum levels 3.5 mcg/ml) were suggested as a possible explanation for the failure of the trial. Alongside this small controlled study, other case reports were published over the following few years (Essa, 1986; Leibovici and Tariot, 1988; Marin and Greenwald, 1989).

In 1990 and 1995 two open label studies (Gleason and Schneider, 1990; Lemke, 1995), both investigating carbamazepine efficacy in the treatment of behavioural symptoms in AD patients, who had failed to respond to prior treatment with neuroleptics, reported more encouraging results. In the first series, five out of nine patients showed clear improvement, according to the Brief Psychiatric Rating Scale (BPRS) score. In the second series, fifteen severely demented patients were treated with carbamazepine alone or in addition to haloperidol (except two patients in whom the treatment had to be discontinued due to severe adverse effects). Following four weeks of treatment, significant improvement was observed, as indicated by the BPRS score.

More recently were published three RCTs (Cooney et al., 1996; Olin et al., 2001; Tariot et al., 1998) and one meta-analysis (Ballard et al., 2009) looking at carbamazepine monotherapy for BPSD. In 1996, Cooney et al. enrolled six AD patients in a small, randomized, placebo-controlled study. Aggressiveness, as measured by the Rating Scale for Aggressive Behaviour in the Elderly (RAGE), was significantly reduced in patients receiving carbamazepine (in doses up to 600 mg daily). A six-week, randomized, parallel-group study, including fifty-one nursing home patients with agitation and dementia, was reported by Tariot et al., in 1998. In this study carbamazepine was administered starting at a dose of 100 mg daily and subsequently increasing by 50 mg every 2-4 days. The modal dose at six weeks was 300 mg daily, the mean serum level achieved was 5.3 mcg/ml and significant short term efficacy was demonstrated (BPRS score decreased 7.7 points in the carbamazepine group vs. 0.9 points in the placebo group; CGI score improved in 77% of the carbamazepine-receiving patients vs. 21% of the placebo-receiving patients). Adverse effects did not occur significantly more often in the carbamazepine group. The authors recommended a carbamazepine serum level of 5-8 mcg/ml when treating elderly patients with BPSD. In 2001, Olin et al. performed a six-week, randomized, double-blind, placebo-controlled, parallel-group trial of carbamazepine in twenty-one agitated AD patients, who had been unsuccessfully treated with antipsychotics. The carbamazepine group (400 mg daily) showed a modest clinical benefit (not statistically significant), as assessed by the Clinical Global Impression of Change (CGIC) score, compared to the placebo group. Significant efficacy of carbamazepine versus the placebo was demonstrated regarding the hostility item of the BPRS score.

As already mentioned in this chapter, several recently published review articles have agreed in indicating that carbamazepine is the most promising anticonvulsant for treatment of BPSD (Amann et al., 2009; Ballard and Corbett, 2013; Konovalov et al., 2008; Pinheiro, 2008; Yeh and Ouyang, 2012). On the other hand, safety concerns and its high potential for drug-drug interaction (especially in patients often treated with polytherapy) are considered major limiting factors. Therefore, since the routine use of carbamazepine in BPSD is not recommended, it is considered reasonable to use it as a second-line treatment in patients who are sensitive or unresponsive to antipsychotics or who have significant cardiovascular risk factors (Yeh and Ouyang, 2012).

Valproate is a simple branch-chain fatty acid with several therapy indications, such as partial and generalized seizures, bipolar mood disorder and migraine headaches. Multiple mechanisms of action underlie the various therapeutic effects of this drug, and include both immediate biochemical activities and long-term genomic modifications. Its immediate biochemical activities include blocking of voltage-dependent sodium channels and calcium T-type channels, inhibition of high-frequency action potential firing (McLean and Macdonald, 1986), and indirect GABAergic effects. Early studies showed that GABA levels were elevated by valproate (Chapman et al., 1983; Chapman et al., 1984) and reports on the structure-function relationship demonstrated consistent results between seizure control and GABA level elevation, induced by different valproic acid analogue compounds (Keane et al., 1983; Tang et al., 1997). The direct inhibition of GABA transaminase (Maitre et al., 1974) and succinic semialdehyde dehydrogenase (Mesdjian et al., 1982), enzymes responsible for GABA catabolism, is thought to account for valproate's GABAergic activities. The increase in GABA levels within the brain is considered of relevance not only for seizure control, but also for the other therapeutic effects of valproate in bipolar disorder (Freeman et al., 2002) and migraine (Lee et al., 1995). As already mentioned, it is worth considering that gene expression is altered by valproate (Bosetti et al., 2005; Tang et al., 2004) and it is very likely that a variety of long-term effects of the drug rely upon this genomic-level mechanism.

Among the first reports on valproate use in treating BPSD, there was one conducted by Mellow et al. in 1993. In this small open-label trial, out of four demented patients treated with sodium valproate, two showed significant improvement and a third had a transient response, over one to three months follow up. Several subsequent case reports, case series and uncontrolled open trials suggested the efficacy of valproate in the treatment of BPSD (Forester et al., 2007; Haas et al., 1997; Herrmann, 1998; Lott et al., 1995; Narayan and Nelson, 1997; Porsteinsson et al., 2003; Sival et al., 2004).

The positive results of open-label trials contrast with conflicting findings derived from controlled trials. Five RCTs looking at the effect of valproate monotherapy in treating BPSD have been published to date (Herrmann et al., 2007; Porsteinsson et al., 2001; Sival et al., 2002; Tariot et al., 2001; Tariot et al., 2005). In 2001, Porsteinsson and colleagues assessed the efficacy and tolerability of divalproex sodium for the treatment of agitation in fifty-six nursing home patients with dementia. The participants were randomized to receive either placebo or individualized doses of rapid-acting divalproex sodium. The initial dose was 375 mg/day, subsequently titrated upward to an average daily dosage of 826 mg (in this trial a non-blinded supervising physician was allowed to alter the drug dosage by 125 mg per day, on the basis of written reports by the blinded reviewers). At the end of the six-week treatment period, no significant difference in the agitation item of the BPRS scale was noted; as mentioned by the authors, only when several covariates were taken into account was there a significant response to the treatment. Moreover, no significant difference in overall response, measured by the CGI scale, was shown by comparing the treated and control groups. In addition, side effects, even if generally rated as mild, occurred more frequently in the treatment group. Therefore, despite some limitations, the authors suggested the possible short-term efficacy and tolerability of divalproex sodium for the treatment of agitation in dementia. Another paper on a six-week, randomized, double-blind, placebo-controlled, parallel-group study was published by Tariot et al. in 2001. Namely, 172 nursing home residents with dementia and secondary mania were enrolled and randomly assigned for treatment either with a placebo or divalproex sodium. The starting dose was 125 mg twice a day, followed by daily 125 mg upward titration to a target dose of 20 mg/kg/day (the maximum dosage reached was 30 mg/kg/day). Regarding the primary outcome, no appreciable difference in efficacy was demonstrated, as measured by means of the Bech-Rafaelsen Mania Scale score. Furthermore, when compared to the placebo, the treated group showed no significant difference in their BPRS scores, but a significant improvement in CMAI total score and verbal agitation subscale, and a significant worsening in the CGI score. As a result of a disproportionate number of withdrawals, primarily due to excessive somnolence in the treatment group, the study was terminated ahead of full enrolment completion. Doses equal to or higher than 15 mg/kg/day were associated with poor compliance. The authors concluded that divalproex sodium did not improve the signs and symptoms of mania associated with dementia, but it did improve symptoms of agitation. In 2002, a randomized, double-blind, placebo-controlled, cross-over study failed to demonstrate the efficacy of sodium valproate on aggressive behaviour in dementia (Sival et al., 2002). Forty-two demented patients were included in the analysis. The treatment with sodium valproate 240 mg twice daily produced no differences compared to the placebo in aggressive behaviour, as measured by means of the Social Dysfunction and Aggression Scale-9 and CGI scores (primary outcome). A significant improvement was shown regarding restless, melancholic and anxious behaviour (secondary outcome). Low doses and the short three-week treatment period were advocated as possible explanations for the negative findings of this study. In 2005, Tariot and colleagues published a randomized, double-blind, placebo-controlled trial investigating the efficacy of divalproex sodium in nursing home residents, with possible or probable AD, complicated by agitation (Tariot et al., 2005). Namely, 110 patients were randomly assigned to receive divalproex sodium at a mean dose of 800 mg/day or a placebo for six weeks. Neither the primary outcome measurements (changes from baseline in the agitation item of the BPRS), nor secondary ones (including assessment of total BPRS, CGIC, CMAI scores) showed any significant improvement in favour of the treatment group. Finally, similar negative results were also reported in 2007 by Herrmann et al. This randomized, double-blind, placebo-controlled, crossover study investigated the efficacy and tolerability of valproate for the treatment of agitated and aggressive behaviour in moderate-to-severe AD patients. Fourteen patients were included in the study; analysis included assessment of the NPI and CMAI scales at baseline and after six weeks of the treatment with valproate and placebo, with a two week interval between each phase. Significant deterioration was observed during active treatment (at a mean dose of 1135 mg daily) compared to the placebo group. Tolerability concerns, with patients treated with valproate experiencing a significantly higher number of adverse events than the placebo group, were also raised, suggesting that the treatment may be poorly tolerated.

A Cochrane systematic review, evaluating whether evidence supports the use of valproate and its analogues for treatment of agitation in demented patients, was published in 2004 (Lonergan and Luxenberg, 2004). To include two additional randomized studies later published, an updated review was released in 2009 (Lonergan and Luxenberg, 2009). Various flaws in the methodology of the studies available and the lack of standardization in the patients' treatments and assessment of their outcome were underscored by the Cochrane reviewers. In particular: in the Porsteinsson study (2001) adequate concealed allocation was undermined by the fact that a non-blinded physician was allowed to adjust divalproex sodium doses on the basis of reports by blinded raters and confidential laboratory reports; in Tariot's study (2001) the premature termination of the study, due to an excessive drop-out rate in the treated group, weakens the author's conclusions; in the report by Sival et al., (2002) concerns regarding the statistical analysis make the results reported questionable. The Cochrane reviewers also underlined that combining results derived from studies that employed short- and long-acting agents and in which the doses vary more than two-fold gives rise to substantial methodological issues. They concluded that the current evidence does not support the use of valproate preparations to control agitation in people with dementia, and suggest on the contrary that valproate therapy is associated with an unacceptable rate of adverse effects. Similar conclusions were also drawn in several other review articles indicating that, according to the available evidence, valproate use cannot be recommended in demented and aggressive elderly patients (Amann et al., 2009; Konovalov et al., 2008; Yeh and Ouyang, 2012).

## References


Alexopoulos GS, Silver JM, Kahn DA, Frances A, Carpenter D (1998) The expert consensus guideline series: treatment of agitation in older persons with dementia. *Postgrad Med.* 26:1–88.

Alexopoulos GS, Streim J, Carpenter D, Docherty JP (2004) Using antipsychotic agents in older patients. *J Clin Psychiatry.* 65 Suppl 2:5–99; *discussion* 100–102; quiz 103–104.

Alzheimer's Disease International (2014) Dementia statistics: numbers of people with dementia. http://www.alz.co.uk/research/statistics.html.

Amann B, Pantel J, Grunze H, Vieta E, Colom F, Gonzalez-Pinto A, Naber D, Hampel H (2009) Anticonvulsants in the treatment of aggression in the demented elderly: an update. *Clin Pract Epidemiol Ment Health.* 5:14.

Ambrósio AF, Soares-Da-Silva P, Carvalho CM, Carvalho AP (2002) Mechanisms of action of carbamazepine and its derivatives, oxcarbazepine, BIA 2-093, and BIA 2-024. *Neurochem Res.* 27:121–130.

American Geriatrics Society, American Association for Geriatric Psychiatry (2003) Consensus statement on improving the quality of mental health care in U.S. nursing homes: management of depression and behavioral symptoms associated with dementia. *J Am Geriatr Soc.* 51:1287–1298.

American Geriatrics Society 2012 Beers Criteria Update Expert Panel (2012) American Geriatrics Society updated Beers Criteria for potentially inappropriate medication use in older adults. *J Am Geriatr Soc.* 60:616–631.

Ancill RJ, Carlyle WW, Liang RA, Holliday SG (1991) Agitation in the demented elderly: a role for benzodiazepines? *Int Clin Psychopharmacol.* 6:141–146.

APA Work Group on Alzheimer's Disease and other Dementias, Rabins PV, Blacker D, Rovner BW, Rummans T, Schneider LS, Tariot PN, Blass DM; Steering Committee on Practice Guidelines, McIntyre JS, Charles SC, Anzia DJ, Cook IA, Finnerty MT, Johnson BR, Nininger JE, Schneidman B, Summergrad P, Woods SM, Berger J, Cross CD, Brandt HA, Margolis PM, Shemo JP, Blinder BJ, Duncan DL, Barnovitz MA, Carino AJ, Freyberg ZZ, Gray SH, Tonnu T, Kunkle R, Albert AB, Craig TJ, Regier DA, Fochtmann LJ (2007) American Psychiatric Association practice guideline for the treatment of patients with Alzheimer's disease and other dementias. Second edition. *Am J Psychiatry.* 164:5–56.

Ballard C, Corbett A (2013) Agitation and aggression in people with Alzheimer's disease. *Curr Opin Psychiatry.* 26:252–259.

Ballard CG, Gauthier S, Cummings JL, Brodaty H, Grossberg GT, Robert P, Lyketsos CG (2009) Management of agitation and aggression associated with Alzheimer disease. *Nat Rev Neurol.* 5:245–255.

Ballard TM, Knoflach F, Prinssen E, Borroni E, Vivian JA, Basile J, Gasser R, Moreau JL, Wettstein JG, Buettelmann B, Knust H, Thomas AW, Trube G, Hernandez MC (2009) RO4938581, a novel cognitive enhancer acting at $GABA_A$ alpha5 subunit-containing receptors. *Psychopharmacology* (Berl). 202:207–223.

Banerjee S (2009) The Use of Antipsychotic Medication for People with Dementia: Time for Action. London, UK, Department of Health.

Barnard EA, Skolnick P, Olsen RW, Mohler H, Sieghart W, Biggio G, Braestrup C, Bateson AN, Langer (1998) International Union of Pharmacology. XV. Subtypes of $GABA_A$ receptors: classification on the basis of subunit structure and receptor function. *Pharmacol Rev.* 50:291–313.

Bjork JM, Moeller FG, Kramer GL, Kram M, Suris A, Rush AJ, Petty F (2001) Plasma GABA levels correlate with aggressiveness in relatives of patients with unipolar depressive disorder. *Psychiatry Res.* 101:131–136.

Bonnert TP, McKernan RM, Farrar S, le Bourdellès B, Heavens RP, Smith DW, Hewson L, Rigby MR, Sirinathsinghji DJ, Brown N, Wafford KA, Whiting PJ (1999) Theta, a novel gamma-aminobutyric acid type A receptor subunit. *Proc Natl Acad Sci USA* 96:9891–9896.

Bosetti F, Bell JM, Manickam P (2005) Microarray analysis of rat brain gene expression after chronic administration of sodium valproate. *Brain Res Bull.* 65:331–338.

Brodaty H, Arasaratnam C (2012) Meta-analysis of nonpharmacological interventions for neuropsychiatric symptoms of dementia. *Am J Psychiatry.* 169:946–953.

Buskova J, Busek P, Nevsimalova S (2011) Gabapentin in the treatment of dementia-associated nocturnal agitation. *Med Sci Monit.* 17:149–151.

Chambers CA, Bain J, Roshottom R, Ballinger BR, McLaren S (1982) Carbamazepine in senile dementia and overactivity: a placebo, controlled double-blind trial. *IRCS Med Sci.* 10:505–506.

Chan D-C, Kasper JD, Black BS, Rabins PV (2003) Presence of behavioral and psychological symptoms predicts nursing home placement in community-dwelling elders with cognitive impairment in univariate but not multivariate analysis. *J Gerontol A Biol Sci Med Sci.* 58:548–554.

Chapman AG, Croucher MJ, Meldrum BS (1984) Anticonvulsant activity of intracerebroventricularly administered valproate and valproate analogues: a dose-dependent correlation with changes in brain aspartate and GABA levels in DBA/2 mice. *Biochem Pharmacol.* 33:1459–1463.

Chapman AG, Meldrum BS, Mendes E (1983) Acute anticonvulsant activity of structural analogues of valproic acid and changes in brain GABA and aspartate content. *Life Sci.* 32:2023–2031.

Christensen DB, Benfield WR (1998) Alprazolam as an alternative to low-dose haloperidol in older, cognitively impaired nursing facility patients. *J Am Geriatr Soc.* 46:620–625.

Coccaro EF, Kramer E, Zemishlany Z, Thorne A, Rice CM III, Giordani B, Duvvi K, Patel BM, Torres J, Nora R (1990) Pharmacologic treatment of non-cognitive behavioral disturbances in elderly demented patients. *Am J Psychiatry.* 147:1640–1645.

Collinson N, Kuenzi FM, Jarolimek W, Maubach KA, Cothliff R, Sur C, Smith A, Otu FM, Howell O, Atack JR, McKernan RM, Seabrook GR, Dawson GR, Whiting PJ, Rosahl TW (2002) Enhanced learning and memory and altered GABAergic synaptic transmission in mice lacking the alpha 5 subunit of the $GABA_A$ receptor. *J Neurosci.* 22:5572–5580.

Cooney C, Mortimer ANN, Smith A, Newton K, Wrigley M (1996) Carbamazepine use in aggressive behavior associated with senile dementia. *Int J Geriatr Psychiatry.* 11:901–905.

Cooney C, Murphy S, Tessema H, Freyne A (2013) Use of low-dose gabapentin for aggressive behavior in vascular and Mixed Vascular/Alzheimer Dementia. *J Neuropsychiatry Clin Neurosci.* 25:120–125.

Covington JS (1975) Alleviating agitation, apprehension, and related symptoms in geriatric patients: a double-blind comparison of a phenothiazine and a benzodiazepine. *South Med J.* 68:719–724.

Cummings JL, Schneider E, Tariot PN, Graham SM; Memantine MEM-MD-02 Study Group (2006) Behavioral effects of memantine in Alzheimer disease patients receiving donepezil treatment. *Neurology.* 67:57–63.

Dalby MA (1971) Antiepileptic and psychotropic effect of carbamazepine (Tegretol) in the treatment of psychomotor epilepsy. *Epilepsia.* 12:325–334.

Dawson GR, Maubach KA, Collinson N, Cobain M, Everitt BJ, MacLeod AM, Choudhury HI, McDonald LM, Pillai G, Rycroft W, Smith AJ, Sternfeld F, Tattersall FD, Wafford

KA, Reynolds DS, Seabrook GR, Atack JR (2006) An inverse agonist selective for alpha5 subunit-containing $GABA_A$ receptors enhances cognition. *J Pharmacol Exp Ther.* 316:1335–1345.

De Vugt ME, Stevens F, Aalten P, Lousberg R, Jaspers N, Verhey FRJ (2005) A prospective study of the effects of behavioral symptoms on the institutionalization of patients with dementia. *Int Psychogeriatr.* 17:577–589.

Essa M (1986) Carbamazepine in dementia. *J Clin Psychopharmacol.* 6:234–236.

Eustace A, Coen R, Walsh C, Cunningham CJ, Walsh JB, Coakley D, Lawlor BA (2002) A longitudinal evaluation of behavioural and psychological symptoms of probable Alzheimer's disease. *Int J Geriatr Psychiatry.* 17:968–973.

Field MJ, Hughes J, Singh L (2000) Further evidence for the role of the α2δ subunit of voltage dependent calcium channels in models of neuropathic pain. *Brit J Pharmacol.* 131:282–286.

Finder VH (2010) Alzheimer's disease: a general introduction and pathomechanism. *J Alzheimers Dis.* 3:5–19.

Forester B, Vanelli M, Hyde J, Perez R, Ahokpossi C, Sribney W, Adkison L (2007) Report on an open-label prospective study of divalproex sodium for the behavioral and psychological symptoms of dementia as monotherapy and in combination with second-generation antipsychotic medication. *Am J Geriatr Pharmacother.* 5:209–217.

Freeman MP, Freeman SA, McElroy SL (2002) The comorbidity of bipolar and anxiety disorders: prevalence, psychobiology, and treatment issues. *J Affect Disord.* 68:1–23.

Garcia-Alloza M, Tsang SW, Gil-Bea FJ, Francis PT, Lai MK, Marcos B, Chen CP, Ramirez MJ (2006) Involvement of the GABAergic system in depressive symptoms of Alzheimer's disease. *Neurobiol Aging.* 27:1110–1117.

Gauthier S, Wirth Y, Möbius HJ (2005) Effects of memantine on behavioural symptoms in Alzheimer's disease patients: an analysis of the Neuropsychiatric Inventory (NPI) data of two randomised, controlled studies. *Int J Geriatr Psychiatry.* 20:459–464.

Gleason RP, Schneider LS (1990) Carbamazepine treatment of agitation in Alzheimer's outpatients refractory to neuroleptics. *J Clin Psychiatry.* 51:115–118.

Grad RM (1995) Benzodiazepines for insomnia in community-dwelling elderly: a review of benefit and risk. *J Fam Pract.* 41:473–481.

Griffin CE 3rd, Kaye AM, Bueno FR, Kaye AD (2013) Benzodiazepine pharmacology and central nervous system-mediated effects. *Ochsner J.* 13:214–223.

Guay DR (2007) Newer antiepileptic drugs in the management of agitation/aggression in patients with dementia or developmental disability. *Consult Pharm.* 22:1004–1034.

Gutierrez A, Khan ZU, Ruano D, Miralles CP, Vitorica J, De Blas AL (1996) Aging-related subunit expression changes of the $GABA_A$ receptor in the rat hippocampus. *Neuroscience.* 74:341–348.

Haas S, Vincent K, Holt J, Lippmann S (1997) Divalproex: a possible treatment alternative for demented, elderly aggressive patients. *Ann Clin Psychiatry.* 9:145–147.

Hawkins JW, Tinklenberg JR, Sheikh JI, Peyser CE, Yesavage JA (2000) A retrospective chart review of gabapentin for the treatment of aggressive and agitated behavior in patients with dementias. *Am J Geriatr Psychiatry.* 8:221–225.

Herrmann N (1998) Valproic acid treatment of agitation in dementia. *Can J Psychiatry.* 43:69–72.

Herrmann N (2001) Recommendations for the management of behavioral and psychological symptoms of dementia. *Can J Neurol Sci.* 28 Suppl 1:S96–107.

Herrmann N, Lanctôt KL (2005) Do atypical antipsychotics cause stroke? *CNS Drugs.* 19:91–103.

Herrmann N, Lanctôt KL (2007) Pharmacologic management of neuropsychiatric symptoms of Alzheimer disease. *Can J Psychiatry.* 52:630–646.

Herrmann N, Lanctot K, Myszak M (2000) Effectiveness of gabapentin for the treatment of behavioral disorders in dementia. *J Clin Psychopharmacol.* 20:90–93.

Herrmann N, Lanctot KL, Rothenburg LS, Eryavec G (2007) A placebo-controlled trial of valproate for agitation and aggression in Alzheimer's disease. *Dement Geriatr Cogn Disord.* 23:116–119.

Herrmann N, Mamdani M, Lanctôt KL (2004) Atypical antipsychotics and risk of cerebrovascular accidents. *Am J Psychiatry.* 161:1113–1115.

Keane PE, Simiand J, Mendes E, Santucci V, Morre M (1983) The effects of analogues of valproic acid on seizures induced by pentylenetetrazol and GABA content in brain of mice. *Neuropharmacology.* 22:875–879.

Kim Y, Wilkins KM, Tampi RR (2008) Use of gabapentin in the treatment of behavioural and psychological symptoms of dementia: a review of the evidence. *Drugs Aging.* 25:187–196.

Konovalov S, Muralee S, Tampi RR (2008) Anticonvulsants for the treatment of behavioral and psychological symptoms of dementia: a literature review. *Int Psychogeriatr.* 20:293–308.

Lanctôt KL, Herrmann N, Mazzotta P, Khan LR, Ingber N (2004) GABAergic function in Alzheimer's disease: evidence for dysfunction and potential as a therapeutic target for the treatment of behavioural and psychological symptoms of dementia. *Can J Psychiatry.* 49:439–453.

Lanctôt KL, Herrmann N, Rothenburg L, Eryavec G (2007) Behavioral correlates of GABAergic disruption in Alzheimer's disease. *Int Psychogeriatr.* 19:151–158.

Layton D, Harris S, Wilton LV, Shakir SA (2005) Comparison of incidence rates of cerebrovascular accidents and transient ischaemic attacks in observational cohort studies of patients prescribed risperidone, quetiapine or olanzapine in general practice in England including patients with dementia. *J Psychopharmacol.* 19:473–482.

Lee WS, Limmroth V, Ayata C, Cutrer FM, Waeber C, Yu X, Moskowitz MA (1995) Peripheral $GABA_A$ receptor-mediated effects of sodium valproate on dural plasma protein extravasation to substance P and trigeminal stimulation. *Br J Pharmacol.* 116:1661–1667.

Leibovici A, Tariot PN (1988) Carbamazepine treatment of agitation associated with dementia. *J Geriatr Psychiatry Neurol.* 1:110–112.

Lemke MR (1995) Effect of carbamazepine on agitation in Alzheimer's inpatients refractory to neuroleptics. *J Clin Psychiatry.* 56:354–357.

Li K, Xu E (2008) The role and the mechanism of gamma-aminobutyric acid during central nervous system development. *Neurosci Bull.* 24:195–200.

Liperoti R, Gambassi G, Lapane KL, Chiang C, Pedone C, Mor V, Bernabei R (2005) Cerebrovascular events among elderly nursing home patients treated with conventional or atypical antipsychotics. *J Clin Psychiatry.* 66:1090–1096.

Livingston G, Johnston K, Katona C, Paton J, Lyketsos CG (2005) Old Age Task Force of the World Federation of Biological Psychiatry: Systematic review of psychological approaches to the management of neuropsychiatric symptoms of dementia. *Am J Psychiatry.* 162:1996–2021.

Lonergan E, Luxenberg J (2004) Valproate preparations for agitation in dementia. *Cochrane Database Syst Rev.* Issue 2:1–16.

Lonergan E, Luxenberg J (2009) Valproate preparations for agitation in dementia. *Cochrane Database Syst Rev.* Issue 3:1–48.

Löscher W, Hönack D, Taylor CP (1991) Gabapentin increases aminooxyacetic acid-induced GABA accumulation in several regions of rat brain. *Neurosci Lett.* 128:150–154.

Lott AD, McElroy SL, Keys MA (1995) Valproate in the treatment of behavioral agitation in elderly patients with dementia. *J Neuropsychiatry Clin Neurosci.* 7:314–319.

Louzada PR, Paula Lima AC, Mendonca-Silva DL, Noël F, De Mello FG, Ferreira ST (2004) Taurine prevents the neurotoxicity of beta-amyloid and glutamate receptor agonists: activation of GABA receptors and possible implications for Alzheimer's disease and other neurological disorders. *FASEB J.* 18:511–518.

Lowe SL, Francis PT, Procter AW, Palmer AM, Davison AN, Bowen DM (1988) Gamma-aminobutyric acid concentration in brain tissue at two stages of Alzheimer's disease. Brain. 111:785–799.

Lyketsos CG, Steinberg M, Tschanz JT, Norton MC, Steffens DC, Breitner JCS (2000) Mental and behavioral disturbances in dementia: findings from the Cache County Study on Memory in Aging. *Am J Psychiatry.* 57:708–714.

Machnicki G, Allegri RF, Dillon C, Serrano CM, Taragano FE (2009) Cognitive, functional and behavioral factors associated with the burden of caring for geriatric patients with cognitive impairment or depression: evidence from a South American sample. *Int J Geriatr Psychiatry.* 24:382–389.

Maitre M, Ciesielski L, Mandel P (1974) Effect of 2-methyl 2-ethyl caproic acid and 2-2-dimethyl valeric acid on audiogenic seizures and brain $\gamma$ aminobutyric acid. *Biochem Pharmacol.* 23:2363–2368.

Maneuf YP, Gonzalez MI, Sutton KS, Chung FZ, Pinnock RD, Lee K (2003) Cellular and molecular action of the putative GABA-mimetic, gabapentin. *Cell Mol Life Sci.* 60:742–750.

Marin DB, Greenwald BS (1989) Carbamazepine for aggressive agitation in demented patients during nursing care. *Am J Psychiatry.* 146:805.

Mattson RH, Rothman DL, Behar KL, Petroff OAC (1997) Gabapentin: A GABA active drug. *Epilepsia. 38*:65–66.

McKhann G, Drachman D, Folstein M, Katzman R, Price D, Stadlan EM (1984) Clinical diagnosis of Alzheimer's disease: report of the NINCDS-ADRDA Work Group under the auspices of Department of Health and Human Services Task Force on Alzheimer's Disease. *Neurology.* 34:939–944.

McKhann GM, Knopman DS, Chertkow H, Hyman BT, Jack CR Jr, Kawas CH, Klunk WE, Koroshetz WJ, Manly JJ, Mayeux R, Mohs RC, Morris JC, Rossor MN, Scheltens P, Carrillo MC, Thies B, Weintraub S, Phelps CH (2011) The diagnosis of dementia due to Alzheimer's disease: recommendations from the National Institute on Aging-Alzheimer's Association workgroups on diagnostic guidelines for Alzheimer's disease. *Alzheimers Dement.* 7:263–269.

McLean MJ, Macdonald RL (1986) Sodium valproate, but not ethosuximide, produces use- and voltage-dependent limitation of high frequency repetitive firing of action potentials of mouse central neurons in cell culture. *J Pharmacol Exp Ther*. 237:1001–1011.

Meehan KM, Wang H, David SR, Nisivoccia JR, Jones B, Beasley CM Jr, Feldman PD, Mintzer JE, Beckett LM, Breier A (2002) Comparison of rapidly acting intramuscular olanzapine, lorazepam, and placebo: a double-blind, randomized study in acutely agitated patients with dementia. *Neuropsychopharmacol*. 26:494–504.

Mellow AM, Solano-Lopez C, Davis S (1993) Sodium valproate in the treatment of behavioral disturbance in dementia. *J Geriatr Psychiatry Neurol*. 6:205–209.

Mesdjian E, Ciesielski L, Valli M, Bruguerolle B, Jadot G, Bouyard P, Mandel P (1982) Sodium valproate: kinetic profile and effects on GABA levels in various brain areas of the rat. *Prog Neuropsychopharmacol Biol Psychiatry*. 6:223–233.

Monroe RR (1975) Anticonvulsants in the treatment of aggression. *J Nerv Ment Dis*. 160:119–26.

Moretti R, Torre P, Antonello RM, Cazzato G, Bava A (2003) Gabapentin for the treatment of behavioural alterations in dementia: preliminary 15-month investigation. *Drugs Aging*. 20:1035–1040.

Mountjoy CQ, Rossor MN, Iversen LL, Roth M (1984) Correlation of cortical cholinergic and GABA deficits with quantitative neuropathological findings in senile dementia. *Brain*. 107:507–518.

Narayan M, Nelson JC (1997) Treatment of dementia with behavioral disturbance using divalproex or a combination of divalproex and a neuroleptic. *J Clin Psychiatry*. 58:351–354.

Nasrallah HA, White T, Nasrallah AT (2004) Lower mortality in geriatric patients receiving risperidone and olanzapine versus haloperidol: preliminary analysis of retrospective data. *Am J Geriatr Psychiatry*. 12:437–439.

O'Connor DW, Ames D, Gardner B, King M (2009) Psychosocial treatments of psychological symptoms in dementia: a systematic review of reports meeting quality standards. *Int Psychogeriatr*. 21:225–251.

Olin JT, Fox LS, Pawluczyk S, Taggart NA, Schneider LS (2001) A pilot randomized trial of carbamazepine for behavioral symptoms in treatment-resistant outpatients with Alzheimer disease. *Am J Geriatr Psychiatry*. 9:400–405.

Olsen RW, Sieghart W (2009) GABA A receptors: subtypes provide diversity of function and pharmacology. *Neuropharmacology*. 56:141–148.

Palop JJ, Mucke L (2010) Amyloid-beta-induced neuronal dysfunction in Alzheimer's disease: from synapses toward neural networks. *Nat Neurosci*. 13:812–818.

Pandey GN, Conley RR, Pandey SC, Goel S, Roberts RC, Tamminga CA, Chute D, Smialek J (1997) Benzodiazepine receptors in the post-mortem brain of suicide victims and schizophrenic subjects. *Psychiatry Res*. 71:137–149.

Petroff OA, Rothman RL, Behar KL, Lamourcux D, Mattson RH (1996) The effect of gabapentin on brain gammaaminobutyric acid in patients with epilepsy. *Ann Neurol*. 39:95–99.

Pinheiro D (2008) Anticonvulsant mood stabilizers in the treatment of behavioral and psychological symptoms of dementia (BPSD). *Encephale*. 34:409–415.

Pinquart M, Sörensen S (2003) Associations of stressors and uplifts of caregiving with caregiver burden and depressive mood: a metaanalysis. *J Gerontol B Psychol Sci Soc Sci.* 58:112–128.

Porsteinsson AP, Tariot PN, Erb R, Cox C, Smith E, Jakimovich L, Noviasky J, Kowalski N, Holt CJ, Irvine C (2001) Placebo-controlled study of divalproex sodium for agitation in dementia. *Am J Geriatr Psychiatry.* 9:58–66.

Porsteinsson AP, Tariot PN, Jakimovich LJ, Kowalski N, Holt C, Erb R, Cox C (2003) Valproate therapy for agitation in dementia: open-label extension of a double-blind trial. *Am J Geriatr Psychiatry.* 11:434–440.

Raudino F, Mascalzi MG, Zagami A (2004) Gabapentin and behavioral disorders in severe Alzheimer disease. *J Clin Psychopharmacol.* 24:459–460.

Regan WM, Gordon SM (1997) Gabapentin for behavioral agitation in Alzheimer's disease. *J Clin Psychopharmacol.* 17:59–60.

Reinikainen KJ, Paljarvi L, Huuskonen M, Soininen H, Laakso M, Riekkinen PJ (1988) A post-mortem study of noradrenergic, serotonergic and GABAergic neurons in Alzheimer's disease. *J Neurol Sci.* 84:101–116.

Reitz C, Brayne C, Mayeux R (2011) Epidemiology of Alzheimer disease. *Nat Rev Neurol.* 7:137–152.

Rissman RA, De Blas AL, Armstrong DM (2007) $GABA_A$ receptors in aging and Alzheimer's disease. *J Neurochem.* 103:1285–1292.

Rissman RA, Mobley WC (2011) Implications for treatment: $GABA_A$ receptors in aging, Down syndrome and Alzheimer's disease. *J Neurochem.* 117:613–622.

Robinson SR, Bishop GM (2002) Abeta as a bioflocculant: implications for the amyloid hypothesis of Alzheimer's disease. *Neurobiol Aging.* 23:1051–1072.

Rossor MN (1982) Neurotransmitters and CNS disease. *Dementia Lancet.* 2:1200–1204.

Ruano D, Cano J, Machado A, Vitorica J (1991) Pharmacologic characterization of $GABA_A$/benzodiazepine receptor in rat hippocampus during aging. *J Pharmacol Exp Ther.* 256:902–908.

Ruano D, Benavides J, Machado A, Vitorica J (1995) Aging-associated changes in the pharmacological properties of the benzodiazepine (omega) receptor isotypes in the rat hippocampus. *J Neurochem.* 64:867–873.

Schneeweiss S, Setoguchi S, Brookhart A, Dormuth C, Wang PS (2007) Risk of death associated with the use of conventional versus atypical antipsychotic drugs among elderly patients. *CMAJ.* 176:627–632.

Schneider LS, Dagerman KS, Insel P (2005) Risk of death with atypical antipsychotic drug treatment for dementia: meta-analysis of randomized placebo-controlled trials. *JAMA.* 294:1934–1943.

Sink KM, Holden KF, Yaffe K (2005) Pharmacological treatment of neuropsychiatric symptoms of dementia: a review of the evidence. *JAMA.* 293:596–608.

Sival RC, Duivenvoorden HJ, Jansen PA, Haffmans PM, Duursma SA, Eikelenboom P (2004) Sodium valproate in aggressive behaviour in dementia: a twelve-week open label follow-up study. *Int J Geriatr Psychiatry.* 19:305–312.

Sival RC, Haffmans PM, Jansen PA, Duursma SA, Eikelenboom P (2002) Sodium valproate in the treatment of aggressive behavior in patients with dementiada randomized placebo controlled clinical trial. *Int J Geriatr Psychiatry.* 17:579–585.

Suh GH, Shah A (2005) Effect of antipsychotics on mortality in elderly patients with dementia: a 1-year prospective study in a nursing home. *Int Psychogeriatr.* 17:429–441.

Suman-Chauhan N, Webdale L, Hill DR, Woodruff N (1993) Characterisation of [3H]gabapentin binding to a novel site in rat brain: homogenate binding studies. *Eur J Pharmacol.* 244:293–301.

Tampi RR, Tampi DJ (2014) Efficacy and Tolerability of Benzodiazepines for the Treatment of Behavioral and Psychological Symptoms of Dementia: A Systematic Review of Randomized Controlled Trials. *Am J Alzheimers Dis Other Demen.* Epub ahead of print.

Tang W, Palaty J, Abbott FS (1997) Time course of α-fluorinated valproic acid in mouse brain and serum and its effect on synaptosomal γ-aminobutyric acid levels in comparison to valproic acid. *J Pharmacol. Exp Ther.* 282:1163–1172.

Tang Y, Glauser TA, Gilbert DL, Hershey AD, Privitera MD, Ficker DM, Szaflarski JP, Sharp FR (2004) Valproic acid blood genomic expression patterns in children with epilepsy – a pilot study. *Acta Neurol Scand.* 109:159–168.

Tariot PN, Erb R, Podgorski CA, Cox C, Patel S, Jakimovich L, Irvine C (1998) Efficacy and tolerability of carbamazepine for agitation and aggression in dementia. *Am J Psychiatry.* 155:54–61.

Tariot PN, Raman R, Jakimovich L, Schneider L, Porsteinsson A, Thomas R, Mintzer J, Brenner R, Schafer K, Thal L (2005) Divalproex sodium in nursing home residents with possible or probable Alzheimer disease complicated by agitation: a randomized, controlled trial. *Am J Geriatr Psychiatry.* 13:942–949.

Tariot PN, Schneider LS, Mintzer JE, Cutler AJ, Cunningham MR, Thomas JW, Sommerville KV (2001) Safety and tolerability of divalproex sodium in the treatment of signs and symptoms of mania in elderly patients with dementia: results of a doubleblind, placebo-controlled trial. *Curr Ther Res.* 62:51–67.

Taylor CP, Gee NS, Su TZ, Kocsis J, Welty DF, Brown JP, Dooley DJ, Boden P, Singh L (1998) A summary of mechanistic hypotheses of gabapentin pharmacology. *Epilepsy Res.* 29:233–249.

Taylor CP, Vartanian MG, Yuen P, Bigge C, Suman-Chauhan N, Hill DR (1993) Potent and stereospecific anticonvulsant activity of 3-isobutyl GABA relates to in vitro binding at a novel site labelled by tritiated gabapentin. *Epilepsy Res.* 14:11–15.

Taylor M, Bhagwagar Z, Cowen PJ, Sharp T (2003) GABA and mood disorders. *Psychol Med.* 33:387–393.

Thompson S, Herrmann N, Rapoport MJ, Lanctôt KL (2007) Efficacy and safety of antidepressants for treatment of depression in Alzheimer's disease: a metaanalysis. *Can J Psychiatry.* 52:248–255.

Trinh NH, Hoblyn J, Mohanty S, Yaffe K (2003) Efficacy of cholinesterase inhibitors in the treatment of neuropsychiatric symptoms and functional impairment in Alzheimer disease: a meta-analysis. *JAMA.* 289:210–216.

Whiting PJ, Bonnert TP, McKernan RM, Farrar S, Le Bourdellès B, Heavens RP, Smith DW, Hewson L, Rigby MR, Sirinathsinghji DJ, Thompson SA, Wafford KA (1999) Molecular and functional diversity of the expanding $GABA_A$ receptor gene family. *Ann N Y Acad Sci.* 868:645–653.

Whitworth TL, Quick MW (2001) Upregulation of gamma-aminobutyric acid transporter expression: role of alkylated gamma-aminobutyric acid derivatives. *Biochem Soc Trans.* 29:736–741.

Yeh YC, Ouyang WC (2012) Mood stabilizers for the treatment of behavioral and psychological symptoms of dementia: an update review. *Kaohsiung J Med Sci.* 28:185–193.

In: Gamma-Aminobutyric Acid (GABA) ISBN: 978-1-63321-838-3
Editors: Josipa Vlainić and Maja Jazvinšćak Jembrek 

*Chapter 10*

# GABA PHARMACOLOGY IN VETERINARY MEDICINE: FROM ANESTHESIA TO PHOBIAS TREATMENT

***Jelena Šuran[1]* and Josipa Vlainić[2]***

[1]Department of Pharmacology and Toxicology, Faculty of Veterinary medicine, University of Zagreb, Croatia

[2]Department of Molecular Medicine, Laboratory of Molecular Neuropharmacology, Rudjer Boskovic Institute, Zagreb, Croatia

## ABSTRACT

As in human medicine, numerous substances that potentiate the effect of GABA on $GABA_A$ receptors are commonly used in veterinary medicine. The indications for the use of GABA positive allosteric modulators, among them benzodiazepines and barbiturates, in animals are very similar to those in humans. Benzodiazepines are clinically used as anticonvulsants, behavioral modifiers, premedicaments, anesthesia inducers and adjuvants in neuroleptanalgesia. Barbiturates are used as anesthetics, anticonvulsants and as euthanasia agents. Sometimes these drugs are administered in combination, mostly for anesthesia or for behavior modification, e.g. for thunderstorm phobia in dogs. Although neither the FDA nor the EMA have approved benzodiazepines for the use in animals, their clinical use in veterinary medicine is increasing, especially for various behavioral disorders. Due to their closeness to humans, companion animals, such as dogs and cats, are frequently diagnosed for separation anxiety, depression and various displacement and self-directed behaviors, which is followed by increased prescription and use of benzodiazepines. Benzodiazepines and barbiturates are considered valuable in veterinary practice, but one must always take into consideration their species-specific pharmacological properties, with the emphasis on adverse reactions and side effects: short-term memory and learning impairment, ataxia, lethargy, somnolence, addiction, paradoxical excitement, anxiety, aggression, excessive vocalization, sleep disturbances, transient apnea, and respiratory and cardiovascular depression. Moreover, it should be noted that severe untoward effects are described within literature, e.g. idiosyncratic

* Faculty of Veterinary Medicine, Heinzelova 55, 10000 Zagreb, Croatia. Email: jelena.suran@vef.hr.

hepatotoxicity has been reported following diazepam administration in cats as well as during phenobarbital treatment in dogs.

**Keywords**: GABA, benzodiazepines, barbiturates, animal, veterinary medicine

## INTRODUCTION

The GABA modulating drugs, such as benzodiazepines and barbiturates, are commonly used in animals. Benzodiazepines and barbiturates enhance the action of the neurotransmitter γ-aminobutyric acid (GABA) at $GABA_A$ receptors (Crowell-Davis, 2006a). Namely, their place of action is a modulatory site at $GABA_A$ receptor that is allosterically regulated. Namely, the postsynaptic chloride channel gating occurs following the interaction of GABA with the $GABA_A$ receptor. The consequent opening of the $Cl^-$ channel and $Cl^-$ influx occurs, as well as hyperpolarization of neuronal membranes and the reduction in neuronal excitability. To be more precise, benzodiazepines, such as clonazepam and diazepam, bind to a site at the interface of an α and γ subunit at the $GABA_A$ receptor. $GABA_A$ receptors are compromised of five subunits (mostly 2α, 2β and 1γ). Upon binding of benzodiazepines to the receptor, an enhancement in the potency of GABA occurs by the increase in the frequency of the chloride channel opening (Crowell-Davis, 2006a).

Barbiturates bind to the β subunit of $GABA_A$ receptors and increase the duration of the chloride ion channel opening – they increase the efficacy of the neurotransmitter GABA. In higher concentrations than those potentiating the action of GABA, barbiturates have the effect on direct gating and/or opening of the chloride ion channel (Rho et al., 1996). This is the reason for the increased toxicity of barbiturates compared to benzodiazepines during overdose.

Benzodiazepines and barbiturates have many indications in veterinary medicine. Benzodiazepine derivatives are usually used as anticonvulsants (clonazepam, lorazepam, midazolam, oxazepam, zonisamide, and diazepam), tranquilizers (diazepam and alprazolam), myorelaxans and for premedication and anesthesia (diazepam, midazolam and zolazepam in combination with tiletamine). Barbiturates, such as methohexital, pentobarbital and thiopenthal, are mainly used as anticonvulsants, anesthetics and for euthanasia. Namely, phenobarbital is the most common antiepileptic drug used in dogs and cats. Moreover, pentobarbital and thiopental are widely accepted as surgical anesthetics. Both of these drugs are also used for euthanasia in small and laboratory animals. Namely, their intravenous administration is followed by respiratory and cardiac arrest, and death.

When using these drugs in animals, one must always consider the species differences in drug metabolism, effectiveness, and safety, and hence - the dose. For example, there are differences between species in diazepam metabolism; in horses, the duration of action is 24-48 h, in cats 5.5 h and in dogs 3.2 h, while the action of its intermediate metabolite, nordiazepam (N-desmethyl diazepam), is 51-120 h, 21 h and 3-6 h, respectively (Overall, 2001).

## PREMEDICATION

In veterinary medicine, premedication is used mainly prior to surgery in order to calm the animal, to facilitate the intravenous application of anesthetics and other drugs, to reduce the dose of anesthetics and possible side effects, and to ensure smooth recovery afterwards. There are several classes of drugs used as pre-anesthetics: anticholinergics, phenotiazines, alpha-2 agonists (xylazine), opioids, the dissociative drugs (ketamine and tiletamine) and benzodiazepines. The latter are used to provide amnesia and muscle relaxation – they do not have any direct analgesic properties. When using these drugs prior to anesthesia, the animal is easier to handle, a much lower dose of the anesthetic drug is needed, and the excitement during drug recovery is reduced.

Diazepam (0.2-06 mg/kg) administered intramuscularly or intravenously is considered as safe premedicant, especially in older dogs with cardiac diseases. Followed by ketamine, it is used to induce anesthesia with 5-22 minutes duration. The recovery from anesthesia characterizes 10-15 minutes of ataxia and incoordination, followed by fast convalescence (Wright, 1982). Diazepam is excessively used in equine practice, in combination with ketamine and xylazine hydrochloride for induction of anesthesia, and alone as a sedative/ataractic/neuroleptic drug. However, it can cause muscle fasciculations, weakness and ataxia even at doses sufficient to cause sedation (Shini, 2000). On the other hand, this drug combination ensures smooth induction and recovery from anesthesia in swine. In goats, diazepam prolongs the period of analgesia, increases muscle relaxation and prevents reflex movements of the limbs when administered 15 minutes after intramuscular atropine, and followed by an injection of ketamine. This combination of atopine, ketamine and diazepam is used in other domestic but also in wild animals. For example, in diurnal raptors (birds of prey), ketamine and atropine could be mixed and administered in the brachial vein. To assure proper anesthesia this drug combination should be followed by diazepam within 5 minutes. Namely, birds become immobilized within 15 seconds and anesthetized within 1 minute. The special attention should be given to owls which are specifically sensitive to anesthetics and require much lower doses of these drugs and greater attention during anesthetization (Gross, 2001). California sea lions, northern elephant seals and harbor seals have been anesthetized for surgical purposes with a combination of atropine and diazepam 5-10 minutes before anesthetic ketamine (Gage, 1984). Combination of diazepam and ketamine has been used in river otters, leopard seal, gray seals and harbor seals (Gales, 1989). Harbor seal pups were sedated with diazepam to facilitate blood and muscle sample collection (Clark 2004, Greig 2003), but in the study by Lapierre and colleagues (2007) the pups experienced mild to severe bradycardia and excessive salivation.

Benzodiazepine diazepam has the broad spectrum of actions and therefore it is widely used; for example, one can use diazepam to restraint the alligators (Spiegel et al., 1984).

Sometimes two drugs are combined in one formulation in order to achieve tranquilization and deeper and safer anesthesia of an animal. Zolazepam, a pyrazolodiazepinone derivative structurally related to the benzodiazepines, is successfully used in combination with tiletamine, a dissociative anesthetic (NMDA antagonist), for rapid induction and anesthesia of wild carnivores and primates. It is relatively safe (Calle, 2005) and has fewer side effects than ketamine (Cattet et al., 1999; Sleeman et al., 2000). It should be mentioned that due to unwanted situations there is sometimes a need for prompt reaction in blocking the effects of the drug used, mostly in cases where animal swallowed a larger number of tablets or even where inappropriate drug dose have been used. In cases of benzodiazepine overdose, flumazenil, a specific and competitive benzodiazepine receptor antagonist, is effective in completely or partially abolishment of the benzodiazepine effects (Roche Pharmaceuticals, Inc. 1997). Besides its use within different animal species such as dogs, cats, monkeys, etc., this antidote has been successfully used even in pinnipeds, to reverse sedation induced by zolazepam, and midazolam (Karesh et al. 1997; Tahmindjis et al. 2003). Nevertheless, it should be emphasized that it has been shown that flumazenil might act as a partial agonist at $GABA_A$ receptors (Pericic et al., 2004; Pericic et al., 2005; Jazvinscak Jembrek et al., 2008).

## Barbiturate Anesthesia

Barbiturates are mainly used for anesthesia in veterinary medicine. Barbiturates as anesthetics depress the cortex activities of the brain, both motor and sensory areas, the thalamus and the reticular activating system (RAS) of the CNS (Scholfield, 1975). It has been reported that they also raise the threshold of spinal reflexes in cats (Branson, 2001).

Pentobarbital sodium is a short-acting barbiturate, frequently used as an intravenous anesthetic in dogs and cats. Nevertheless, rapid intravenous administration can be lethal. Since it has a narrow therapeutic index, when injecting pentobarbital intravenously, it is recommended to administer only half of the dose initially and then, after a few seconds, to administer the remainder of the dose gradually until the anesthetic effect is achieved (Papich, 2011). During this 2-4 minute period, the reflexes and respiration of the animal should be observed until the desired depth of anesthesia is reached. It is extremely important to monitor the respiration rate carefully through anesthesia, because depression of respiration may occur. In addition, some individuals, mainly dogs, can have symptoms of delirium or excitement during the recovery phase, manifested by whining, barking, attempts to stand or walk, and leg padding movements (Branson, 2001). Female cats are more susceptible to pentobarbital than male and thus require a lower dose (33 mg/kg in comparison to 40 mg/kg, respectively). According to Sis and Herron (1972) barbiturates should not be used in kittens, since the depth of anesthesia is difficult to control and recovery time is significantly prolonged in comparison to other anesthetics. For example, thiopental has a shorter duration of action and it is not associated with excitatory side effects. However, like pentobarbital, it has a narrow therapeutic index and is not recommended for anesthesia that will last longer than several dozen minutes. Moreover, thiopental, as well as other barbiturates, should be used only when it is possible to monitor cardiovascular and respiratory functions of patient, in this case animal. Besides being used as anesthetics barbiturates, namely thiopental, are often used for induction of anesthesia in animals premedicated with atropine. Pentobarbital is used as an anesthetic in horses, cattle and swine. It can also be used as a sedative drug (1-4.4 mg/kg) in combination with a local anesthetic, for operations in large animals. Nevertheless, special attention should be given since following intravenous administration of pentobarbital alone. Namely, when used as an anesthetic it may produce prolonged periods of recumbence and excitement during recovery. This is potentially and especially dangerous in large animals, as they try to stand up before regaining control over their locomotion. Likewise, thiopental alone is not recommended for use in horses because the recovery period is marked by excitement and incoordination. Better results are obtained when thiopental is given in combination with guaifenesin or when used following premedication with xylazine or acepromazine (Branson, 2001). One should also note that thiopental elevates blood glucose and induces leucopenia in horses (Branson, 2001).

Pentobarbital is used as an anesthetic for castration procedures in boars. It can be injected intratesticulary (1.5-20 ml of a 30% solution) (Branson, 2001). Boars will become uncoordinated in a few minutes, with recumbence at 5-15 minutes following administration. Anesthesia is checked by pricking the scrotal skin with a needle. For longer surgical procedures for example in swine, premedication of atropine (0.07-0.09 mg/kg), meperidine (1-2 mg/kg) and promazine (2 mg/kg) can be used prior to barbiturate anesthesia (Branson, 2001). Nevertheless, swine need a longer period (than humans, dogs and some other species) to recover from barbiturate anesthesia, possibly due to large amounts of adipose tissue. Therefore, when using thiopental in swine endotracheal intubation is necessary to provide respiration.

In goats and sheep barbiturates are rapidly metabolized and duration of anesthesia is much shorter than in other species. Thus, in small ruminants pentobarbital is useful for induction of anesthesia, for example to catheterize the jugular vein for injections of additional drugs, to perform intubation, etc.

Rabbits have a narrow margin between surgical anesthesia level and respiratory arrest, and they vary individually in response to anesthetic used; in a similar manner, their recovery may vary from 1 to 10 hours (Murdock, 1969). Therefore, thiopental may be used as the anesthetic of choice – the animals usually recover within 15 minutes (Murdock, 1969; Wood, 1978).

Due to the narrow margin of safety, pentobarbital may not be an anesthetic of choice in chickens. However, it can be used if oxygen and adequate ventilation are provided. In birds, atropine should be used as premedication to prevent bronchial secretion. Induction of anesthesia in birds occurs in about 2 minutes, surgical anesthesia lasts approximately 30 minutes and the animal recovers within 90 minutes (Branson, 2001).

Barbiturates have been used successfully in other species as well, such as monkeys and chimpanzees (Domino et al., 1969), guinea pigs, gerbils, laboratory rodents and wild animals. According to Branson (2001) frogs can be anesthetized with 60 mg/kg of pentobarbital administered through the dorsal lymph sac. Surgical anesthesia occurs in 30 minutes and lasts for about 9 hours.

Pentobarbital use is contraindicated in large cats since they are not able to metabolize it, so anesthesia may last for 7 days probably due to drug deposition in adipose tissue. Thus, ultrashort-acting barbiturates, such as thiopental sodium, are a drug of choice (animal will sleep from 6 to 24 hours).

Beside for anesthesia, pentobarbital could be used as an anticonvulsant during status epilepticus, and as premedicament in order to induce euthanasia.

Among animal species, cats have marked susceptibility of respiratory function following barbiturate administration, which implies that RAS in cats sends signals or impulses to the medullar control centers governing respiration. Subanesthetic doses of barbiturates accelerate respiration rates in many animals, while large doses act as depressant to the respiratory center in the medulla (Branson, 2001). Therefore, when barbiturate as anesthetic is used, special attention should be given to the animal's respiration, assuring adequate airway maintenance and ventilation. During anesthesia, there is an increased risk of hypothermia and consequently ventricular fibrillation, which occurs in all animals following administration of pentobarbital, and in half of the animals anesthetized with thiopental (Branson, 2001). Sensitivity of animals to uremia may be also increased and consequently the barbiturate sleeping time may be prolonged. When barbiturates are administered to a patient with impaired renal function, there is a risk of severe depression of vital functions and death. Additionally, birds eliminate barbiturates via renal excretion so slowly that there is a high risk of coma from respiratory failure (see earlier). According to Sinn (1994), phenobarbital, methohexital, thiobarbiturates and barbital should not be used in companion birds because they have a low margin of safety and produce prolonged violent recoveries.

Since the rate of metabolism of barbiturates varies among different animal species, there are differences in their action and the special attention should be given to the amount of adipose tissue since it can make large variations in the utilization and consequently drug metabolism. Most laboratory animals as well as domestic animals metabolize barbiturates faster than humans. Cats are an exception – they require more time to metabolize these drugs. Namely, dogs metabolize pentobarbital at the rate of 15% per hour, horses at 50% per hour, sheep at 49% per hour. In comparison, humans metabolize pentobarbital at the rate of 4% per hour (Branson, 2001). These variations are the leading cause of the differences in the duration of action within the species. There are also variations within the breeds – barbiturates induce longer anesthetic effects in Greyhound dogs than in mixed breeds, due to their low percentage of body fat and slower liver metabolism of drugs (Robinson et al., 1986).

It is interesting to notice that even the type of litter upon which we hold an animal contributes to variations in duration of the anesthesia. Namely, softwood bedding may increase liver enzymes levels and hence reduce the duration of anesthesia (Branson, 2001).

When anesthetics, and among them of interest barbiturates, are used in combination with neuromuscular agents and antibiotics, such as aminoglycosides, the margins of safety in view of neuromuscular transmission should be considered. In cats anesthetized with pentobarbital and treated with neomycin, complete neuromuscular paralysis occurred due to neomycin binding to $Ca^{2+}$ receptive sites at the motor end plate of the skeletal muscle (Adams, 1976).

## SEIZURE MANAGEMENT

Epilepsy is the most commonly diagnosed neurological disorder in companion animals, but seizures have also been noted in other animals, such as horses, cattle and goats. In veterinary literature epilepsy is defined as the recurrence of seizures (Knowles, 1998), a chronic recurrence of seizures without a demonstrable substrate (Jaggy and Heynold, 1996) or as two or more recurrent seizures (Berendt, 2005). Seizures, the clinical result of a rapid, excessive neuronal discharge in the brain, are classified as primary (genetic) or secondary (acquired), and as generalized and focal. Generalized seizures are more common in small animals and the incidence is greater in dogs than cats (Boothe, 2001). Canine epilepsy is defined as recurrent seizures for which no underlying abnormality can be identified (Knowles, 1998). In contrast to humans, with more than forty epileptic syndromes and related conditions, canine epilepsy is not differentiated into syndromes, mainly due to the lack of proper diagnostic procedures in veterinary practice (e.g. EEG). The most common seizure types in canine epilepsy taxonomy are generalized tonic-clonic convulsions and grand mal (Schwartz-Porsche et al., 1985).

Epilepsy could be caused by an acquired organic lesion (brain tumor or trauma), toxicosis, hypoglycemia, renal failure, liver disease or electrolyte imbalance (acquired or secondary epilepsy), but most canine patients are classified as having idiopathic - genetic or inherited, primary epilepsy (Schwartz-Porsche, 1994). The hereditary component of epilepsy in dogs has been shown in pedigree studies on several breeds. This is the case in Beagles (Bielfelt et al., 1971), German Shepherd Dogs (Falco et al., 1974), Labrador Retrievers (Jaggy et al., 1998), Golden Retrievers (Srenk and Jaggy, 1996), Bernese Mountain Dogs (Kathmann et al., 1999), Belgian Tervuerens (Famula and Oberbauer, 2000), Viszlas (Patterson et al., 2003), Keeshonds (Hall and Wallace, 1996) and English Springer Spaniels (Patterson et al., 2005). Moreover, a mutation in the *Epm2b* gene has been proven cause in so-called Lafora disease in miniature wirehaired Dachshunds, which is an autosomal, recessive, progressive myoclonic epilepsy. This was the first genetic mutation identified in a canine epilepsy syndrome, and is expected to contribute to the understanding of the aetiopathogenesis of the disease. However, it is likely that genetic mechanisms in epilepsy vary across breeds, and possibly across bloodlines within the same breed (Licht et al., 2002). Some authors recommend the use of the International League Against Epilepsy (ILAE) guidelines, with some modifications, to classify the seizures in dogs (Berendt and Gram, 1999; Licht et al., 2002; Podell, 2004; Schwartz-Porsche, 1994).

The four stages of seizure (prodrome, aura, ictus and post-ictal phase) as in humans are recognized in dogs and have been used commonly within veterinary literature. However, it is always a great challenge for veterinary practitioners as well as for owners to determine aura as a sensory focal seizure, and to notice subtle changes in behavior, that may be used as a warning sign before the progression of the seizure. Most cases of canine epilepsy start with the first seizure between 6 months and 6 years of age (Holliday, 1980). Although these seizures are mainly described as generalized tonic-clonic, recently more focal seizures have been recognized as well (Berendt and Gram, 1999; Jaggy and Bernardini, 1998; Licht et al., 2002), with focal onset preceded by an aura-like event. In addition, many veterinary patients with focal seizures have focal intracranial pathology similar to humans (Pitkanen and Sutula, 2002; Podell, 1995).

Epilepsy pathophysiology can be viewed as a fundamental imbalance between excitatory and inhibitory neurotransmitter levels; the blockade of GABAergic inhibition may produce seizures, with concomitant increase in glutamate activity. In addition, altered extracellular potassium and calcium concentrations and changes in neuronal membrane function can lead to excessive depolarization (Boothe, 2001). Fortunately, these mechanisms are conducive to pharmacological manipulation. On the other hand, although the underlying mechanisms have been extensively studied in humans and rodents, knowledge on pathophysiology of canine and feline epilepsy is scarce. Namely, a decrease in GABA and an increase in glutamate levels in the cerebrospinal fluid of canine patients have been observed only in several studies (Ellenberger et al., 2004; Loscher and Schwartz-Porsche, 1986; Podell and Hadjiconstantinou, 1997). However, in Labrador Retrievers with genetically determined epilepsy, a decrease in GABA and glutamate levels have been observed (Ellenberger et al., 2004).

There are only several reports on canine temporal lobe epilepsy in the veterinary literature; these specific seizures include phenobarbitone responsive hypersialosis (Stonehewer et al., 2000), and episodic dyscontrol (rage) syndrome (Dodman et al., 1992). In addition, Buckmaster and colleagues (2002) failed to prove that dogs refractory to medication have temporal lobe epilepsy, which is typical in humans with same onset.

Regarding therapy, only a few antiepileptic drugs (AED) are suitable for dogs, because the elimination half-life of most of them is too short in dogs, and frequently, multiple dosing is not practical for veterinary patients and their owners. As in humans, epilepsy is only controlled, not cured, and treatment has to be administered daily over a lifetime (Frey, 1986). AEDs commonly used in veterinary medicine are phenobarbital sodium and potassium bromide. These drugs can be used concurrently, but in lower individual doses. Phenobarbital, considered as a "broad-spectrum" anticonvulsant, is still the drug of choice in dogs and cats, although there are many newer antiepileptics available. It is effective in 60-80% of dogs (Farnbach, 1984; Schwartz-Porsche et al., 1985). Its lack of efficacy is actually more often due to inappropriate use of the drug (inadequate dose, failure to monitor serum levels, lack of owner compliance) than to pharmacoresistance of epilepsy (Chandler, 2006). It depresses the motor centers of the cerebral cortex, therefore having excellent anticonvulsant properties. Additionally, it is the most effective anticonvulsant inhibiting the progressive intensification of the seizure activity that may accompany epilepsy. Namely, phenobarbital enhances responsiveness to the inhibitory postsynaptic effects of GABA. Additionally, phenobarbital inhibits glutamate activity and calcium fluxes across the neuronal membrane.

The initial dose of phenobarbital is 2.5 mg/kg orally every 12 h (Podell, 2004). Monitoring the patient`s blood levels of phenobarbital is advisable; since the therapeutic range for dogs may vary between 15 to 45 (Farnbach, 1984), for cats 23-38, and for horses 15-20 μg/ml (Papich, 2011). These broad therapeutic ranges may differ for animals that are concurrently treated with bromide; for example, for dogs this range can additionally vary between 9-36 μg/ml (Trepanier et al., 1998). Phenobarbital has a high bioavailability, with maximal plasma concentration reached 4-8 h after administration. Elimination half-life in dogs is 56-102 h, while it takes 2-3 weeks to reach a steady state (Boothe, 2001) and during this period, the serum levels of phenobarbital should be monitored. According to Chandler (2006), the dose should be increased until a serum concentration of 30-35 μg/ml is reached, and each time the dose is changed, the serum concentration needs to be measured 10-14 days after the dose change. To avoid a large decrease in phenobarbital serum levels, it is important to administer phenobarbital at the same time, at a 12 h interval. If seizure control remains inadequate, potassium bromide could be added at 30 mg/kg once daily or 15 mg/kg twice daily. However, there is variability regarding this drug's metabolism and elimination, mainly due to differences in the hepatic metabolism. Its half-life differs not only between and within species, but also in the same animal. Phenobarbital is a potent inducer of hepatic microsomal enzymes, and is capable of increasing the rate of clearance of other drugs metabolized in the liver, as well as increasing its own metabolism rate. At serum concentrations above the 35 μg/ml, phenobarbital is hepatotoxic. Moreover, since phenobarbital increases the activity of microsomal enzymes, it also increases metabolism of endogenous hormones, so estrogens, androgens, progestational, adrenocortical steroids and thyroid hormones levels may be decreased.

In addition, phenobarbital has several side effects that can influence owner compliance with the therapy and most of them are present during the first two weeks of treatment. These side effects include ataxia, sedation, polydipsia, polyuria and polyphagia. During chronic therapy with phenobarbital, physical dependence occurs, so abrupt discontinuation of the therapy may cause withdrawal seizures (Podell, 2004).

Sometimes primidone is used to treat epilepsy in domestic animals. Primidone is metabolized to phenylethylmalonamide (PEMA) and phenobarbital. Both of these metabolites have anticonvulsant activity, but primidone's efficacy is probably mainly due to phenobarbital effects.

Potassium bromide, the oldest AED, can be used as first-line treatment of epilepsy or in addition to phenobarbital. It increases GABAergic inhibition in rat hippocampus and cortex slices (Meierkord et al., 2000), so its anticonvulsant activity could be explained by its effect on the GABAergic system. Its use in humans has significantly declined over the years due to its common side effects such as skin lesions (dermatitis, acne), gastrointestinal (nausea/emesis) and neurological symptoms (depression, lethargy, tremor, ataxia, paresis etc.).

The half-life of potassium bromide in dogs is 15-20 days (March et al., 2002) and it reaches a steady state levels after 100-200 days of use (Chandler, 2006). Thus, a loading dose of bromide is 450-600 mg/kg over five days, plus the recommended daily dose. Nevertheless, one must be aware that salt levels in the diet can affect bromide serum levels by increasing bromide renal elimination. As it is well tolerated, potassium bromide is mainly used in animals with liver disease, in which the treatment with phenobarbital is unadvisable, or as a concurrent therapy along with phenobarbital.

Since benzodiazepines promote the inhibitory action of GABA in both the brain and spinal cord, they do not only decrease seizure spread but also block the arousal and centrally depress spinal reflexes. When epileptic animal continue to have seizures regardless of its phenobarbital and/or bromide therapy, diazepam may be given intra rectum. This is also the first choice for emergency treatment of status epilepticus and cluster seizures, especially because absorption of diazepam given intra rectum is greater than the oral administration or intramuscular injection (Mealey and Boothe, 1995). According to Dowling (1999), diazepam may be administered per rectum when the animal experiences an initial generalized seizure or when a second or third generalized seizure occurs within 24 h from the initial one. Diazepam is not an AED of choice for chronic administration in dogs, since tolerance to the anticonvulsant activity of diazepam develops within one week (Pericic et al., 2007; Svob Strac et al., 2008; Vlainic and Pericic, 2009). However, diazepam may be used for the long-term treatment in cats having epilepsy resistant to phenobarbital therapy.

Some studies suggest that gabapentin may be effective in the treatment of seizures refractory to potassium bromide or phenobarbital therapy (Chandler, 2006). It is an analogue of the neurotransmitter GABA, but it does not interact with $GABA_A$ or $GABA_B$ receptors, although it seems that it may enhance GABA synthesis and GABA synaptic concentration, along with the interaction with voltage-sensitive calcium channels in cortical neurons and reduction of the monoamine neurotransmitters release. In dogs, an initial single dose of 10 mg/kg and then 10 mg/kg three times a day is recommended (Podell, 2004). Pregabalin is very similar to gabapentin since it is not an agonist or antagonist for the GABA receptors; hence, its anticonvulsant effect occurs via the inhibition of the calcium channels in neurons. Half-life of pregabalin in dogs is 7 hours, compared to 3-4 hours for gabapentin. Pregabalin is considered as an AED and is commonly introduced in therapy when the seizures become refractory to other drugs. Pregabalin is used mainly in conjunction with other anticonvulsants, because it reduces seizure frequency in refractory patients when combined with phenobarbital and/or potassium bromide.

Other AED that may be used in veterinary medicine for the control of seizures, although their primary mechanism of action is not GABAergic modulation, are phenytoin, levetiracetam, felbamate and zonisamide. Nevertheless, one should notice that dogs metabolize phenytoin much more quickly than humans, which makes it ineffective as an antiepileptic. Also, due to drug interaction and hepatotoxicity, it`s concurrent administration with phenobarbital should be avoided. Phenytoin is considered toxic and generally unacceptable as an anticonvulsant in cats (Schwartz and Porsche, 1989).

In human medicine there are several GABAergic drugs that are recently introduced in anticonvulsive therapy, such as imidazopyridine zolpidem (Pericic et al., 2008), which will probably be used in veterinary medicine especially due to its safety in older animals (Vlainic and Percic, 2010).

## Pharmacological Treatment of Behavioral Disorders

Stress has been identified as a state in which an animal reacts to an endogenous or exogenous threat and focuses its energy on coping with a dangerous situation (Belpedio, 2010). Noise, immobilization, novelty, transport, restricted housing can cause arousal, fear and frustration in animals, which leads to a stress response that manifests itself through behavioral, cardiovascular and endocrine reactions (Beerda et al., 1999). Fear and aggression in dogs, anxiety, and even urine spraying in cats, can be the manifestation of a behavioral stress response. These behavioral problems may lead the owners to consider various pharmacological treatments, although guidelines advise not to use them without consultation with the specialist (Overall, 2011). Currently there is an increasing trend of diagnosing the psychological disorders in companion animals, such as various anxiety disorders followed by an increased demand for psychopharmacological medication. However, these drugs have not been approved for veterinary use and their use for the treatment of behavior problems in animals remains off-label. Namely, only clomipramine for separation anxiety in dogs, and selegiline for cognitive dysfunction in elderly dogs have been approved for the use (in USA) in mentioned indications. It is the veterinarian`s responsibility to examine the patient, to interview the owner, and to determine whether the off-label use of the medication is appropriate and will be beneficial. At the same time, he is obligated to inform the owner about the meaning of the off-label status of the drug. Additionally, first a valid veterinarian-owner-patient relationship must be established.

According to many authors, psychotherapeutic agents, along with behavioral and environmental interventions, provide better and faster treatment outcomes (Dodman et al., 1996; Hewson et al., 1998; King et al., 2000; Moon-Fanelli & Dodman, 1998; Overall, 1994; Overall, 2001). According to Overall (2001), it is important to emphasize the importance of several guidelines for clinicians treating animals with the problematic behavior: to clearly formulate the diagnosis, to have an insight into the neurochemistry of the condition, to understand the side effects of the chosen drug(s), and to monitor behavioral changes caused by the drugs(s). The latter can help clinician to reject any hypothesis about underlying neurophysiological mechanisms, especially if very specific behavioral changes emerge. These changes are caused by alterations in the neurotransmitters: acetylcholine, serotonin, noradrenaline, dopamine, excitatory amino acids, and GABA. Benzodiazepines (alprazolam, clonazepam, diazepam and oxazepam), which are widely used for behavioral problems, such as aggression in dogs or spraying in cats. Their calming effect is possibly due to their influence on he limbic system and the reticular formation effects, without impairment of cortical function, in comparison to barbiturates (Overall, 2001). In order to facilitate daytime functioning and excitement tempering, benzodiazepines may be given at low doses. Moderate doses are given for their anxiolytic effect and easier social interaction, while higher doses will facilitate sleep. However, in some animals, benzodiazepines are not effective in alleviating fear-related aggression, but instead cause a paradoxical increase in such behavior (Johnstone, 2005). Some benzodiazepines, such as clonazepam, have a muscle relaxation effect at lower doses than those needed for behavioral effects (Overal, 2001).

Benzodiazepines are essential for the treatment of sporadic events involving profound anxiety or panic (e.g. thunderstorms, fireworks, panic associated with departure of humans, signaled by an external indicator, e.g. an alarm clock), but they must be given to the animal at least 1 h before the anticipated stimulus or minimally before the patients exhibit signs of distress (Overall, 2001). This timing allows repeat dosing and permits concomitant use of the tricyclic antidepressants (TCA) or selective serotonin reuptake inhibitors (SSRI) (Overall, 2001). When using benzodiazepines, one must consider their amnesic effect and the interaction with learning. Thus, they may be more useful in situations in which the control of intense fear is more important than ongoing learning (Crowell-Davis, 2006b). The optimal doses in the treatment of behavioral disorders in animal may vary greatly. Animals should be closely monitored for several hours after administration of a benzodiazepine test dose in the low range of the dosage schedule, in order to see if there are side effects, such as paradoxical excitement or sedation (Crowell-Davis, 2006b). According to Crowell-Davis (2006b), paradoxical excitement occurs at a specific window of dosage, and if it occurs, the dose should be increased. In some dogs, excitement or agitation may also occur (Papich, 2011), while in some cats, diazepam can cause the irritability and aberrant behavior (Gross, 2001). If sedation occurs, the dose should be lowered. If no side effect occurs, the dose should be tested and tackled in the fear-inducing situation. In addition, it is not advisable to provide prescription medication for behavior problems in companion animals without regular checkups of the patient, at least every three months. At that point, therapy progress can be assessed and reevaluated, changed or continued (Crowell-Davis, 2006b).

Two phenomena that occur during prolonged use of benzodiazepines are physical dependence and tolerance (Crowell-Davis, 2006b; Pericic et al., 2007; Vlainic and Pericic, 2009). The latter implies that steadily increasing doses of benzodiazepines will be needed to achieve the same behavioral effect. Withdrawal of the drug in animals that have used benzodiazepines for more than a few weeks should be gradual, over a period of at least one month. This allows the assessment of the need for further therapy of problem behavior. Abrupt termination of the therapy often results in a rebound – the resumption of the symptoms that may be worse than before the treatment (Crowell-Davis, 2006b). Some of the described rebound symptoms in dogs are tremor, rigidity, decreased food intake, anorexia, hyperthermia, and tonic-clonic convulsions (McNicholas et al., 1983). Lorazepam withdrawal abstinence syndrome is much less intense in dogs and has a shorter latency to onset than diazepam abstinence syndrome, which also includes clonic and tonic-clonic convulsions, and was reported to have been lethal in two dogs (McNicholas et al., 1983).

Long term use of diazepam in cats should be also avoided because of a risk of the liver toxicity. Cases of fatal idiopathic hepatic necrosis have been reported (Papich, 2011).

Benzodiazepines (diazepam, oxazepam, temazepam, alprazolam etc.) are sometimes abused to tame race and in show horses.

Diazepam is considered as a good tranquilizing agent for swine (Gross, 2001) as well as other animal species. It can be used to prevent anxiety and aggressiveness in mink. Moreover, it can also be used to improve mating in hereditarily deaf white mink (Hedlundstrain), because females of this strain refuse to mate during their estrus, becoming aggressive, vicious and even deadly toward other animals. An oral dose of 1 mg of diazepam per animal for two successive days, followed by a maintenance level of 0.66 mg per animal daily, successfully reduces that aberrant behavior (Gross, 2001).

Diazepam and oxazepam are very effective as appetite stimulants in cats and goats, through the induction of the GABAergic neurotransmission and a central inhibition of the satiety center in the hypothalamus (Gross, 2001; Macy and Gasper, 1985). On the other hand, benzodiazepines are not effective as appetite stimulants in dogs (Gross, 2001).

Another benzodiazepine, chloridazepoxide hydrochloride, can be used to tame wild animals. It reduces aggression and promotes docile, even friendly behavior (Hentschele, 1961). Nevertheless, the calming effect is fastest in mule deer (few minutes), while European lynx, dingo or sea lion become calm within 2-4 hours. Additionally, it has been shown to be effective in Guinea baboons, California sea lions, Burmese macaques, red kangaroos, white bearded gnu, gerenuk and golden marmosets (Hentschele, 1961). However, chlordiazepoxide failed to produce the desired effect in a Sumatran tiger, Hensel`s cats, South American tapirs and klipspringers (Hentschele, 1961).

## References

Adams HR, Mathew BP, Teske RH, Mercer HD (1976) Neuromuscular blocking effects of aminoglycoside antibiotics on fast- and slow-contracting muscles of the cat. *Anesth Analg*. 55:500-7.

Beerda B, Schilder MBH, Van Hooff JAR, Devries HW, Mol JA (1999) Chronic stress in dogs subjected to social and spatial restriction. I. Behavioral responses. *Physiol Behav*. 66:233–42.

Belpedio C (2010) Understanding Kennel Stress in Canines (Canis lupus familiaris) — A Review of the Literature. *JACAB* 4:7-14.

Berendt M, Gram L (1999) Epilepsy and seizure classification in 63 dogs: a reappraisal of veterinary epilepsy terminology. *J Vet Intern Med*. 13:14–20.

Berendt M (2005) Epilepsy. In: Vite CH, Braund KG (Eds.), *Braund`s Clinical Neurology in Small Animals*. International Veterinary Information Service, Ithaca, NY, USA.

Bielfelt SW, Redman HC, McClellan RO (1971) Sire- and sex related differences in rates of epileptiform seizures in a purebred beagle dog colony. *Am J Vet Res*. 32:2039–48.

Boothe DM (2001) *Anticonvulsant drugs and analeptic agents. In: Veterinary Pharmacology and Therapeutics*. Eds: Adams RH. 8th ed., Blackwell Publishing Professional, Ames, Iowa. 372-392.

Branson KR (2001) Injectable anesthetics. In: VeterinaryPharmacology and Therapeutics. 8th ed., Eds: Adams RH. *Blackwell Publishing Professional,* Ames, Iowa. 213–268.

Buckmaster PS, Smith MO, Buckmaster CL, LeCouteur RA, Dudek FE (2002) Absence of temporal lobe epilepsy pathology in dogs with medically intractable epilepsy. *J Vet Intern Med.* 16:95–99.

Calle PP (2005) Zoo animals. In:*The Merck Veterinary Manual.* 9th ed. Eds: Kahn CM. Merck & Co, Inc. Whitehouse station, U.S.A. 1658-66.

Cattet MR, Caulkett NA, Polischuk SC, Ramsay MA (1999) Anesthesia of polar bears (Ursus maritimus) with zolazepam-tiletamine, medetomidine-ketamine, and medetomidine-zolazepam-tiletamine. *J Zoo Wild Med.* 30:354–60.

Chandler KE, Princivalle AP, Fabian-Fine R, Bowery NG, Kullmann DM, Walker MC, (2006) Plasticity of GABA(B) receptor-mediated heterosynaptic interactions at mossy fibers after status epilepticus. *J Neurosci.* 23:11382–91.

Clark, CA (2004) Tracking changes: Postnatal blood and muscle oxygen store development in harbor seals (Phoca vitulina). *Master's thesis.* University of Alaska, Anchorage, AK. 82 pp.

Crowell-Davis SL (2006a) Amino Acid Neurotransmitters: Glutamate, GABA, and the Pharmacology of Benzodiazepines. In: *Veterinary Psychopharmacol.* Wiley-Blackwell, 25-34.

Crowell-Davis SL (2006b) *Benzodiazepines.* In: VeterinaryPsychopharmacology. Wiley-Blackwell, Eds: Cowell-Davis, S.L., Murray, T., 2006. Wiley-Blackwell, pp. 34-71.

Dodman NH, Miczek KA, Knowles K, Thalhammer JG, Shuster L (1992) Phenobarbital-responsive episodic dyscontrol (rage) in dogs. J. Amer. Vet. Med. Ass. 201:1580–1583.

Dodman NH, Donnelly R, Shuster L, Mertens P, Miczek K (1996) Use of fluoxetine to treat dominance aggression in dogs. *J Amer Vet Med Ass.* 209:1585–7.

Domino EF, McCarthy DA, Deneau GA (1969) General anesthesia in infrahuman primates. *Fed Proc.* 28:1500-9.

Dowling PM (1999) Update on therapy of canine epilepsy. *Can. Vet. J.* 40, 595-598.

Ellenberger C, Mevissen M, Doherr M, Scholtysik G, Jaggy A (2004) Inhibitory and excitatory neurotransmitters in the cerebrospinal fluid of epileptic dogs. *Am J Vet Res.* 65:1108–1113.

Falco MJ, Barker J, Wallace ME (1974) The genetics of epilepsy in the British Alsatian. *J Small Anim Pract.* 15:685–92.

Famula TR, Oberbauer AM (2000) Segregation analysis of epilepsy in the Belgian tervueren dog. *Vet Rec.* 147:218–221.

Farnbach GC (1984) Serum concentrations and efficacy of phenytoin, phenobarbital, and primidone in canine epilepsy. *J Amer Vet Med Ass.* 184:1117–1120.

Frey HH (1986) Use of anticonvulsants in small animals. *Vet Rec.* 26:484-6.

Gage LJ (1984) Restraint and anesthesia in pinnipeds. *Proc. Annu Meet Am Assoc Zoo Vet.* 31.

Gales N J (1989) Chemical restraint and anesthesia of pinnipeds: A review. *Mar Mamm Sci.* 5:228–56.

Greig JE (2003) *Vasoactive hormone concentrations during development of the harbour seal, Phoca vitulina.* M.Sc. thesis, University of Waterloo, ON. 47 pp

Gross ME (2001) *Tranquilizers, α-adrenergicagonists and related agents. In: Veterinary Pharmacology and Therapeutics.* 8th ed., Eds: Adams RH. Blackwell Publishing Professional, Ames, Iowa. 299-342.

Hall SJ, Wallace ME (1996) Canine epilepsy: a genetic counselling programme for keeshonds. *Vet Rec.* 138:358–360.

Hentschele WP (1961) Chlordiazepoxide for calming zoo animals. *J Amer Vet Med Ass.* 139:996-998.

Hewson CJ, Luescher A, Parent JM, Conlon PD, Ball RO (1998) Efficacy of clomipramine in the treatment of canine compulsive disorder. *J Amer Vet Med Ass.* 213:1760–6.

Holliday TA (1980) Seizure disorders. Vet Clin North Amer Small Anim Pract. 10:3–29.

Jaggy A, Heynold Y (1996) *Idiopathic epilepsy in the dog.* Schweiz Arch Tierheilkd. 138:523–531.

Jaggy A, Bernardini M (1998) Idiopathic Epilepsy in 125 dogs: a long term study. Clinical and electroencephalographic findings. *J Small Anim Pract.* 39:23–29.

Jaggy A, Faissler D, Gaillard C, Srenk P, Graber H (1998) Genetic aspects of idiopathic epilepsy in Labrador retrievers. *J Small Anim Pract.* 39:275–280.

Jazvinscak Jembrek M, Svob Strac D, Vlainic J, Pericic D (2008) The role of transcriptional and translational mechanisms in flumazenil-induced up-regulation of recombinant GABA(A) receptors. *Neurosci Res.* 61:234–241.

Johnstone I (2005) *SystemicPharmacotherapeutics of the Nervous System. In: The Merck Veterinary Manual.* 9th ed. Ed: Kahn CM. Merck & Co, Inc. Whitehouse station, U.S.A. 2019-2031.

Karesh WB, Cook RA, Lim M (1997) South American pinnipeds: Immobilization,telemetry, and health evaluations. *Proc Annu Meet Am Assoc Zoo Vet.* 291–295.

Kathmann I, Jaggy A, Busato A, Bartschi M, Gaillard C (1999) Clinical and genetic investigations of idiopathic epilepsy in the Bernese mountain dog. *J Small Anim Pract.* 40:319– 325.

King JN, Simpson BS, Overall KL, Applby D, Pageat P, Ross C, Chaurand JP, Heath S, Beata C, Weiss AB, Muller G, Paris T, Bataille BG, Parker J, Petit S, Wren J (2000) Treatment of separation anxiety in dogs with clomipramine: results from a prospective, randomized, double-blind, placebo controlled, parallel-group, multicenter clinical trial. *Appl Anim Behav Sci.* 67:255–75.

Knowles K (1998) Idiopathic epilepsy. *Clin Tech Small Anim Pract.* 13:144–151.

Lapierre JL, Schreer JF, Burns JM, Hammill MO (2007) Effect of diazepam on heart and respiratoty rates of harbor seal pups following intravenous injection. *Mar Mamm Sci.* 23:209-217.

Licht MH, Harper KM, Lin S, Curtin JJ, Hyson LL, Willard K (2002) Clinical presentations of naturally occurring canine seizures: similarities to human seizures. *Epilepsy Behav.* 3:460–470.

Loscher W, Schwartz-Porsche D (1986) Low levels of gammaaminobutyric acid in cerebrospinal fluid of dogs with epilepsy. *J Neurochem.* 46:1322–1325.

Macy DW, Gasper PW (1985) Diazepam-induced eating in anorexic cats. *J Am Anim Hos Assoc.* 21:17-20.

March PA, Podell M, Sams RA (2002) Pharmacokinetics and toxicity of bromide following high-dose oral potassium bromide administration in healthy Beagles. *J Vet Pharmacol Ther.* 25:425–432.

McNicholas LF, Martin WR, Cherian S (1983) Physical dependence on diazepam and lorazepam in the dog. *J Pharmacol Exp Ther.* 226:783-9.

Mealey KL, Boothe DM (1995) Bioavailability of benzodiazepines following rectal administration of diazepam in dogs. *J Vet Pharmacol Therap.* 18:72-74.

Meierkord H, Grunig F, Gutschmidt U, Gutierrez R, Pfeiffer M, Draguhn A, Bruckner C, Heinemann U (2000) Sodium bromide: effects on different patterns of epileptiform activity, extracellular pH changes and GABAergic inhibition. *Naunyn-Schmiedebergs Arch Pharmacol.* 361:25–32.

Moon-Fanelli AA, Dodman NH (1998) Description and development of compulsive tail chasing in terriers and response to clomipramine treatment. *J Amer Vet Med Ass.* 212:1252–7.

Murdock HR Jr (1969) Anesthesia in the rabbit. *Fed Proc.* 28:1510-6.

Overall KL (1994) Use of clomipramine to treat ritualistic motor behavior in dogs. *J Amer Vet Med Assoc.* 205:1733–41.

Overall KL (2001) Pharmacological treatment in behavioral medicine: the importance of neurochemistry, molecular biology and mechanistic hypotheses. *Vet J.* 162:9-23.

Papich MG (2011) Saunders Handbook of Veterinary Drugs: Small and Large Animal, 3rd Edition, Elsevier Saunders, St. Louis, Missouri, USA.

Patterson EE, Mickelson JR, Da Y, Roberts MC, McVey AS, O`Brien DP, Johnson GS, Armstrong PJ (2003) Clinical characteristics and inheritance of idiopathic epilepsy in Vizslas. *J Vet Intern Med.* 17:319–325.

Patterson EE, Armstrong PJ, OBrien DP, Roberts MC, Johnson GS, Mickelson JR (2005) Clinical description and mode of inheritance of idiopathic epilepsy in English springer spaniels. *J Amer Vet Med Ass.* 226:54–58.

Pericic D, Lazic J, Jembrek MJ, Strac DS, Rajcan I (2004) Chronic exposure of cells expressing recombinant $GABA_A$ receptors to benzodiazepine antagonist flumazenil enhances the maximum number of benzodiazepine binding sites. *Life Sci.* 76(3):303-17.

Pericic D, Lazic J, Strac DS (2005) Chronic treatment with flumazenil enhances binding sites for convulsants at recombinant alpha(1)beta(2)gamma(2S) GABA(A) receptors. *Biomed Pharmacother.* 59(7):408-14.

Pericic D, Strac DS, Jembrek MJ, Vlainic J (2007) Allosteric uncoupling and up-regulation of benzodiazepine and GABA recognition sites following chronic diazepam treatment of HEK 293 cells stably transfected with alpha1beta2gamma2S subunits of GABA (A) receptors. *Naunyn Schmiedebergs Arch Pharmacol.* 375(3):177-87.

Pericic D, Vlainic J, Svob Strac D (2008) Sedative and anticonvulsant effects of zolpidem in adult and aged mice. *J Neural Transm.* 115:795-802.

Pitkanen A, Sutula TP (2002) Is epilepsy a progressive disorder? Prospects for new therapeutic approaches in temporal-lobe epilepsy. *Lancet Neurol.* 1:173–181.

Podell M (1995) The use of diazepam per rectum at home for the acute management of cluster seizures in dogs. *J Vet Intern Med.* 9:68–74.

Podell M, Hadjiconstantinou M (1997) Cerebrospinal fluid gammaaminobutyric acid and glutamate values in dogs with epilepsy. *Am J Vet Res.* 58:451–456.

Podell M (2004) Seizures. In: *BSAVA Manual of Canine and Feline Neurology.* Eds.: Platt S, Olby N, BSAVA, 97–112.

Rho JM, Donevan SD, Rogawski MA (1996) Direct activation of $GABA_A$ receptors by barbiturates in cultured rat hippocampal neurons. *J Physiol.* 497:509-22.

Robinson EP, Sams RA, Muir WW (1986) Barbiturate anesthesia in greyhound and mixed-breed dogs: comparative cardiopulmonary effects, anesthetic effects, and recovery rates. *Am J Vet Res.* 47:2105-12.

Roche pharmaceuticals, INC. (1997) *Valium® (brand of diazepam) injection.* Nutley, NJ.

Scholfield CN, Harvey JA (1975) Local anesthetics and barbiturates: effects on evoked potentials in isolated mammalian cortex. *J. Pharmacol Exp Ther.* 195:522-31.

Schwartz-Porsche D, Loscher W, Frey HH (1985) Therapeutic efficacy of phenobarbital and primidone in canine epilepsy: a comparison. *J Vet Pharmacol Ther.* 8:113–9.

Schwartz-Porsche D, Kaiser E (1989) Feline epilepsy. *Probl Vet Med.* 1:628-49.

Schwartz-Porsche D (1994) Seizures. In: *Clinical Syndromes in Veterinary Neurology.* Ed: Braund KG, St Louis, MO, Mosby, 234–251.

Shini S (2000) A review of diazepam and its use in the horse. *JEVS* 20:443-9.

Sinn LC (1994) Anesthesiology. In: *Avian medicine: principles and application.* Eds: Ritchie BW, Harrison GJ, Harrison LH. Wingers Publishing, Lake Worth, Florida.

Sis RF, Herron MA (1972) Anesthesia of the newborn kitten. *Lab Anim Sci.* 22:746-7.

Sleeman JM, Cameron K, Mudakikwa AB, Nizeyi JB, Anderson S, Cooper JE, Richardson HM, Macfie EJ, Hastings B, Foster JW (2000) *Field anesthesia of free-living mountain gorillas (Gorilla gorilla beringei) from the Virunga Volcano region,* Central Africa J Zoo Wild Med. 31:9–14.

Spiegel RA, Lane TJ, Larsen RE, Cardeihac PT (1984) Diazepam and succinylcholine chloride for restraint of the American alligator. *J Am Vet Med Assoc.* 185:1335-6.

Srenk P, Jaggy A (1996) Interictal electroencephalographic findings in a family of golden retrievers with idiopathic epilepsy. *J Small Anim Pract.* 37:317–321.

Stonehewer J, Mackin AJ, Tasker S, Simpson JW, Mayhew IG (2000) Idiopathic phenobarbital-responsive hypersialosis in the dog: an unusual form of limbic epilepsy. *J Small Anim Pract.* 41:416–421.

Svob Strac D, Vlainic J, Jazvinscak Jembrek M, Pericic D (2008) Differential effects of diazepam treatment and withdrawal on recombinant $GABA_A$ receptor expression and functional coupling. *Brain Res.* 1246:29-40.

Tahmindjis MA, Higgins DP, Lynch MJ, Barnes JA, Southwell CJ (2003) Use of a pethidine and midazolam combination for the reversible sedation of crabeater seals (Lobodon carcinophagus). *Mar Mamm Sci.* 19:581–589.

Trepanier LA, Van Schoick A, Schwark WS, Carrillo J (1998) Therapeutic serum drug concentrations in epileptic dogs treated with potassium bromide alone or in combination with other anticonvulsants: 122 cases (1992-1996). *J Am Vet Med Assoc.* 213:1449–53.

Vlainic J, Pericic D (2009) Effect of acute and repeated zolpidem treatment on pentylenetetrazole-induced seizure threshold and on locomotor activity: comparison with diazepam. *Neuropharmacol.* 56:1124-30.

Vlainic J, Pericic D (2010) Zolpidem is a potent anticonvulsant in adult and aged mice. *Brain Res.* 1310:181-8.

Wood C (1978) Anesthesia in rabbits. *Vet Rec.* 102:386.

Wright M (1982) Pharmacologic effects of ketamine and its use in veterinary medicine. *J Am Vet Med Assoc.* 180:1462-71.

# EDITORS' CONTACT INFORMATION

**Dr. Josipa Vlainić, DVM, Ph.D.,**
Laboratory of Molecular Neuropharmacology
Division of Molecular Medicine
Rudjer Boskovic Institute
Bijenicka 54
10000 Zagreb, Croatia
Tel: +385-1-4571268
Fax: +385-1-4561010
Email: josipa.vlainic@irb.hr

**Maja Jazvinšćak Jembrek, Ph.D.,**
Laboratory of Molecular Neuropharmacology
Department of Phychology
Croatian Catholic University
Zagreb, Croatia
Email: jazvin@irb.hr

# INDEX

## A

## B

## C

## D

## E



## F

## G



## H

## I



## J



## K



## L

## M

## N



## O

## P

## T

## U



## V



## W



## Y



## Z